spectives,
ures and
navigating
in sought
approach
. Without
onceiving,
lihood, a
st-person
tive to the
mothers
any stripe
tive) think
parents so
sures. The
dmission.
enhanded
tion.

my Myth)
h College
MA, USA

important for each woman and to use that understanding to inform our care. Reading this book provides a unique view of pre-conception, pregnancy, birth and parenting not as a purely medical, mechanical event, but as a complex physical and emotional, social and spiritual experience.

Why Didn't Anyone Tell Me? offers every professional involved with the health of women and their families a wealth of practical information and insight. The stories, wisdom and evidence-based information are a unique and perfect mix of personal experiences and science that are well researched and informative, making the book a pleasure to read.

Put simply, this book is a must-read for all expectant parents and health care professionals.

Leasa Green
Registered Nurse/Midwife, New South Wales

Rebecca Griffin's book Why Didn't Anyone Tell Me? *is an excellent resource now available for pregnant woman and their partners. It is a fresh approach to conception, pregnancy, birth and parenting issues, using real stories about these subjects by real people. The stories provide excellent insight into other people's experiences and help normalise the reader's own experiences. Some of the stories are very moving, many issues are covered and the medical issues raised are also discussed in the book after each story.*

The information contained in the book is up to date, accurate and easy to understand. It is also refreshingly unbiased about birth and parenting choices for women. A joy to read!

Tania Davies
Bachelor of Nursing, Flinders University, South Australia
BSc (Honours) Midwifery, City University London

When I had my first child I was filled with excitement, but that excitement was tinged with fear: 'What if I am not a good mother?' and 'What if I get it wrong?' Then she was born and our home was filled with an endless run of feeding problems, sleep deprivation and mother guilt. I was sure that others were thinking 'She isn't doing it right' or 'Why is she doing that all wrong … What a bad mother.'

The snatches of wisdom and experiences that we shared, sometimes reluctantly (occasionally accidentally) once a week at my first mothers' groups were my saving grace. The relief that I was not alone going through 'these things', not the only one scared of being seen as a bad mother and filled with guilt for not being perfect was liberating. These women, by sharing their stories, reassured me that my daughter and I were 'just fine'.

This book is a collection of dozens of parents' experiences of pregnancy, birth, adoption, IVF, sleep deprivation and fatherhood. It is your 'Oh, it isn't just me' moment on the bookshelf.

Sue Phillips, *Someone Else's Child*

WHY DIDN'T ANYONE TELL ME?

*Collective wisdom
on creating a family
from conception to
birth and beyond*

REBECCA GRIFFIN

ACER PRESS

For Gordon, my partner in crime

For my children, Sarah, Zoë and Oliver

Ad eorum memoriam quos valde amo

First published 2010
by ACER Press, an imprint of
Australian Council *for* Educational Research Ltd
19 Prospect Hill Road, Camberwell
Victoria, 3124, Australia

www.acerpress.com.au
sales@acer.edu.au

Edited by Elisa Webb
Cover and text design by ACER Project Publishing
Cover image copyright © Anna B Photography 2010
Typeset by ACER Project Publishing
Printed in Australia by BPA Print Group

National Library of Australia Cataloguing-in-Publication data:

Author:	Griffin, Rebecca.
Title:	Why didn't anyone tell me? : collective wisdom on creating a family from conception to birth and beyond / Rebecca Griffin.
ISBN:	9780864318787 (pbk.).
Notes:	Includes bibliographical references and index.
Subjects:	Families. Conception. Pregnancy. Childbirth. Parenting. Child rearing.
Dewey Number:	306.85

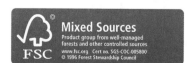

This book is printed on Master Laser Paper derived from
well-managed forests and other controlled sources certified by the
Forest Stewardship Council, a non-profit organisation devoted to
encouraging the responsible management of the world's forests.

Foreword

Although books on the subjects of pregnancy and parenting are all somewhat different in various ways, they share one important feature: they all appear to have been written by experts. The issue of reproduction is one of the most emotive in the field of human endeavour and this is in part due to the way the 'managers' of pregnancy, childbirth and parenting all trumpet their beliefs as being the best and often the only ones to follow. In doing so, alternative points of view are generally either ignored or denigrated, resulting in pictures that are black and white with no shades of grey. First-time mothers and fathers are frequently confused right from the start of their journey, as they will have heard from family and friends a variety of experiences which often seem at variance with what their midwife, obstetrician or paediatrician would have them believe.

As a result of a host of factors—such as the evolution of hospitals, the increase in professionally trained midwives and obstetricians, the elimination of previously fatal childhood illnesses, etc.—having a baby and bringing it up has never been safer. Despite this, competition frequently exists between midwives and obstetricians that is quite unnecessary and seldom has any scientific basis. Parents too become easily attached to a belief or a practice, giving no credence to the possibility that there may be other ways of doing something.

In this book we find a very broad spectrum of experiences, indicating clearly that although many of the fundamental principles are unquestioned, there are numerous different journeys through pregnancy, childbirth and parenting. None automatically exclude or include particular beliefs and nor are any of them perfect for all. They make for fascinating reading whether you are a prospective or current parent, or a professional midwife or obstetrician.

One of the unique features of this book is the inclusion of men, and not just as a token gesture. Men often find they are paid little or no regard other than as the providers of sperm, emotional support and money, but their stories are fascinating. Here we read some of their experiences and as a professional I certainly learnt a lot from them—information I could have done with at the start of my own obstetric journey 40 years ago.

If midwives and obstetricians in training read one book outside the scientific texts required by their schooling, this should be it. An understanding and acceptance of equally valid but different points of view will undoubtedly make them better practitioners, and may even result in a reduction in the number and fierceness of current quarrels which are often based upon a refusal to accept that alternative views may have validity. Parents will also learn from the breadth of experiences so clearly observed here; there is wisdom and honesty in all of them and the shared advice may be very helpful.

I am pleased to have been asked to write the foreword to this book, as I believe it will be an outstanding success. Rebecca has done a fine job collating these varied experiences and her written contributions are exceptional. She deserves to be as proud of this 'baby' as she is of her own three. I congratulate her and commend *Why Didn't Anyone Tell Me?* to tomorrow's parents, midwives, obstetricians and paediatricians.

Michael J Bennett
MBChB, MD, FCOG(SA), FRCOG, FRANZCOG, DDU
Emeritus Professor of Obstetrics and Gynaecology
School of Women's and Children's Health
The University of New South Wales

Contents

Foreword   v
List of information boxes   ix
Acknowledgements   x
Introduction   xii

Chapter One   **Conception isn't always
                  straightforward**   1
                  IVF   4
                  Donor conception   9
                  Surrogacy   13
                  Adoption   17
                  Fostering   23

Chapter Two   **Pregnancy**   27
                  Feelings   28
                  Pregnancies with health risks   43
                  Body image   47
                  Sex   52

Chapter Three **Birth and post-partum**   59
                  Vaginal births: Delivery suites in hospitals 60
                  Vaginal births: Birth centres   67
                  Vaginal births: At home   72
                  Vaginal births: After caesareans (VBAC)   75
                  Caesarean births: Elective and emergency 77
                  Caesarean births: Requested   85
                  Partners' perspectives   87

Chapter Four **Babies**   94
                  Feeding: Breast and bottle   95
                  Sleeping and settling   105
                  Coping without support   116
                  Coping with sick or premature babies   118
                  Coping with sleep deprivation   123

Chapter Five   **Motherhood**   **129**
                   Identity   131
                   Working mums and stay-at-home mums   136
                   Mother guilt   142
                   Postnatal depression and anxiety   149
                   Reflections on motherhood   156

Chapter Six   **Fatherhood**   **165**
                   Identity   167
                   Working dads and stay-at-home dads   171
                   Relationships   178
                   Reflections on fatherhood   187

Chapter Seven   **Families come in all shapes
                   and sizes**   **197**

                   Epilogue   217

Appendices

                   A Research   218
                   B How to start a support group   225

                   Glossary   230
                   Resources   238
                   References and further reading   265
                   Index   287

Information boxes

Common causes of infertility 3
When to seek help getting pregnant. 9
What is third party reproduction? Unravelling the terminology 13
Same sex parenting: ART, adoption and fostering 16
Tips for adoptive parents 20
What is Intrauterine Growth Restriction? 30
Can men get postnatal depression?. 34
Can finding out the sex of the baby affect women?. 37
What is stillbirth and how common is it? 40
How can the loss of a baby affect subsequent pregnancies and
    birthing decisions? 42
Bleeding in pregnancy 45
How do I know what medications are safe to take during pregnancy? 47
Is it safe to exercise during pregnancy?. 49
Food cravings. 52
How soon after delivery can I have sex? 54
Can fear affect childbirth? 62
What are the risks and side effects of epidurals?. 65
What will happen to my vagina?. 66
What is a TENS machine? 69
Mother guilt in birth 71
Are homebirths safe? 74
VBAC: What are my chances? 77
Are caesarean sections safe?. 79
What is pre-eclampsia? 82
Does the number of caesareans you have increase your risk of danger? 87
What is a post-partum haemorrhage? 89
What are breastfeeding rates in developed countries? 97
How to find breastfeeding support. 99
Breastfeeding is 'natural', so it must always be easy, right? 102
Breastfeeding, formula-feeding and bonding. 105
Commonly used methods for helping your baby to sleep 107
How much sleep does my baby need? 109
What is comfort settling? 112
Is there a link between poor infant sleep and postnatal depression? 115
Where can I find extra support?. 117
How to cope with persistent crying 120
First aid for babies and children. 122
Co-sleeping safely 124
Is it normal to feel so overwhelmed? 136
How much money is a stay-at-home mum worth?. 138
Tips for returning to work. 141
When guilt has a purpose. 145
Finding support for mental health issues 152
Postnatal depression 154
Motherless daughters: Finding a connection 162
How many dads choose to stay at home?. 174
Tips for single or divorced dads. 186
Domestic abuse: What it is and what you can do about it 201
Same sex parents. 208

Acknowledgements

So many people helped me with writing this book; I hope I remember to acknowledge and thank them all. This book would never have come to fruition without the steadfast belief in me from some amazing people. Firstly, my husband Gordon, who actually made me believe that I was a good writer— and who put his money where his mouth was. Not only did he look after our children and bring me endless cups of coffee, he constantly reminded me how important this book was and that I was the one to deliver it. That's pretty hard to top. Then, of course, my children, who understood on some level that their mother had to spend spurts of time without them so that she could write. And while it must have been frustrating for you at times, remember this: you were the inspiration for this book. It is my gift to you.

There were people in the industry who looked at my manuscript and championed it. Terri Cornish, a life-long friend, got my foot in the publishing door and was so utterly kind and patient with me. Annemarie Rolls, General Manager of ACER Press, took the time to read my manuscript and went out on a limb to see it published. She has been a wonderful guide and mentor.

The team at ACER Press, under the guidance of Annemarie, were astonishing. Elisa Webb is an editor whose skills, in my eyes, are unparalleled. If I could walk around in life with an 'undo' button and Elisa at my side, censoring my conversations and tweaking my words, I would be one happy camper. Yana Gotmaker worked so hard to get our cover just right and provided much needed reassurance before big media interviews. And Amanda Pinches' organisational skills make my head spin.

It seems I have had help from friends and family everywhere I turn. Andrew Marshall (of www.thinkprimed.com) read my manuscript and developed my website with Ian Shying (of www.eandl.com). Professor Bennett, Dr Campbell, midwife Leasa Green and midwife Tania Davies all set aside large chunks of time to ensure my medical facts were correct. My father, Dr Peter Reay-Young, not only checked my medical facts but also proofread many editions, as did Ruth Ryder. My friend Dr Rachael Glasson wrote a whole section for the book, which I think will greatly benefit parents. Amy Metzger, Jennifer Power, Trevor Elwell, Peter West, Claire Hughes, Joseph Waugh and Evan Ruth all checked various content for accuracy and gave me great feedback.

Of course, where would a woman be without her cheerleaders? Thanks to Natanya Mandel, Jo 'Two Pages!' Johnson, Sue Phillips, Gordon Ramsay (not the chef, the cool guy), Jaki Josef, Soraya Yardley, Kaylee Price, Seamus Heaney (Nobel Laureate; gentleman), Aimée Wood, Christina Cox, Joy Cornish, Kristen Watts, Trish Mangan and Amy Hourigan. I would also like to acknowledge and thank Anna Street for working with me in the beginning stages of this project.

Lastly but by no means least, I thank the contributors, who hailed from all over the globe and who turned this idea into reality. I thank you for your honesty, enthusiasm and insight. The credit for this book goes to you, of course.

Introduction

Why should you read *Why Didn't Anyone Tell Me?* when there are so many other books on parenting? The most important reason is that this book tells the truth. It is not a prescriptive book by an 'expert'; in these pages, you will read stories from everyday parents who tell it like it is. Having read and spoken to all manner of authorities and put their advice into practice with varying degrees of success, the parents who share their experiences here have day-to-day knowledge of the joys and hard yards of parenting, and are a unique source of wisdom and honesty.

Why Didn't Anyone Tell Me? is filled with ideas and insights from parents who share their stories on topics ranging from conception, pregnancy and birth, through to the transition to parenthood and beyond. Woven between the stories are tips, tricks and advice from parents, as well as evidence-based facts sourced from current, peer-reviewed journals. The advice and approaches shared in the book are there for the taking—but equally can be ignored if they do not fit with your views.

If you are in any way involved with pregnancy, birth or parenting, then this book is for you. If you are about to become a parent or are thinking of having children, the stories you will read may give you some insight about the process, both physical and emotional, and may help you along your own path to bringing a child into the world. If you are already a parent and now want to process your experiences through hearing other stories, you may well find this book helpful in your search for meaning or connection. If you are in the profession, either directly (such as a midwife, obstetrician or paediatrician) or indirectly (such as a psychologist or social worker), you have an obligation to listen to the experiences of both men and women. Whether you do this by listening to your patients or attending further training, this book may be a useful adjunct for you.

Nobody's perfect

All parents hope (and worry) that they are doing a good job and many are concerned that they are not living up to the idea of what a 'perfect' parent should be. This kind of thinking is facilitated by a society in which competition is rife, particularly in the parenting arena. It is easy to denigrate your skills as a parent or to second-guess your decisions when you try to live up to unrealistic expectations.

Nearly every mother and father on the planet has picked up the wrong yardstick at some point and measured themselves against it. 'Perfect parent thinking' is widespread in our society and it's only made worse when parents try to measure themselves against something that is completely unrealistic. In this book, you will find stories from both men and women that tell you exactly what is going on behind closed doors, whether it's good, bad or indifferent.

There is no single or 'right' way to raise a child. Of course, there are fundamental principles of care required for babies and children to grow and to thrive. But beyond this, the approaches, techniques, strategies and methods used are an individual choice. This book aims to promote understanding and respect for the choices other mums and dads have made. There is an enormous amount of competition and controversy surrounding parenthood. It is natural to have opinions and it is natural to feel strongly about them. But wouldn't it be nice if everyone took a step back and tried to see things through the eyes of other parents? In reading these stories, I hope that parents view them with curiosity and an open mind, rather than with judgement.

Aims of this book

Why Didn't Anyone Tell Me? does not promote any particular style of parenting. I do not want to convert anyone's beliefs. I do not have an agenda to push. What the book endeavours to do is simply to share honest and detailed accounts of how women and men are parenting today.

I hope that by reading these stories, parents will feel supported and connected to one another. Some may have an 'Ah, I'm not the only one going through this' moment and realise they are not alone. When people have a chance to connect with others, there is a greater sense of support and a reduction in feelings of isolation. Narrative is a powerful tool, and I feel that sharing real stories of everyday parents will help not only to reduce these feelings of isolation but also to increase parental confidence. Through reading such honest accounts of parenting and all the messy emotions and thoughts that can surround it, parents can challenge any 'perfect parent' thinking they may have and recognise that they are not alone in finding raising children a tough gig at times.

I also hope that some of the competition and quarrelling that surrounds parenting is reduced. Parents and professionals need to really listen to what others have gone through—particularly to the stories espousing approaches that may not fit with their own views. Let's face it, while it is easy and comfortable to be surrounded by people who share your values and attitudes, it also means you miss out on connecting with wonderful people who see the world a little differently.

Things you need to know

Hundreds of men and women were interviewed for this book and hundreds more sent in their own stories. Because the nature of parenthood is often intimate, only first names have been used. In some instances, first names have been changed to further protect the identity of an individual or a family. Each story in this book is a true and personal one—it is therefore unique to that person and representative of his or her own personal beliefs, opinions and experience. Some people were quite expressive in describing their feelings about their health care providers. Despite some professionals being depicted harshly, this information has been retained (although identifying information has been removed), as it is an important part of the experience of parenting.

Information boxes have been included to draw out some issues that are currently being debated. Technical terms are highlighted in bold font, and are listed in a glossary at the back of the book.

You are encouraged to take nothing at face value but rather research and read further until you are satisfied with the information you have. A good starting point is the Resources and Reference sections at the end of the book. For a guide on how to conduct high-quality research, see Appendix A: Research on page 218.

More books to come

Why Didn't Anyone Tell Me? is the first in a series of books based on narrative. If you have any stories you wish to contribute to forthcoming books or you would like to find out more about this series, please visit my website at <www.becgriffin.com>.

In a nutshell

Why Didn't Anyone Tell Me? is a book that lifts the lid on parenthood. In it, you will find stories that will make you laugh, weep, be shocked, and ultimately absorbed. Most of all, you will find *Why Didn't Anyone Tell Me?* a cracking read—enjoy!

CHAPTER ONE

Conception isn't always straightforward

'The bond that links your true family is not one of blood, but of respect and joy in each other's life.'

Richard Bach (1998)

If you look up 'conception' in the dictionary, you will see that the definition includes fertilisation and the act of pregnancy. Look more closely and you will see that it refers to a design or a plan. Many people who have children plan for them and many don't; either way, millions of children are conceived without too much effort. But what about the men and women who are unable to conceive without the assistance of technology? And what about the men and women whose only option (or whose preferred option) is to adopt or foster a child? For them, design and planning are paramount.

Assisted reproductive technology (ART) has helped millions of people in the world who would otherwise not have been able to do so to have biological children. Who has benefited from these technologies? Naturally, your first thought might be heterosexual couples who are unable to conceive on their own—and you would be right. However, there are other people who have also benefited from ART: single women, single men, lesbian, gay, bisexual and transgender **(LGBT)** couples and LGBT individuals. According to the International Committee for Monitoring Assisted Reproductive Technology (ICMART) et al. (2009), by 2002, more than three million babies had been born worldwide using ART since the 1980s.

While these relatively new technologies have created wonderful possibilities, they also generate a need to consider issues concerning health, ethics, law and policymaking. According to Galpern (2007), key concerns include:

lack of access; health effects on women and children; potential for devaluation of the lives of people with disabilities; limitations on use by [LGBT] individuals and couples; dangers of selecting characteristics of children; the commercial environment surrounding ART; and the nature of regulation in the US and other countries. (p. 1)

The Gender, Justice, and Human Genetics Program of the Center for Genetics and Society (Canada) has collaborated with key community organisations and delivered a set of principles in its reproductive rights framework that resonate with many groups and individuals worldwide. These principles support equal access to ART, particularly for people with disabilities, and LGBT individuals and couples. While these principles are to be applauded for their equity, law- and policymakers around the world tend not to incorporate them. Therefore, many people who wish to create their own families through ART, adoption or fostering are unable to do so by law, even though it remains a fundamental human right.

In this chapter, you will read stories from people who are in heterosexual relationships and who have used **IVF** (**in-vitro fertilisation**—a form of ART) to conceive their babies and you will hear from people in same sex relationships who have used ART. As you read these stories, you will begin to see the emotional, logistical, financial and legal complexities facing everyone who requires reproductive assistance. You will also hear from people who decided to adopt or foster children, instead of (or in addition to) having their own biological children.

What you may notice is this: all of these babies are fiercely loved. All of these children were meticulously planned; their parents went to great lengths to bring them into their families. And so, while parents are undoubtedly grateful beneficiaries of ART, adoption and fostering, perhaps the greatest beneficiaries of all are the children. For while these parents have fulfilled a lifelong desire to create a family of their own, it is the children who are rewarded with loving family homes. As evidenced by recent empirical research (see Pawelski et al. 2006; Siegel et al. 2008; van Londen et al. 2007), these children know that they are deeply wanted and loved, and form secure bonds with their parents.[1] What greater start to life could a child wish for?

---

1 Foster children often display emotional and behavioural problems but these should be viewed in a wider sociological context. For further information on foster caring, please see page 240 of the Resources section.

Common causes of infertility

In women, the most common causes of infertility are **endometriosis** (25 per cent), tubal problems (12 per cent), and lack of **ovulation** (15 per cent) (Wisot & Meldrum 2004). Endometriosis is the presence of the endometrium (the normal tissue lining in the uterine cavity) growing anywhere outside the uterus. Some people don't know they have endometriosis, while others have strong symptoms, such as severe menstrual pain (especially before menstruation), and pain with intercourse. Tubal problems can be caused by diseases such Gonorrhoea and **Chlamydia**. If left untreated (or inadequately treated), these diseases can damage the function of the fallopian tubes by causing partial or complete obstruction. This in turn can lead to infertility or **ectopic pregnancies**. **Anovulation** (lack of ovulation) can occur on three basic levels in the female reproductive system: the ovaries, the reproductive centres in the brain and pituitary, and malfunction in the interactions among parts of the reproductive system.

Other causes of infertility in women are attributed to **luteal phase** problems (7 per cent), **cervix** or mucus problems (5 per cent), uterus problems (2 per cent) and other/unexplained problems (16 per cent) (Wisot & Meldrum 2004). Luteal phase problems occur when an insufficient amount of **progesterone** is released during the second phase of the menstrual cycle. Cervical problems can include blockages of the cervical canal or deficiencies in the cervical mucus necessary to transport the sperm across the cervix. Uterine problems include **fibroids** or other growths in the uterus that block implantation. Infertility in women is a complex issue and these are only some of the more common causes.

In men, the combined causes of infertility contribute overall to 18 per cent of infertility problems. Problems in men include low sperm counts, weak sperm (sperm that aren't good 'swimmers'), varicocoeles (abnormally dilated veins that cause temperature changes in the testicles), damaged **sperm ducts**, hormonal deficiencies, testicular failure and sperm antibodies. Testicular failure can be caused by tumours, drugs, viral infections (most commonly 'mumps'), trauma and some sexually transmitted diseases. When sperm antibodies are identified, it indicates that the antibodies produced by a female partner incapacitate and kill sperm (Higgins 2006).

The above list of problems may appear daunting but many are treatable and have good outcomes. When women go for testing, their health history will be recorded and they will have a physical examination (this will probably involve **palpation** of the vagina, cervix, uterus, fallopian tubes, ovaries and rectum). Cervical cultures and **pap smears** may also be taken. Other tests may include ovarian reserve testing (assessing ovarian function), testing for ovulation and an examination using ultrasound. Men will have their sperm tested. These tests are not finite; your specialist will decide what tests are most suitable for you (and when) and should talk you through each test and why they intend to perform it.

Before you go for your initial assessment, you should consider gathering as much information as possible. The Resources section on page 241 has a list of websites, books and organisations that can help you find information and form a list of questions to ask. Some questions are obvious, such as cost, while others may not be so obvious, such as what qualifications your specialist has. The best place to find help is on the internet, through specific discussion forums.

IVF

In-vitro fertilisation—or, as it is more commonly known, IVF—is a process by which egg cells are fertilised by sperm outside of the womb. The words 'in vitro' are Latin for 'in glass', hence the term 'test tube baby'. The process of IVF involves controlling the ovulation process with the use of injections and/or nasal sprays, taking eggs (ova/**oocytes**) from the woman, placing them in fluid and fertilising them with sperm. When the egg is fertilised, it is known as a 'zygote' and is transferred to the woman with the hope of establishing a pregnancy.

While this is a useful (if basic) description of the IVF process, it cannot account for the gamut of emotions that go hand in hand with the IVF journey. When couples resort to IVF, it is an acknowledgement that their bodies cannot produce babies without assistance from reproductive technologies. There is a certain grief in this acknowledgement for many women and men and this is reflected in the stories that follow. IVF is often referred to as a roller-coaster ride: hormones run high and emotions dip and weave as couples anxiously await news of pregnancy. It can also be a financial drain; IVF is not cheap by any stretch of the imagination.

While the IVF process is successful for many women, the overall success rate differs due to varying factors and it is important to remember that IVF doesn't always work. Figuring out how many attempts to make is a personal dilemma and is a choice that can only be made by you.

Riding the roller-coaster: Staying positive about IVF

Lisa and her husband decided to investigate when, after trying to conceive for three years, she hadn't fallen pregnant. Lisa tells us why she couldn't conceive without IVF and how her positive attitude helped her remain calm and confident throughout the process.

Lisa's Story

We tried to conceive naturally for three years before finally admitting that we needed help to get pregnant. The first test performed was a sperm analysis, as it was the quickest and easiest way to find out if there was a problem with my husband's sperm. My darling husband doesn't partake in solo pleasure so getting his head around what he needed to do took a long, long time. After months of conversations about it, we decided that I'd take time off work to go to the clinic to 'assist' him. Well, let's just say that it could have been one huge ego bruising for me because I was practically naked, trying all sorts of fun and games (and dance!) to arouse him, however the room was so sterile and we could hear traffic passing up and down the corridor right outside the room we were in, so my attempts were in vain. Months later, after quite a heated discussion, he went and got the job done (twice) and as it turned out our infertility did not lie with him.

*Our infertility falls under the 'explained' category. It was firstly established that I was not ovulating, which was fixed with the use of **clomid** (clomid is often a first line treatment to induce regular **ovulation**), then after six failed cycles, my mucus was examined and declared 'hostile' and therefore my husband's little swimmers weren't getting through the gate, so to speak. To combat that, we next tried three cycles using intra-uterine insemination (IUI), which is when the sperm is deposited straight into the woman's uterus through artificial means. This procedure is timed with blood tests and internal ultrasounds to catch the egg upon ovulation. There was no reason established why this did not work for us, so **IVF** was the next logical step.*

When we finally sought help after three years of trying to get pregnant naturally, we both had very optimistic attitudes. It was obvious that we could not do this on our own so we both had some feelings of relief that we'd finally put our egos aside and asked for assistance. We knew that IVF created babies and we didn't doubt that it would work for us. Finally, we saw a light at the end of the tunnel and we knew that IVF was going to get us to that light. We had friends who had two beautiful girls through IVF, so, obviously, the technique works for some. Never did we envisage IVF not working for us; it just didn't come up in conversation, ever. To us, it was now a matter of 'when', not 'if'. Also, walking into the fertility clinic as often as we did (for example, blood tests) and seeing the number of other women in the waiting room was comforting. I wasn't pleased that they were having fertility issues, but it made me feel like I wasn't alone and it really opened my eyes as to how common infertility is, so I didn't feel so alienated.

Fortunately, I'm not squeamish with needles, so I was fine with injecting myself in my stomach. My husband, on the other hand, is hopeless around needles and was extremely apologetic that he couldn't watch or hold my hand when I had to do it each morning. He couldn't even be in the same room. I did have a few mood swings due to the hormones but my husband remained very patient with me (in his words: 'It's the least I can do') as his input into the whole IVF procedure was minimal.

Financially, I think we were approximately A$5000 out of pocket (after health care rebates). We were fortunate in that we both worked and had a manageable mortgage *but in all honesty, the cost of the procedure wasn't even a discussion point before going ahead with IVF. We found out the prices after we'd already decided to try IVF.*

Finally getting pregnant was the most exciting thing for both of us. When searching for information on infertility, I came across an online parenting forum. The forum was a great source of support and information when I went through the IVF procedure, however, it was also sad and extremely hard to see how many women suffered from early miscarriages. So as excited as I was that I finally had a little baby in my belly, I was also so aware how precious my tiny little baby was and I guess, for both of us, our parenting instincts kicked in from day one because my husband wrapped me so tightly in cotton wool, it was hard to breathe. We both wanted this baby so much, so keeping me relaxed, calm and safe was now the priority.

My husband told me it was my job to look after baby, while his job was to look after me. While I knew about how common miscarriage was, I don't think my husband or I ever doubted holding our baby in our arms one day. We'd been on this journey for far too long and had cried too many tears for our baby not to be born one day. Yes, we were nervous and cautious, but we felt in our hearts that we were going to be parents in nine months' time, and we couldn't wait.

Lisa's Wisdom	IVF can be a roller-coaster ride, and it will depend on your personality as to how you view that ride. For us, we 'went with the flow'. We didn't ask too many questions and went about it in an almost business-like fashion, trying to take the emotion out of it. However, if you are more of an emotive person, have the tissues handy because all the hormones and the actual procedure itself can take its toll.
	Emotionally, keep the lines of communication open with your partner. IVF can be a very lonely and isolating journey so keep talking to each other. Also, don't be embarrassed to seek support from outside your immediate circle. Fertility clinics usually offer support groups, and as previously mentioned, I found the support I received from the online forum absolutely invaluable. It's very useful to talk to other women going through the same experiences as yourself.

Never say never: Having a baby at 40 through IVF

Bronwyn had always thought she would get married and have children, but when she married at the age of 23, she was eager to experience life before settling down. It wasn't until Bronwyn reached her mid-30s that she and her husband started trying for a baby. However, as 40 approached with no signs of a pregnancy, Bronwyn began to recognise that there might be infertility problems.

Bronwyn's Story

I remember being on our honeymoon in 1991 at the tender age of 23 and my biggest fear was having a honeymoon baby. I needn't have worried. Seventeen years later, at the age of 40, I finally fell pregnant for the first time and gave birth to our beautiful boy, Lachlan.

As a child, I had always thought I would one day get married and have three children. Funnily enough, when I was finally married, I knew that when children did come along that life would change dramatically, so I tried to extend my freedom. Having married fairly young, I wanted to make sure that I travelled the world and 'followed my heart' for as long as possible. It wasn't until I was about 34 that I thought, 'I guess I'd better get on to the baby thing now!' Time went by and as I neared my late 30s, I started to get worried that it wasn't ever going to happen. It had never occurred to me that having a baby would be a problem, as everything else had always come to me pretty easily in life. I had considered **IVF** *but always ruled it out. It was simply something that I was never going to do. The thought of injecting drugs scared me greatly.*

Just before my 39th birthday, I consented to having **laparoscopic surgery** *to find out why I had been unable to get pregnant. I was amazed at what the surgery revealed. It turned out that my ovaries had been stuck down for the past 25 years. Infection and scar tissue from an appendix removal operation that I had at the age of 14 was the culprit. It had also caused some damage to one of my fallopian tubes, making it very unlikely that I could conceive naturally. My gynecologist was also surprised to find six large, benign polyps in my uterus, which were removed in two* **hysteroscopy** *procedures. His verdict was that there was a 'chance' that I could fall pregnant naturally but my best option was IVF. By now, at the age of 39, I was getting very concerned about never having children, so I finally decided to put aside my fears and begin IVF treatment.*

I actually became quite eager to get started. I even thought that I might be able to get away with having just one pregnancy by having twins! I can't tell you how many hours I spent searching the internet for forums containing personal IVF stories. Many people were quite negative, describing how awful the medication made them feel. The thing that I was most afraid of was feeling nauseous. When I finally started the treatment, I was pleasantly surprised that I had very few reactions to the medications, apart from regular headaches from the nasal spray. I was relieved to discover that the injections you have to self-administer were in an easy-to-use pen that wasn't really painful at all.

Finally, after about four weeks of taking medication, I was ready for egg collection. This process was one that I was very nervous about. I had only ever had two operations before—both had made me very sick afterwards—and I was dreading feeling the same way again. But I was pleasantly surprised. I was only under anesthetic for about 25 minutes and I felt absolutely fine afterwards. I was able to go back to work the next day.

By embryo transfer day, we had three **blastocysts**. *One was implanted, and two frozen. Despite everyone saying that embryo transfer is painless and quick, I actually found this to be the hardest part of the whole IVF cycle (unfortunately not painless at all for me). The two-week wait before my pregnancy test was another difficult time that was full of analyzing every tiny twinge in my body. 'Is this a pregnancy symptom, or is it PMS?' As it turned out, my period was three days late but when I had my pregnancy blood test at the clinic, I was told that although there were low levels of pregnancy hormones in my blood,* the embryo had only implanted lightly and not survived. Sad about the result, we had a follow-up visit to the gynaecologist who said that despite the failed attempt, my embryo quality was very good for my age and we had a very good chance of pregnancy if we attempted a couple of IVF cycles.

When the next transfer date arrived, we decided to have two embryos transferred. I was still eager to have twins and was excited about our prospects. Sadly, after the two-week wait, the pregnancy test came back negative.

Disappointed that I would have to go through the whole process of injections again, not to mention fork out another several thousand (US) dollars, we signed up for a second IVF cycle. This time ten eggs were collected; nine were fertilized and we still had six viable embryos on the day of transfer. Two were implanted and the other four observed overnight to see how they grew. The next day I received a phone call from the scientists to say that the remaining four were no longer viable. I was very upset about not having any left to freeze, and as the week progressed, I became convinced that this cycle had not worked. At this point, I became emotional, thinking that I didn't really want to have to do another stimulated cycle again and wondered if we could actually afford to do another cycle. The money would have to come out of extra payments that we had put into the mortgage.

I'll never forget the day that I was at work and received the call from the clinic to say that I was actually pregnant. After convincing myself that this cycle had failed, I tried very hard to hold back the tears as the nurse told me the wonderful news. Finally, I was pregnant for the first time in my life. I wanted to squeal and tell everybody at work but had to restrain myself. I rang my husband straight away, who was just as elated. After 17 years of marriage, it almost felt a bit unbelievable.

Even though I was 40, I had a great pregnancy with no morning sickness. I did develop **gestational diabetes** in the third trimester and was put on a strict, healthy diet which I believe actually gave me extra energy at a stage when many women feel very tired. Lachlan was born by caesarean section at nearly 39 weeks. He's the most beautiful little boy, happy, and with an infectious little chuckle. He brings joy to every day and I can't describe how wonderful it is to have him in our lives.

If I knew everything that I know today, I guess I would have begun the whole IVF process a lot earlier, but to be honest, I really wasn't ready until I was 39. We are now trying for another baby. As I write, I am just about to go for my third egg collection. It is a little scary being 41 and trying to beat the odds statistically, but my gynecologist says that my chances for success are high, so I just have to hold onto that hope and keep trying.

Bronwyn's Wisdom
I think a very important thing that I've learned through this whole process is to keep your life in balance and appreciate the wonderful things that you have in your life now; to live in the moment and live life to the full while you're on the journey. When you do that, rather than focus on what you do not yet have, all of the disappointments along the way are a lot easier to handle.

Postscript: Bronwyn is happy to report that she has given birth to her second child.

When to seek help getting pregnant

According to Higgins (2006), if you are healthy, have regular menstrual cycles and time your intercourse to coincide with ovulation, yet you still cannot conceive, you should consult your doctor after one year if you are younger than 35 and after six months if you are older than 35. She notes that the media stories of celebrity mothers who have babies in later life have given many women a false sense of security. You might put off pregnancy due to your career, your desire to travel and to experience life or you may not have found a suitable partner. Whatever your reasons, you should take into account the fact that by the age of 36–40, a woman's remaining supply of eggs rapidly loses the ability to be fertilised. In women younger than 36, 20–25 per cent of embryos conceived are chromosomally defective, and these embryos either fail to implant or are miscarried (often unnoticed by the woman). However, in women over the age of 40, the incidence of anomalies rises to 50–80 per cent.

If you have always dreamed of having a family, it is a good idea to have yourself checked out by your doctor to ensure your body is able to conceive. Many women like Bronwyn do not realise there is a problem until they start trying to get pregnant. If this problem is detected early, it might be treatable. Additionally, if you discover you may have problems conceiving, this might be an influencing factor as to when you decide to start trying for a baby. It is natural to want to wait until you find the right partner for you but if you find that your 'clock' is ticking or you know that you have certain time constraints due to problems already detected, you may like to consider 'going it alone', whether you are female or male. For more information and a list of helpful organisations, please see page 241 of the Resources section.

Donor conception

The decision to have a baby using donated sperm, eggs or embryos—like any other form of assisted conception—is necessarily imbued with emotions and implications. To begin with, if you are choosing this path because you have not found the right person to have children with or because you cannot have a baby with the partner you love, you may experience feelings ranging from self-doubt and grief to a sense of resignation. However, if you are in a same sex relationship, you will have likely known for a long time that you would need to use donated sperm, eggs or embryos to have a baby. Either way, it is important to talk through your feelings with a counsellor before you embark on this process, as you will not only need to deal with your own emotions, you will need to address questions about what you will tell your children and when. This is an individual choice and while you should obviously discuss it with your partner (if you have one), you should consider consulting with a professional counsellor who specialises in donor conception.

Not just a roll in the sack: Conceiving in a same sex relationship

Yumi and her partner decided to use donor sperm from someone they met through a parenting forum on the internet. They chose this option over anonymous donation, as they wanted their child's father involved in their family life.

Yumi's Story

*All things considered, I think that we had a pretty easy time conceiving our son. I have friends who had spent years trying to conceive their babies with varying degrees of success. One couple I know ended up spending A$70 000 on **IVF**, so I didn't assume we would conceive straight away, but there was definitely a part of me that was hoping it would be that easy.*

As lesbians, conception is obviously way more complex than a roll in the sack. There are many times I have thought to myself 'If only it was that easy!' To create a whole new little person just by having sex would be so cool! Funny how not being able to do that puts a whole new perspective on what people have been doing for millennia.

Lesbians manage to conceive babies though all sorts of means. I have friends who used anonymous sperm from a clinic and others who asked their best male friend to 'donate'. I even know one woman whose heterosexual best friend volunteered her husband's sperm (luckily, the husband was obliging and my friend now has a happy three-year-old).

When we first started thinking about babies, we didn't know any men who we would have wanted to be our sperm donor, or who we felt comfortable asking. We were also pretty sure we wanted our baby to have a father—someone involved in his life that he could develop a relationship with. So anonymous sperm was out. Luckily, we didn't have too much trouble meeting a guy through a parenting forum on the internet. This guy was a great match for us in terms of what our expectations were and the boundaries we wanted to set. About a year after first meeting this guy, we were all ready to start trying to get pregnant. I won't go into detail about how we actually got to this point but we had worked through all the necessary health checks, legal negotiations, personal discussions and so forth.

People are always fascinated to know how the 'deed' is actually done between two people who presumably aren't having sex with each other. But in my experience, even the most fascinated people are not sure how to ask this sort of personal question (fair enough too). So, I am glad you asked! This is how it was done.

The father of our baby-to-be (I'll call him Joe) lived in a different state. So in order to conceive, one of us had to make the interstate trip at exactly the right time every month.

Fortunately, my body obligingly ran to a regular 28-day cycle. I even ovulated on a Saturday, so we could make this trip on the weekends.

When my partner and I made the trip, we would check into a hotel that was conveniently located across the road from Joe's house. We got so good at this that we even knew how to pick this particular hotel from the 'mystery hotel' selections on a travel website, making it much cheaper.

We usually pre-arranged the times we would 'try', to ensure Joe was available. I had read on the internet that the best quality sperm is to be found in the mornings, so we usually tried early in the day.

I don't have the details of what went on from Joe's end (it's probably fairly obvious), but we would meet him in our hotel foyer at the pre-arranged time to receive the jar of sperm. He always wrapped it up carefully to keep it nice and warm for the journey across the road. The handover moments were always a bit hilarious. I am sure it looked as though we were doing some illicit drug deal as the whole thing had to happen quite quickly. More than once we have laughed at the thought of what would have happened if anyone did get suspicious and asked us to explain ourselves or the content of our jar. But that never happened.

We used a large-barrel syringe to inject the sperm into me trying as best as possible to coat the **cervix**. *This was very low-tech* **artificial insemination**. *But it seems sperm is much hardier than you might think when a baby is waiting to be born.*

All up, we repeated this process seven times over the course of a year. In hindsight, seven times doesn't seem that much. But at the time, I found it very stressful. A whole month could be consumed by monitoring **ovulation**, *preparing for possible conception and waiting to do a pregnancy test. I became obsessed with online advice about how to conceive and possible signs of early pregnancy. Every month I had phantom pregnancy symptoms.*

Funnily enough, the time I actually did conceive I was convinced I wasn't pregnant. We had just returned from a month in Thailand and I was due to start a new job. So I had it in my mind that we would try one more time then take a break for a while so I could get into my new work. About ten days after we had 'tried', I had a little bit of bleeding which I assumed was my period starting. I actually felt a bit relieved that I wouldn't have to explain to my new employer why I was four months pregnant only three months into my contract. Also that week I had to go away on a pretty relaxed work trip that involved cocktails on the beach and spa baths in my 'free upgrade' hotel suite (remind me again what they tell you not to do when you are pregnant … I am pretty sure drinking alcohol and having spa baths are on that list).

It was a week or so after that trip that it finally dawned on me my period had never properly appeared and I was feeling a bit light-headed. I suggested to my partner that maybe we should try a pregnancy test just in case. She raced out and bought one straight away.

It took about three seconds for the second line to appear on the pee-stick. By that stage, I was close to four weeks pregnant so my hormones were well and truly in gear. There was no mistaking it; that was definitely a positive pregnancy test. Nonetheless, I did a few more just to be sure. I still have those tests sitting in my sock drawer.

Eight months and a very long labour later my son was born—all 9.2 pounds of him—happy and healthy.

Yumi's Wisdom

So what I have learned from this experience? Firstly, when it comes to lesbian conception a sense of humour is a must. Doing things like negotiating sperm handovers or screening men who could potentially be the father of your child is surreal. Embarrassment is not an option so laughter definitely helps.

But mostly I have learnt that you just don't have total control over what your body will do, no matter how hard you try. It's so easy to get frustrated and angry with yourself when pregnancy doesn't happen and so much harder to just relax and take the attitude of 'what will be, will be'. This is particularly the case with artificial insemination, which is all about thinking and planning (rather than sex and fun). I genuinely feel like the best thing we did to help our conception was to take a trip overseas and refocus on other things. I am sure that when I actually did conceive it was in part because I was relaxed.

As discussed in 'Same sex parenting: ART, adoption and fostering' (page 16), third party reproduction is incredibly complex and the laws surrounding it are either non-existent or differ from country to country (and even within countries). It is therefore crucial that all parties involved seek legal advice before embarking on this journey. The options available through third party reproduction provide many couples with the opportunity to turn their dream of parenthood into reality. This method is gaining momentum and as it becomes more widely used, there is increased understanding of the moral, ethical and legal issues involved. As aptly stated by the American Society for Reproductive Medicine (2006):

> *The ultimate goal of physicians, mental health professionals, and attorneys specializing in reproductive law is to enable this process to move forward as smoothly as possible and bring joy and satisfaction to all parties involved in ensuring the conception and delivery of a healthy child. (p. 15)*

If you are considering using any of the methods in this chapter to conceive a child, talk to people who are experienced in the process and who have travelled the same complex (and at times, confusing) path. The best place to do this is through support groups (both face-to-face and online). For a list of groups, websites and legal organisations, please refer to the Resources section on page 242. To learn how to start your own support group, see Appendix B on page 225.

Surrogacy

Surrogacy is a complicated process that raises complex ethical, moral and legal issues. Both heterosexual and same sex couples use surrogacy; here we read the story of two men in a same sex relationship who used donated eggs, their sperm and a **gestational carrier** to fulfil their dream of becoming parents.

What is third party reproduction? Unravelling the terminology

The term 'third party reproduction' is an umbrella term that refers to the use of eggs, sperm or embryos that have been donated by a third party ('the donor') in order to enable an individual or a couple ('the recipient/s') to become parents. Donors can be anonymous or known (this is obviously a choice to be made by both parties). The term also refers to 'traditional surrogacy' and 'gestational carrier' arrangements. Traditional surrogacy involves a woman using the sperm of the recipient (or from a donor) to conceive. She therefore has a genetic link to the pregnancy, as her own eggs are fertilised. A gestational carrier (also known as 'gestational surrogate' and 'uterine carrier') carries the pregnancy for the recipient. Her eggs are not used and she does not have a genetic link to the pregnancy. Instead, donor eggs and sperm are used to create an embryo, which is then implanted in the woman who will carry the baby.

Two men and two babies: Fathering children through surrogacy

Trevor and Pete embarked on a long and exhilarating journey that ultimately led them to India and the birth of their twins, Evelyn and Gaia.

Trevor's Story

Both Pete and I had always wanted to have a family. I had previously been in a 12-year relationship with a solicitor who was equally adamant that he did not want a family. When I met Pete, I raised it as a 'deal breaker' two weeks into our relationship and he said he also wanted to have children.

It took us three years of research. Every time I learned something that really showed we could do this, Pete got more nervous and excited. We really thought we were one generation away from being able to do this. We initially looked into the United States, which ultimately became too expensive as we needed to have resources for education and raising the children in reserve. However, the States gave us a mature framework to tackle India. In the States, they asked us what ten traits we would like to see in our children (from the egg donor). While thinking about this, we made a decision that we did not want to have 'pasty poms' and were looking at Hispanic egg donors so the children had some protection from the hot Australian sun. As this was the case, I looked to South America to see if we could go there, but that wasn't possible. But I came across an Israeli couple who had delivered their baby with a clinic in India just a few weeks earlier.

We talked a lot about it, and asked for feedback from one of Pete's sisters and a very close aunty of mine. We did not require their validation—but their excitement and positive comments on us being dads were wonderful. We asked a friend who is a doctor in Mumbai to check out the clinic and after some good initial feedback, we started the process. Looking back, I cannot believe how naive we were. This is why we are so active in our Gay Dads group and have put a lot of energy into helping others get through this.

We didn't choose surrogacy—surrogacy chose us. We cannot adopt in Australia as a same sex couple. We had seen many examples of co-parenting that had not worked out. Our worst fear would be a co-parent changing the rules. We even had offers of eggs from a friend that donates eggs altruistically in Australia to help couples conceive but the fear that someone can or may have something over you legally to take the children away was just too scary. Surrogacy was the easiest of all the hard options and the biological connection enables us to have rights ... of a sort. The non-biological father has no rights to the children under current Australian law. If it was legal or had been straightforward, we would have adopted from a developing country and given a home to children who are in desperate need of one.

Once we made up our minds, we decided to implant two surrogates and have two babies with both of us being bio-dad (biological fathers) to one of the children each. We wanted to be the youngest fathers possible.

Our UK egg donor is young and gorgeous and has mixed English and Pakistani heritage. She sings like an angel and can play multiple instruments and speak several languages—we hoped that some of this would go through to the children, as well as her big sub-continental eyes. We liaised with the UK clinic, started her hormonal treatments and linked her into our clinic. The whole process of getting clinics talking to clinics in other countries proved to be very difficult. Doctors could not co-ordinate themselves and the added issue of her Pakistani heritage caused issues with an Indian visa. We forget how easy it is for us to travel on UK and Australian passports. The final 'kick-off' injection supplied by the clinic in the UK was taken on the plane to India and when she arrived, they said it could not be used because it was not 'temperature controlled'—£700 wasted! When her eggs were collected there were not enough to allow us to fertilise half each. This meant we still had to find another egg donor to complete our original intentions to have a child each (even though they would not be biologically connected as was our original intention). The clinic had an egg donor collection earlier that day and they offered us 'first choice' on an egg donor who looked very similar to our friend. We had 40 minutes to make a decision on whether to move forward with both lots of eggs, so we asked them not to tell us whose sperm was mixed with which eggs.

To discuss **gestational carriers**, we need to look at titles. Within our Gay Dads group, people have different views on the term 'mother'—some believe their children have a genetic mother and a birth mother. Pete and I decided that the title 'mother' implied nurture, so we use the terms 'egg donor' and 'gestational surrogate'. When you consider that the surrogate has no genetic link with the children and the egg donor has no involvement in *the raising of the children, the term 'mother' does not sit well with us. There are many wonderful mothers who have no genetic link to the children they raise. My own sister-in-law has been the most wonderful mother to my niece who was from a previous relationship my brother had. To me she is a mother, and I can only reconcile the core principles and importance of the term 'mother' to someone who does the hard work of decades of love, nurture and support. The biggest problem we have with 'surrogate', 'step' and 'blended' families is the different mix of terminology and agreed language used to describe them.*

We did not choose our gestational surrogate and many couples—both straight and gay—are making the same decision. With India being less mature than the US system in terms of process, you have less information. We have worked with a new hospital in Delhi to make sure that more information is provided (like personal interests of the egg donor), as well as getting them to agree that an egg donor can only work with one couple per country.

I don't know of any male same sex couples that do not plan for a child each as a preferred option. In helping gay fathers, we now recommend they both leave sperm samples (even if they are only trying to conceive one baby first) so that a second egg collection can be carried out in a few months using the same egg donor and then the embryos can be frozen until the couple are ready to have a second child. There are no guarantees the egg donor will be available but this kind of planning means their children will have the genetic half-sibling link, further protecting the families. We may over-plan these things, but showing our intent in creating a family is all we can do for now, until the law catches up. Only when we are allowed to marry will our children be protected in the same manner as the children of heterosexual couples.

Words cannot describe the overwhelming emotions that cascade through you once the nurse hands you your baby for the first time. It is something that only a new parent could understand. We are welling up just reliving that moment. We feel all children need a mixture of male and female energy. Pete is far more nurturing than a number of women we know. Dads don't get the recognition they deserve. There are many fantastic dads out there but try counting the storybooks that talk about dad and child—there are not that many. They do need to have women in their lives, and the girls have an abundance of women who spend time and energy with them. Everyone wants the best for them. People just want assurances that the girls are healthy and are well looked after. Our neighbour has three boys and turns up for her 'girlie fix', the girls' five older female cousins visit often and their grandmother is about to arrive from the UK for a three-month stay.

We get asked a lot about Mother's Day. What we have decided to do is make it a day about the incredible women who came before them and whose blood runs through their veins. My aunts are writing letters with stories about my grandmother who passed last year, and they have their cousins and aunts to talk about Pete's mum who passed at Christmas. They will also get onto Skype and speak to their great aunts in the UK, so they can talk about their great grandmother and her life. We think it's important for them to know where they come from, and of course we will encourage them to embrace their Indian heritage if they so desire.

We are constantly judged by people in the community, as well as on blogs and parenting websites. But we talk to strangers all the time and to date, no one has said anything negative directly to our face. I know we will make mistakes and there will be things we can do better but we will give our children the best beginning we can. Being a father is the most wonderful thing a man can be. Gay rights are the civil rights of our generation and no one is making our family sit at the back of the bus. Our children will be told what black people went through, what women went through and what we went through to have them in our lives, and our hopes are that when they are young adults this will all be academic.

Trevor's Wisdom	Communicate with your partner and understand the roles you will both play. I encourage all gay men to work out what they would do if they were to split and write down an agreement of what an 'ideal' separation would be. We have an agreement and it revolves around the children, not us. The fact we did this made us understand our relationship and roles more—a double whammy for the children. Lastly, try not to listen to too many people … you'll go mad.

Same sex parenting: ART, adoption and fostering

In the case of LGBT couples and individuals, ART may or may not be required. For example, ART is the only way in which male couples can conceive biological children. Some lesbian couples also use ART when the egg of one of the partners is used with donor sperm and transferred to the other partner. But two women in a same sex relationship who wish to conceive may use fresh semen samples (as in Yumi's story on page 10).

If you are considering this option, you should proceed with some caution; you need to be fully satisfied that the sample you receive does not have a sexually transmitted infection, for example. If you prefer to ensure the 'safety' of the sperm you use, you should obtain your sperm from a registered donation clinic. Sperm donated to clinics undergo rigorous testing. The sperm donor and the sperm will be screened and tested for diseases. Furthermore, most reputable clinics quarantine the sperm for a period of six months to ensure the donor is free of HIV before the sperm is thawed and used.[2] In addition to the aspect of safety, many female couples obtain sperm from a fertility clinic for **ease of access** and so that the sperm can be stored for future use if necessary. If you know someone who is willing to donate sperm, you can ask them to do this through a fertility clinic (for reassurance, convenience and future access).

In 2009, the Ethics Committee of the American Society for Reproductive Medicine reviewed the issue of same sex couples who wish to become parents. It concluded that: 'ethical arguments supporting denial of access to fertility services on the basis

---

2 Positive men (men living with HIV) who wish to have children may have access to a technique called '**sperm washing**', a process that concentrates and separates the fertilising sperm from infectious seminal fluid. This technique is still relatively new and, while recent reports indicate high success rates (i.e. no transference of the virus to the woman carrying the pregnancy or to the baby), safety cannot yet be 100 per cent guaranteed (Sauer et al. 2009).

of marital status or sexual orientation cannot be justified' (p. 1). This conclusion was based on the fact that there is no persuasive evidence that children are harmed or disadvantaged solely by being raised by unmarried parents, single parents or LGBT parents (for a full discussion on this issue, please see 'Same sex parents' on page 208). However, as Jones (2010) points out, 'the law trumps ethical considerations' (p. 302). Same sex couples wishing to access ART are bound by the laws of their country, and laws not only differ from country to country—they also differ within countries. This is exemplified by United States legislation, where laws regarding same sex couples and ART differ from state to state. For relevant legislation, please refer to page 267 of the References section.

Legislation is also pivotal for same sex couples considering adoption and/or fostering. In 2008, the European Court of Human Rights established a principle that European countries could no longer exclude LGBT individuals from applying for child adoption. The same principle holds true for the United Kingdom and South Africa. As with ART, adoption legislation differs within countries, including the United States, Australia and Canada.

As declared in Article 16(1) of the Universal Declaration of Human Rights (1948), 'Men and women of full age, without any limitation due to race, nationality, or religion, have the right to marry and found a family.' While some countries and states/territories are beginning to legislate in alignment with this article, same sex couples (both male and female) are still discriminated against and remain more vulnerable as parents than traditional, married, heterosexual couples.

If you are in a same sex relationship and find yourself in the position of needing ART or you are looking to adopt (or foster) a child, you should familiarise yourself with the legislation in your country. The best way to start is to talk to other people who have been through a similar process and you can easily do this online. You might also like to consider contacting a free legal service in your area if one is available or you can look up the relevant legislation on the internet (some relevant legislation is also listed in the References section of this book). If you have the means, you might consider paying a lawyer for a consultation to discuss your legal rights. Additionally, there are many LGBT lobby groups that you can phone or email for further information. For a list of blogs, websites, lobby groups and community forums please see page 242 of the Resources section.

Adoption

Adoption for many people (both couples and singles) is a last resort after coming to terms with infertility and the inability to conceive using IVF.

However, people adopt for many other reasons. Some adopt to add to their own biological family. Some adopt to give children who are living in poverty (usually in a developing country) a better chance at life, otherwise known as 'inter-country' adoption. Yet others are in a same sex relationship or are single and choose to adopt instead of going through the process of ART. Whatever the reasons for adopting, it is always a complex process.

From Russia with love: Adopting a baby from a foreign country

Karen met her husband later in life and when they decided to have a baby, they were shocked to discover that their chances of doing so were very small. Karen had originally ruled out foreign adoption, but a meeting with a Ukraine woman changed her mind—and her life.

Karen's Story

When my husband and I married in July of 1996, we referred to ourselves as 'late bloomers'; he was 38 and I was 36. We knew we wanted children, so after just a few months, we talked with a fertility physician. Unfortunately, after several rounds of medication, he informed us that our chances for children were slim to none and we'd best consider adoption.

Obviously, there is a certain amount of grieving that a couple experiences when told such news. The visions you have in your mind of what your children will look like have to fade, or at least, be closed away in some closet in your heart and mind.

After a time, Gary and I started the arduous process of adoption. We agreed we'd rather adopt domestically. We picked an agency, pulled our home study together, made our photo album and letter, and began advertising. Suddenly, becoming a parent meant marketing ourselves to prospective birth mothers. We networked, we prayed, we traveled to birth mothers' homes and met them in hospitals.

We came close several times. Three times, in fact—yet no one saw us as 'the right' parents. In those losses, Gary and I grew closer; however, I can assure you, a heart truly does break. Four years of married life and we were still not a 'family' but thank goodness we had each other.

We considered foreign adoption as time passed. We had even chosen an agency but it just did not feel right. It was expensive. It seemed risky. The paperwork was overwhelming. Gary was always up for an adventure to another country. I was always hesitant. I had traveled abroad 20 years earlier but now the world seemed in turmoil. I just had so many misgivings.

Then we met this wonderful woman from the Ukraine who had made it her life's mission to connect Russian children with American parents. Her agency was just a fledgling but she was so heart-warming, we knew if we adopted internationally, it would be with her. Finally, after a very heartening phone call from a cousin sharing yet another wonderful international adoption story, we decided to give her a call. It was April 2001.

At the very first meeting, this amazing, lovely woman told us of twin baby boys not even on the adoption register yet. They were from Murmansk—almost at the top of the world. They were six months old. We said we were interested. She said her husband, an attorney, would handle most of the paperwork. She sent us medical information and a video of one of the boys. Physicians reviewed their medical profiles and assured us the boys were healthy.

I showed the tape to my sister and tiny niece and nephew. They immediately fell in love with Igor, who would soon be Thomas Andrew. My sister said very resolutely, 'Go get those precious babies.'

Just six weeks later, we did. We were off to Moscow and from there, Murmansk. After all the years of struggle and the pain of disappointment, our international adoption was to be a smooth and flawless process. On our flight from New York to Moscow, I talked with a mother who was with a group of teens headed to Russia on a mission trip to build a park for an orphanage. She pointed to her son who would serve as translator for the group. She and her husband had adopted him from Russia just three years prior to the trip. As I watched him joke with his friends, I hoped that my sons would grow up to be as cute, outgoing and bright as he was.

Our guide took us to the orphanage the day after we arrived. It was very run down, as were many of the buildings in Murmansk. But once inside, it was bright, cheery, clean and cosy. The nursery was full of babies and we instantly spied Igor (Thomas) sitting in one of the cribs. Kyrill (Joseph) was still asleep, so his caregiver woke him and brought him to us. They let us spend time with them in another room. Both boys were very friendly and curious. They did not make many sounds but smiled and smiled. I was amazed that even small babies ate porridge. Igor (Thomas) practically jumped into his food and was quite a mess by the end of the meal. Kyrill (Joseph) let his food come to him and was a much 'neater' eater. They washed down their porridge and smashed apple with a cup—yes, a cup—of tea. I remember thinking at the time they were very sweet but definitely all boy (I still feel that way!). The orphanage must only use diapers on special occasions because we noticed our boys were wearing rags between their legs. We bought diapers for the orphanage and many other supplies.

On the 14th of June we went to court. It was very formal. We explained why we wanted to adopt the boys. We found out that their birth parents were not living together and that the boys had two older sisters (aged 10 and 15). The judge left, returned 15 minutes later and told us we were granted the adoption of Thomas Andrew and Joseph Patrick.

Once back in Moscow, there were all kinds of appointments and paperwork to ensure that the boys could travel with us. Thanks to recent law changes, once we as American citizens had adopted the boys, they were automatically granted citizenship. This expedited the process.

Finally, it was time to fly home. Thomas screamed for the first ten minutes on the flight. Then he settled down and was great the rest of the time. Joe seemed to view it as an adventure. He tried ice cream. He laughed at himself in the mirror of the plane's restroom. I still marvel at how trusting and brave these little babies were. They were taken from the warm, secure cocoon of the orphanage and thrown into the noisy, uncomfortable world with two people they had barely gotten to know. They are to this day just as brave and confident about new things. They continually amaze me.

After the ten hour flight from Moscow to New York, we literally ran with the boys in their strollers to catch our connecting flight to Cincinnati. From Cincinnati (another flight we barely made), we made the last leg to Indianapolis to be greeted by at least 30 family and friends who could wait no longer to meet the boys.

The boys, although exhausted, went to everyone and smiled for all. When we at last arrived home and put them in their cribs, Joey looked around the room and at me and just sighed blissfully—what a moment. I cried and thought to myself, 'These little guys now have parents. I'm their mom, Gary's their dad. We're a family!'

Karen's Wisdom	Both practically and emotionally, I would say, be patient. I've learned that all things happen for reasons and they occur only when it is time. Tolerate each step—whether it is paperwork or disappointment. Be sure to network with everyone because this can lead to great joy. Finally, trust. For me, personally, going to Russia was a tremendous leap of faith. To be honest, I was more than hesitant. However, I believed this was what we were supposed to do—and it was.

Tips for adoptive parents

If you are planning an inter-country adoption, make sure that you are aware of the laws in both your country and the country you intend to adopt a child from. If you are granted adoptive rights, it's a good idea to collect as much memorabilia from that country as you can, as your child will come to treasure it in the future. It is always a good idea to foster a sense of culture and pride in your child (although you shouldn't force this on them), as well as acknowledging and discussing why they look different to the rest of the family. These are just a few of the many issues you need to consider when adopting a child from another country. As always, it is very helpful to talk to those who have gone before you and you can seek out adoptive parents quite easily on the internet. A great place to start for inter-country adoption is page 239 of the Resources section.

Excuse me, I'm over here: Sam's plan to adopt his parents

Joe and his wife attempted fertility treatment several times before deciding to cease and look into the process of adoption. Here Joe tells us about the 'marketing' aspect of adoption in the United States and how couples have to prove that they are capable and fit to raise children.

Joe's Story

'I can't do this anymore.' I attempt to give my wife an injection to make her ovulate or maybe it is to delay **ovulation**. *I cannot keep them straight. In the three years since our marriage, we have progressed in our efforts to conceive a child as far as we can. So bruised and swollen is her hip that the oversized needle bounces off her skin. 'If it doesn't work this time, I don't think I can either', she replies.*

Several days after Cathy's eggs were taken, we receive a call from the fertility specialist: 'They're not the best quality but I'd like to implant them anyway.' At our first appointment after the eggs are implanted, he confirms that our second attempt at **in-vitro fertilization** *has failed. 'But don't be too discouraged', he says. 'We're going to get you a baby'.*

Several weeks later, a leading fertility specialist at Vanderbilt University lays our file down and stares across his desk at us. 'Stop spending your money. You will not conceive your own child.' We're exhausted; from the drive, from the stress, from more tests. His words come like a punch in the gut. We sit in silence. A routine the doctor has no doubt been through many times. He waits and watches as the initial shock turns to frustration, then anger, sadness, then, strangely, a sense of relief. Relief from the burden of wondering if, had we tried one more time, would it have worked? We are relieved of the responsibility of making that decision.

'Have you considered adoption?' he asks. 'No', I reply. Adoption meant accepting that we would not have our own child. He shares some information with us, just in case we change our mind.

Three months later, an expectant mother tells us that she will keep her child and not adopt her baby to us. The doctor was right. Our desire to be parents overcame our need to bear our own child. We completed the social work process. We passed a battery of tests, surveys, background checks and interviews. We are declared 'fit' to be parents. For nothing. We are prepared emotionally and financially. Our home is ready. We persist, and invest more time and money—and hope—and complete the legal aspects of adoption. Six months later, it happens again. We return the baby items because an empty crib is too difficult.

I send an email message to friends, asking that if anyone hears of a potential adoption, they keep us in mind. One Friday afternoon I get a call from a lawyer friend. He was contacted by an expectant mother who was with an adoption agency but became uneasy about the arrangements. She believed it was too late to change, having already had an early labor false alarm. She looked in the Yellow Pages *under adoption attorneys and called the first listing—my friend's legal firm.*

'Joe, are you still interested in adopting?' he asks. He explains the situation. 'She's coming in this afternoon. You'll be one of several couples we present. I need some information on you and your wife. Do you have anything?'

'An agency just returned our portfolio yesterday. Will that work?'

'A portfolio?'

'Yes. It includes everything about us, including the process we've been through.'

'Perfect.'

Fifteen minutes later I deliver it to his office. At four o'clock that afternoon, I receive another call. 'She selected you', he informs me.

'Are you serious?'

'She picked you because you seemed ready.'

Two weeks later our son is born. I want to name him Sam. It is a good 'barber shop' name like Gus and Ed and Bill. My wife was not so sure. At church the Sunday before, the sermon was about Hannah. Hannah was barren, yet she was given a son. He was named Samuel: 'Gift from God'. Our son's name is Samuel.

Suddenly, it all makes sense. In hindsight, never before has a plan appeared so obvious. The plan worked. Sam is a miracle. Sam is my son and I'm his father.

We never say 'Sam is adopted', like he has some incurable condition. We adopted him; and he adopted us. We tell him about the process we went through and how long it took for us to find each other. 'The whole time,' I tell him, 'you were out there saying, "Excuse me, I'm over here".' To that, he falls out of his chair laughing.

As Sam's parents, it's our responsibility to teach him, to help him find happiness; to the best of our ability, remind him why he's here on this earth. It's our privilege to explain how he came to us; that we chose each other. Sometimes those roles are reversed.

Joe's Wisdom

Though difficult during such an emotional time, it is important for anyone considering or experiencing infertility treatment or adoption to be realistic. Educate yourself on what your infertility condition might be, the success rate for treatment, and the cost involved. While undergoing infertility treatment, a friend who had been through this process told me to skip directly to **IVF**. He and his wife started with the basic hormone treatment like we did, and his wife eventually gave birth to triplets but only after attempting all options leading up to, and including, IVF.

In denial, I took the unrealistically positive fertility specialist's words to heart and ignored my friend's practical advice. But I learned that three years of progressing up the treatment ladder is more costly—in time, money, and emotion.

Find support from others who share your situation. As with so many life events, difficulty conceiving a child, and adoption, are only really understood by those who have experienced it. They will avoid telling you that if you just relax, you'll get pregnant. They know that less than 10 per cent of adopting couples actually get pregnant afterward.

Be prepared; it becomes a business transaction. Those with money and an effective marketing plan find the most success. The sanctity of becoming parents, along with pride and privacy, are sacrificed by the mother during countless invasive tests. Fathers collect sperm samples in public facilities as unknowing patients bang on the door, only to deliver them to insensitive nurses. Emotionless sex happens on a schedule.

During adoption screening, your life is revealed to strangers whose job it is to judge your capability to be a parent. Countless tests are implemented to determine your suitability—tests that so many biological parents would have difficulty passing.

Fostering

Fostering is caring for someone else's children in your own home. The baby, child, or teenager is placed in your care, either short or long term, depending on their circumstances. They may require foster care because of a serious illness in their family or they may need foster care because of serious abuse. Because of this, many foster children are distressed and therefore foster parents work closely with social workers and counsellors to ensure the emotional wellbeing of the child they are fostering. As with adoption, people foster for many different reasons. Many people foster if they have been unable to adopt a baby or child and many people foster purely to help children in need. If you are interested in fostering a child, please refer to page 240 of the Resources section.

Can we have breakfast tomorrow? The joy and heartbreak of fostering

Laura always knew she wanted a large family—a combination of her own biological children and foster children. She freely admits to entering the fostering process without much knowledge of what to expect, and while it has been challenging, Laura and her family have been enriched by all the children they have welcomed.

Laura's Story

Fostering kids was always in our life path; it was never a set 'when, where or why', more a given that at some point it was something that we'd both dearly love to do. We both work in child-related fields and have three young children of our own, so it seemed a natural progression once our family had moved into a settled state.

Many people thought that we went in too early, and that the experience would be detrimental to our three children. We took the opposite view, contemplating how wonderful it would be to give our kids a sense of perspective of what can actually happens in a child's life, and encourage empathy, tolerance and all the other essential life skills that go along with sharing your family with unfamiliar little people.

There was obviously also the fact that there were hundreds, if not thousands, of children needing somewhere warm and safe to sleep that were no less important or special than our own. The most common comment we receive when people ask about our fostering is, 'I couldn't do that, I couldn't give them back.' The second most common response is along the lines of, 'Don't you think you're inviting other people's problems into your family?' The third is always, 'But what about your own children, shouldn't you wait until they're older?'

We were very naive entering into fostering and have had our ups and downs because of it but we do still foster—our children (now a little older) are beautifully empathetic and giving towards all our visitors, and we couldn't be prouder of them. We have also had the pleasure of caring for and making a difference in eight children's lives to date.

Probably foolishly we didn't do a great deal of research prior to becoming carers. Growing up, several of my friends were in care, and for as long as I can remember it was just something I was going to do. My husband is also very family oriented and was 100 per cent supportive and in all honesty was actually the one who made all the phone calls and got the ball rolling.

We went with an agency that had been recommended to us by a friend of a friend who worked in a hospital. She had fostered for some time, and stressed to us the importance of having support ourselves as carers. There is quite a bit of discussion out there regarding the pros and cons of fostering with agencies as opposed to the Department of Community Services (DoCS). In hindsight I can see both sides, however at the time the agency seemed the right way to go.

From our experience, the general process seems quite similar among the different agencies in Australia. We initially made phone contact and were sent out an information package outlining the different types of care available. We then sent in our application, a complete life history of ourselves and had several home visits. We also did the Shared Lives Training Program, updated our first aid certificates and sent through insurance information. Our doctors were required to complete questionnaires and we both had police checks done. There was also a home inspection, and our three children were interviewed by two agency workers. While some parts of the process were a little intrusive, I remember thinking at the time that it seemed too easy—information was taken at face value and I was a bit uneasy about some of the soon-to-be carers we did our training with.

The biggest hurdle we faced initially was the time it would take to become carers. The only reason we decided against going with DoCS was that we were told it would take 12 months to qualify. With the demand for foster carers so high, we were astounded that it could take so long, when really, if the process was streamlined, it should only take 6–8 weeks.

From the very beginning, I have found the system to be quite challenging. The kids themselves are wonderful, but it is difficult to see how these children can have positive outcomes, given the amount of bureaucracy and procedure their lives are governed by.

To date, all the children we have cared for come from parents who themselves were raised in care. Fifteen to twenty years ago, they were these kids. All the kids we have cared for have suffered unimaginable abuse and neglect and all come from parents who love them and fight desperately to have them returned. All the kids we have been involved with thus far have gone onto long-term placements.

There have been many times that we have professed that we'll never put ourselves through this again. Our family has been pulled, pushed and prodded in every way. My children have been put at risk by 'decision making' people deciding while a child was living with our own three children that we didn't need to know about his long history of sexualised behaviours. The very same decision makers then suggested that we discuss the matter at 'next month's case meeting' while the child continued to share the house with my three children.

We also learnt not to trust what we were told, especially after having a 2-, 4-, 5- and 6-year-old arrive from the police station for a 'week-long' emergency placement that lasted 7 months. Those four children were in desperate need of stability, love and support, and any behaviours that they had were absolutely no fault of their own. They were all delightful little beings. The flipside of this was having one of those children accuse us of unimaginable acts only to retract the accusation the following day, suggesting that they were upset that they weren't able to live with us forever.

This accusation was followed closely by the removal of two delightful, settled and happy little children, an investigation, a sincere apology for the way in which the matter was handled and two weeks of listening to our six-year-old cry herself to sleep because she wasn't able to say goodbye to her two foster sisters. Naturally, the case workers' priority is for the children they are responsible for, but we believe that there should be a certain level of consideration for the biological children of carers.

Having said that, new arrivals are always exciting. We are a routine family and to date, all our kids have settled in very quickly. Everyone seems to kick into gear and assume their roles. My absolute must each day is to have uniforms ready on beds, homework and bags packed and everything organised before going to bed.

I am continually surprised by how adaptable these kids are. One minute they are with their parent(s), and the next minute they are delivered to an absolute stranger—by strangers—and expected to cope. We can't reassure them with any information, because we have no information. We have been fortunate that all our kids have settled very quickly, and in all honesty, only one little boy from our first placement had difficulty settling at night. He would play, chat and sing happily during the day, then scream, kick and punch anything he could at bedtime. He was so angry. All we could do was be there for him and sit with him until he fell asleep. After a week or so he settled, but still slept with his fists clenched.

As I type this, there are two little boys sleeping soundly in our spare room with clean clothes, full tummies and mountains of love and support until their own families are settled and ready to care for them. One is two years old and arrived with maybe two words and the darkest, dullest eyes I've seen on a child. After the first week, he was running around like a madman and now chats and sings continually and has lovely bright blue eyes. His brother is six and is also delightful. He has some additional needs that we are in the process of working out, and he too has beautiful big blue eyes. They are both happy and settled boys; however they are both very keen to be able to get back to live with mum. As I tucked the six-year-old in tonight he asked me if we could have breakfast again tomorrow — such as a heartbreaking thing to hear from a child.

Laura's Wisdom	Initially, I actively encouraged friends and family to look into fostering. There are so many kids that need caring homes, even for respite. We live in a lovely community and at the time, I couldn't understand why more people didn't do it. Now with hindsight, I understand that we have no control over any situation involving the foster care system and are actively inviting heartache at any moment into our family.
	We figure that we've been through so much and have heard so many horrible things that literally nothing could shock us now. We were thrown in at the deep end and anything less than seven kids at a time is a walk in the park! We also get huge amounts of satisfaction and while

at this point, we cannot fix the system, we can make a little difference in a few children's lives, and that is enough.

The only advice I could possibly give is be prepared, good luck and good on you!

Why didn't anyone tell me that ...

- Doctors don't know everything! After being told we could never conceive children on our own, we went on to have two beautiful children.

- When you have fallen pregnant easily once, the second or subsequent times may not happen so easily.

- You can get pregnant the first month off the pill, even if you have been taking it for years and are trying to get your body back in a normal rhythm.

- Mothers can sometimes tell the moment they conceive—don't let someone tell you differently!

- You can ovulate from two sides.

- My husband would only have to look sideways at me and I would be pregnant!

- After having spent three years trying to conceive, as a male, I thought that was enough. It wasn't until after baby number one was born that my wife started the discussion of having a sibling. This had never occurred to me and was a real blow, having just reached what I thought was our goal. I wasn't prepared at all for that.

- You can get pregnant while breastfeeding.

- You may face tough decisions about what to do with remaining frozen embryos. Do you let them defrost for laboratory research? Give them to nurses to practise with? Give them to research? Or do you give them to another couple? That's quite a moral dilemma.

- The press would go mad over our use of surrogacy. They are always using terms such as 'rent-a-womb', which is very hurtful to us and to other women and men who are doing this because it is the only way for them to create a family.

CHAPTER TWO

....

Pregnancy

'Whether your pregnancy was meticulously planned, medically coaxed, or happened by surprise, one thing is certain—your life will never be the same again.'

Catherine Jones (Bagamary & Iglesias 2008)

Planned or unplanned, pregnancy signals a huge transition in a woman's life; a transition that leaves us almost in a state of limbo for nine months. As Maushart so eloquently puts it, 'Pregnancy is kind of a no-woman's land, in which one is not quite yet mother, but no longer other' (1997, p. 80).

Consider this fact: the average human pregnancy lasts 6480 hours. During these hours, *all* women will experience changes, both physical and emotional, that cause significant impact, not only for themselves but probably for their partners also. It's interesting that for the first 2000 hours of pregnancy, many couples (and individuals) choose not to tell anyone that they're pregnant; a concept that is completely counter-intuitive for many who are dying to shout the news from the rooftops. When asked why, many parents-to-be explain that they don't want to 'jinx' anything or fear having to tell people of a miscarriage. Hence, the magic '12 weeks' is a true signifier for many that the pregnancy is real: a baby will be born.

In the following stories, you will read about the cocktail of emotions felt by women about their pregnancies, ranging from overwhelming delight, to sheer terror; with many swinging between the two extremes. You will read about women who planned their pregnancies, yet still felt shock and disbelief that they actually had a baby growing inside them; you will hear from women who did not plan their pregnancies and struggled to make the right choice for themselves *and* their babies. You will also hear how men cope with pregnancy and how especially in the area of **postnatal depression**, their emotions can mimic those of their female partners.

We look at one woman's story of miscarriage and another woman's story of pregnancy that ended in the stillbirth of her baby. These stories have not been included to frighten you (as you will see, stillbirth is quite rare in developed countries) but to honour all of the parents and their babies who were born sleeping. Stories about pregnancies with health risks are also included in this chapter.

Body image is a huge part of any woman's life and this is no different in pregnancy. In this chapter, we explore how a few women coped with their rapidly changing bodies. Some embraced the shape of their new body and showed off their bump with tight-fitting clothes. Others lamented the 'sexual armour' of pregnancy and the resultant lack of male attention that had once been an important and validating element of their sexuality. We also hear how pregnancy has impacted on couples' sex lives, and how they have adapted to their new priorities.

Feelings

Pregnancy is a life-changing event. Feelings during pregnancy are obviously different for everyone. When you first discover you are pregnant, you can be worried, ecstatic, devastated, confused, angry, caught off guard, delightfully surprised, teary and/or ambivalent. As the pregnancy progresses, not only are you at the mercy of your fluctuating hormones, you also have the impending birth to consider. Some people eagerly anticipate birth, while others are anxious about the unknown (even for women who have previously given birth, as each birth is different). As well as the hormonal changes, physical changes (such as the softening of ligaments or the obviously growing belly) can cause discomfort, ranging from mildly irritating to outright painful.

It is little wonder, then, that many women enter this stage of life with some trepidation. In this section, we take a look at how women felt about their pregnancies. Some women, like Shell, were elated when they discovered they were pregnant. Others, like Aviva, were horrified. We hear from Helen, whose pregnancy triggered depression in her partner and also from Khrishna, who was shocked to find out she was having a baby boy, instead of the girl she had dreamed about. All of these women grappled with difficult emotions, yet all of them ultimately came to terms with their decisions.

When reality hits: Second thoughts that last for seconds

Shell had desperately wanted a baby and had tried for over a year before her dream became a reality. Like so many newly pregnant women, however, Shell became overwhelmed with the reality of having a baby. Luckily for Shell, this was short-lived and despite some pregnancy scares, everything went well.

Shell's Story

My partner and I had been trying to conceive for about a year when we found out I was pregnant. We had been using **ovulation** *predictors and had been trying so hard, we decided to give ourselves a break and just stop. And that's when it happened. I had been really quite tired for a week or so, and one evening I threw up the glass of water I drank at bedtime. I didn't think much of it but when telling colleagues at work the next day, it dawned on me that I could possibly be pregnant. One of my close colleagues also remarked on the size of my bust and I resolved to do a pregnancy test that evening.*

When I got home, I was shocked to see the positive result. No matter how much I had dreamed of that moment, and how excited I had expected to be, a very big part of me was so very scared. I thought to myself 'Hold on, this is actually happening now! What have we done? Is this a good idea?' My partner was ecstatic. I was partly ecstatic and partly scared. I was scared of losing the life I had lived up until that point and having to share my partner with someone else. These were all things we had discussed before trying to get pregnant but once we were pregnant, it all became real and terrifying.

I was very tired in the first trimester and suffered moderately from morning sickness. I was able to work and cope with daily life thanks to some anti-nausea medication. Physical changes included breast tenderness and a notable change in breast size, which was quite upsetting for me, as I was already an E cup. I also had quite low blood pressure and was often dizzy. I hated these physical symptoms but knew that they were happening because I was pregnant.

In the second trimester, my morning sickness and dizziness abated a little and I started to feel less tired. It was quite fun until I started experiencing **sacroiliac pain** *midway through the second trimester. Every movement was painful and I started to get quite down. After many physiotherapy appointments and the fitting of a back brace, I was able to again embrace being pregnant with less pain.*

The third trimester was full of excitement and impatience for the impending birth. This was when I really got stuck into the nursery and started nesting! I loved it and while the birth couldn't come quickly enough, I now really miss being pregnant. I lost a lot of weight in the third trimester and the doctors were concerned our baby had **Intrauterine Growth Restriction (IUGR)**. *They scanned us at 32 weeks and, thankfully, he didn't have it.*

Despite the initial shock, pregnancy was generally a great time for me emotionally. I kept expecting to turn into a real cow due to my hormones running amok. I did get a bit teary and emotional when I was in pain with my hips, and also when awaiting the test results. Aside from that, I was able to work up until 36 weeks and I loved it. It was just so exciting for me to incubate this new life and await his arrival.

Shell's Wisdom

Every pregnancy is different, just as each woman is different—and subsequent pregnancies for the same woman can be different. For me, pregnancy wasn't all roses all of the time. It is OK to lose the plot occasionally. And don't ever think you're alone, because—guaranteed— if you're experiencing it, someone else is experiencing it too. I would encourage you to seek out other women who are in the same situation.

Try to relax and enjoy the pregnancy as much as you can, because it generally only lasts nine months and it's the last real chance for you to rest (as much as possible) before the birth of your baby. Take time out to take care of yourself. Housework can wait! Rest when you feel tired and take care of *yourself*. Oh, and ask for help if you need it!

What is Intrauterine Growth Restriction?

Intrauterine Growth Restriction (IUGR) is a term to describe a condition in which your unborn baby is smaller than expected for its gestational age. Much like growth charts for newborns and young children, IUGR is diagnosed using gestational growth charts, based on gestational age. Gestational age is calculated either by using the date of your last menstrual period as a reference point or through ultrasound measurements. If your unborn child is thought to be below the 10th percentile for its gestational age, this may be considered a diagnosis of IUGR.

The causes for IUGR are most commonly attributed to placental insufficiency (for example, there may be a decreased flow in the uterus and placenta or the placenta may be low-lying). If the cause is due to maternal factors, it could be that you have high blood pressure or diabetes. Substance misuse and/or smoking cigarettes are also known causes of IUGR. Lastly, the cause may lie with the baby. For example, it may have a chromosomal abnormality or a congenital infection. There are many causes of IUGR and management is different for each individual, depending on their unique circumstances.

IUGR has a prevalence of 10 per cent for all pregnancies. However, that figure varies in different populations, with rates of 3–5 per cent for healthy mothers and rates of 25 per cent and even higher for some high-risk groups (for example, mothers with high blood pressure). The outcome for babies with IUGR varies and will depend on your own set of circumstances. Try not to be overly worried, as most congenitally normal babies will go on to grow normally in infancy and childhood. It is very important, however, to arm yourself with information about your diagnosis. If your doctor is considering a diagnosis of IUGR, ask them why they think so, how they plan to manage it (i.e. bed rest, early delivery, etc.) and what the short- and long-term prognosis is for your baby. You should also look up some of the organisations and websites listed on page 245 of the Resources section for more information and support.

Reunited: When pregnancy reconnects you with your body

Neither of Aviva's babies were planned and when she discovered (both times) that she was pregnant, she was shocked and worried. Aviva was in a fairly dark place when she became pregnant with her first baby and was very confused about what to do.

Aviva's Story

I would love to be able to say that I felt elated when I discovered I was pregnant, but horrified would describe it better. I was in a pretty bad place at the time; just beginning to find my way out of the worst depressive episode of my life, recently separated from being married, and having a fling with someone I shouldn't have been seeing. Why, then, did I go ahead with the pregnancy?

Well, I had already had a termination when I was 22 and that time I hadn't hesitated; I was at university and it was a mistake. But now, well, I was 28 and I didn't feel that I could go through with a termination a second time. But I agonised. I made a pros and cons list. On the one hand, I wasn't financially set up and neither was the father, and we had only been seeing each other for three months. On the other hand, I felt that being the ripe old age of 28 enabled me to care for a child. There were lots of things on my pros and cons list but I really can't bring myself to think about it, as the thought of not having my children now is just too awful.

My actual pregnancy was a breeze, really, especially compared to some. I did suffer continual nausea for the first four months, which was only partially assuaged by incessant nibbling. Pregnancy was the first time I really felt connected to my body. In the past I had treated it as a totally separate entity from my mind—a nuisance that required feeding, sleep and other bothersome things and I tried as much as possible to ignore its demands. Now I felt that I was my body, and I was being driven to take care of it in a way I never had before. For the first time, I was kind to my body because now there was not just me to consider; there was a tiny, innocent life depending on me.

I have always suffered pretty badly from insomnia and some time before becoming pregnant, I had picked up a book on the subject and flicked through its pages. I was surprised to see pregnancy listed as one of the remedies, but at the time it was just a sort of a mental 'Oh, really?' I know from speaking to friends that many pregnant women don't have this experience, but, especially in the first trimester, sleeping was ridiculously easy for me. As an insomniac, it was heavenly being able to sleep so easily. I vividly recall an occasion when my partner and I had argued during this sleep-filled trimester and he had stormed off. Normally I would have been feeling anxious and going over things in my head but on this occasion I remember thinking 'I really need to have a nap now', and falling asleep.

My second pregnancy was much less enjoyable than my first, as my body's requirements for food and sleep were the same as the first time but I was unable to satisfy *them (particularly the sleep one) in the same way. I wasn't sure I wanted to indulge my food temptations, as I had put on 18 kilos during my first pregnancy and only lost the last of the pregnancy weight through the rather dramatic step of having **peritonitis** (caused by a burst appendix).*

Number two was not a planned pregnancy either. I suspected I was pregnant before I had missed a period. The indicator: the smell of coffee had changed from a deliciously enticing aroma to a nauseating one. I wish my pregnancies had been planned. I love the idea of being married to a man you love, both desirous of having children. I wonder how often it happens like that? In my case, once again there was a pros and cons list, as by this stage my partner and I were not getting on well, but really, when you have had a child already, it is even harder not to go ahead with it. I'm glad I did.

Aviva's Wisdom	The only wisdom I could say I gained from being pregnant is: listen to your body and trust it. The only advice about labour: all fours.

Tables turn: When pregnancy triggers depression in dad

Helen had decided from a fairly young age that she never wanted children and was content and at peace with her decision. Helen's career was her main focus in life and that brought her much satisfaction. So when she found out she was pregnant, she had a termination. However, when she became pregnant again, she was not prepared to endure another one and felt that she could be a good mother to her baby. Unfortunately, her husband developed postnatal depression.

Helen's Story

I was always terrified of childbirth and disinterested in being a mother. I was a career girl, on my way up. It is fair to say I made up my mind I was not going to have children when I was around 27.

Then, one day, I became pregnant. I was in a comfortable relationship but my partner reacted very strangely. He was clearly stricken with some kind of fear. The way he expressed it didn't feel normal and I felt from his reaction it wasn't the right time for a child, so after much soul-searching, I had a termination. One of my close friends flew all the way down to Sydney from Brisbane with her young baby to try to talk me out of it.

Whether because of this or not (I think not), the experience of the termination was dreadful. I will never forget waking up from the anaesthesia in a room full of women who just seemed to cry spontaneously. There was a 13-year-old whose mother had sent her in. There was a Greek Orthodox girl who was engaged to be married to someone she loved, but could not reveal an unplanned pregnancy to her family before the marriage. Her fiancé was there for moral support. There were other women like me, who were in their mid- to late 20s who just weren't ready, or who had already had three or four children and couldn't do it again.

I cried too. I felt wretched and after a few days of healing, I didn't feel any better emotionally. It was because of this experience that I made my mind up that if I ever became pregnant accidentally again, I would go ahead and have the baby. Being a mother might be hard and I certainly didn't plan it but it would not have felt so strange and unnatural as the termination had felt to me.

Sure enough, around two years later, it happened again. I announced to my partner that I was pregnant, that I was going to have the baby, but that he could make up his own mind about whether he wanted to stay with me or not. I promised him he would always be welcome to spend time with his child. This was a relationship that was really more of a close friendship. It was not, in my mind, marriage material but I had a deep affection for my partner and probably a closer sense of family than I had with any other relationship. I trusted him and I knew he wasn't afraid of commitment or duty. But something was amiss. He reacted very badly again. Not unwilling—something else I couldn't put my finger on.

My partner asked me to marry him, and while I felt warmed, it was strange. He smiled and said all the right things but I felt he was just going through the motions. Outwardly, we appeared to be a normal, happy, middle-class couple, albeit on the 'arty' side—he was a designer and I was in advertising. Both my parents and his were delighted with the union. But after our first child was born, my partner became catatonic. He was later diagnosed with severe depression and it has never left him. My being pregnant (signalling the serious commencement of adulthood for him) apparently triggered it.

I was terrified and completely uncertain about many things when I was pregnant, except the fact that I was going to be a mother. I was certain about that and I was certain that I would do the best job I could. I was mothered very well myself and I wanted to be a great mum.

I was not comfortable with my body at all. I didn't like feeling large and unwieldy and I didn't like it that men didn't look at me at all. Being looked at by men was something I always took for granted—it was part of the tapestry of my life. Then suddenly, with a baby bump, they looked right through me. It was as if I didn't exist at all. I am not Elle McPherson, but I was an attractive twenty-something. It was a strange experience.

To complicate things, I was extremely horny. This was a raging kind of feeling that was way more intense than anything I had ever experienced before. My partner was romantic but not all that sexy and I think my constant demand for sex really put him off a bit. He was a bookish, retiring kind of gentleman and the idea of a pregnant partner who was always wanting sex took him by surprise. I think he expected me to be sitting in a corner knitting booties or doing breathing exercises or something.

So, sadly, it was a time of my life when I felt more alone than I ever had before. I felt improper approaching my partner for sex. It was absolutely awful. The fluid retention, the morning sickness, the getting bigger every week, the huge, massive boobs. Feeling at my most unattractive, while at the same time being hornier than ever before was like a conflicted hell. You can't possibly just go out and 'get some' in that condition! I bit my lip and smiled on many occasions, feeling completely at odds with the world and wondering all the time if I had made the right decision to stay with this man. I still wonder. He is still here.

Helen's Wisdom

Becoming a parent with a partner who suffers from depression is an extremely challenging experience. If there is plenty of understanding family support and finances are not an issue it is certainly possible, and it might be made somewhat more comfortable. However, one should not expect the depressed parent to 'change' through the event of becoming a parent, and it should not be expected that life will be 'normal'.

Depression, when it grips the sufferer, does not leave room for others, even needy and vulnerable children. It isn't selective. The antidote is for at least one parent to be able to give fully to the child; to remain upbeat, calm, consistently loving and responsible, attentive, perceptive and communicative, and always able to provide age-appropriate care. The best antidote of all is to have plenty of other stable, happy people around who have room to give and time to listen to the children and their needs.

You should seriously consider having a counsellor—not just for your depressed spouse, but for yourself. You will need professional support and advice, often. An extended family environment would be ideal. A nuclear family situation with no other supports should be avoided. Nobody is strong enough to take on such a challenge alone. You either need a strong, happy supportive family who is willing to take this on, or enough money to be able to afford a small army of professional helpers.

Can men get postnatal depression?

Absolutely. Because it is women who carry and deliver babies, it is automatically assumed by many that postnatal depression (PND) is the domain of women only. However, evidence suggests that around one in fourteen men will experience PND, with some evidence suggesting that the figure is as high as one in three.

It is often maintained that men experience PND as a reaction to their partner's PND, and while this is often the case, it is not the only cause of male PND. A study conducted by Condon et al. (2004) argues that men may have gender-specific factors for psychological distress and that this distress may manifest itself differently than PND in women. They noted that men tend to have fewer support networks; the responsibility of providing financial support can lead to increased work stresses; and that many men lack good role models for fathering. Additionally, men are known to be more reluctant in seeking help with emotional problems.

The Post and Antenatal Depression Association (www.panda.org.au) describe how some men experience PND. Some fathers feel as though they are trapped and unable to get out of their 'cage'; some fathers feel overcome with anger and rage. These men tend to lash out at family members and are often shocked by their own behaviour. Some men (like women) feel completely overwhelmed by their new situation and feel helpless and hopeless at the same time; and some men feel as though they are a 'disappointment' as a father and have let their family down. These feelings are very similar to those felt by women experiencing PND.

If you or your partner experience any of these symptoms, it's very important to seek help. A good starting point is talking to your partner about what you are feeling. You might like to also look up the Resources section of this book and make an appointment with the social worker from your local hospital or community centre. If that is not an option, a visit to your local doctor is always a good starting point.

Boy or girl? When gender affects a mother's feelings in pregnancy

Pregnancy for Khrishna was nothing short of a nightmare. She was not ready for a baby, and when she found out she was pregnant, the one thing that kept her spirits up was that she 'knew' she was having a girl. When she found out that she was in fact having a boy, her world started to spiral out of control.

Khrishna's Story

Growing up, I knew I didn't want kids. I wanted a career and an easy, free life. I had four cats and a dog and that was it. I never wanted to add to that.

*I was living with my partner, in an abusive relationship, working 60 hours a week. I had recently had an **Implanon** put in, so when I started feeling very sick, I figured it must be that. I was throwing up daily, was dizzy, had headaches and was so tired. I also had some odd cramping in my stomach. I lived on ibuprofen for two weeks—I was up to about ten tablets a day; well over the recommended dose. I thought that the Implanon didn't agree with me, so I decided to have it removed. Even though the doctor suggested I leave it for a while longer, I refused.*

Strangely, even though I went through with it, the illness continued. I'm a bit of a drama queen, so I assumed I had a terminal illness. Two weeks after it was removed, I went back to the doctor. My regular doctor wasn't in, so I saw a male. He asked if there was any chance I could be pregnant and I replied 'Well, maybe, but I hope not.' He did a pregnancy test. He was chatting away with me and entering data into my files while we waited for the test to work. He glanced down at the test and said 'Oh, yep, it's positive'. I felt the blood drain from my face and said 'What?' 'Yes, you're pregnant', he replied. I stared at him for a beat and burst into tears. 'Well, what the hell am I supposed to do now?' I shook my head and left.

Once in the car, I cried for about half an hour before I felt I could drive home. On the way home, things went through my head—what are my options? Abortion, adoption, letting the child's father raise it … I just didn't know the answers to anything. I thought about the few kids I knew—they were noisy, loud, annoying, expensive, messy ... and I just didn't want that in my life.

My partner was ecstatic, which made me feel worse. I researched abortions online and I really didn't want to go through that. So I resigned myself to the fact that I was going to have to carry this baby. I admit there were times that I just hoped I'd miscarry. Then it wouldn't be my fault, and the situation would be out of my hands. I realised I had absolutely no idea how pregnant I was, so I made an appointment with my regular doctor. She organised an ultrasound for me.

The minute I saw that little blob on the ultrasound, it felt more like a baby to me. I started thinking 'Well ... OK, this wasn't in my plans. Maybe I can do this. It will be a girl! Most of the kids I know are boys; a girl will be different! It won't be so noisy, smelly and annoying!' How naive. I continued and had the **nuchal scan** *at 12 weeks. At 14 weeks, the morning sickness miraculously stopped.*

My second trimester was good physically. I hated my stomach expanding, however. I was a size six before pregnancy and weighed 50 kg. I had odd cravings—I wanted ice all the time, and one night I had to have a steak sandwich. Another night it was hazelnut gelato. I didn't want any other ice cream. It had to be gelato and it had to be hazelnut. My partner wasn't so sympathetic to my aches and pains and the constant exhaustion. Sex was the last thing on my mind and he wasn't happy about this either, so our already fragile relationship crumbled further.

At 19 weeks, I had the big ultrasound. I was excited—I wanted to find out the sex, although I knew it was a girl. I just knew it! We went to the ultrasound appointment and I was chatting happily with the technician while he took his measurements. I finally said 'So what sex is it?' He said 'Can't you tell?' I didn't know what I was looking at, so I said 'Nope'. My partner said quietly 'It's a boy.' My whole world crashed down and I looked at the technician. He nodded and I started crying. The technician said 'Oh ... I take it you wanted a girl?' I nodded and he replied 'Oh well, you can try for a girl next time'. I gritted my teeth and said 'I am not having more—I didn't want this one.'

We left, and in the car park my partner and I had a huge screaming match. I clearly recall him saying 'Why don't we just call this kid "unwanted bastard child" because that's what you think he is.' My mum was calling to find out about the scan and I ignored her calls as we were driving home. I was still crying. After the eighth call, I answered and she asked how it went.

'Fine.'

She wanted more. 'Well? Is it a boy or a girl?'

I said flatly 'boy'.

She was thrilled.

'I don't want it.'

She said 'God, Khrishna, there are people out there who would want any baby, boy or girl!' I replied 'Fine, then they can have it, because I don't want it.' I hung up on her.

I posted and asked for a help on an internet forum and all I got was abuse. This made things worse. I completely shut down, although I did use one of the suggestions. I went into a children's clothing store the next day and tried to buy an item of blue clothing. I lasted two minutes and after staring at all the pink, ran out in tears. Over the next few weeks at work, whenever a customer with a daughter walked into the store, I walked out. My mother sent me a card with a blue jumpsuit. I threw the jumpsuit away.

My ambivalence towards the pregnancy and baby didn't improve over the next few months. I once again weighed up the idea of abortion, but couldn't face it.

My obstetrician sent me to a social worker at the hospital to discuss my feelings about the baby. She was a wonderful woman and I will always be grateful to her. Through her, I worked out that I thought that if I had a boy, he would turn out like his father, who was far from Prince Charming. She asked what my dad and grandfathers were like. 'They're all great!' I said, surprised. 'Why?' She smiled and said, 'What makes you think your son won't be like them?' She was right.

I had my son by scheduled caesarean section at 39 weeks and the instant he was placed into my arms, I fell totally in love with him. He was absolutely exquisite and perfect. It didn't matter that he wasn't a girl, he was my son.

Khrishna's Wisdom	The only advice I can give is a trite old adage—enjoy your pregnancy as much as you can. I hated every moment of mine and wouldn't even allow photos to be taken of me—I had put on 21 kilos by the end. It took me a year but I did eventually lose the baby weight. The pains and aches and constant tiredness seemed never ending, but there is a light at the end of the tunnel. And really, when they put that baby in my arms, I thought 'What pains?'
	And for the record, I had a daughter a couple of years after my son. My son is a clean freak and hates getting dirty (takes after his mum) and my daughter is an absolute grot. Her day carer said that she could get dirty sitting still!

Can finding out the sex of the baby affect women?

Yes, very much so. A recent study by de Tychey et al. in the *Journal of Clinical Nursing* (2008) set out to determine if the gender of a baby could play a significant role in postnatal depression in women. Interestingly, they discovered that gender expectations did influence PND in women and went on to suggest the importance of these results on early intervention programs and psychotherapeutic care.

While many pregnant women may not admit it to themselves, they often secretly have a preference for a girl over a boy or vice versa. If, like Khrishna, you find out your baby's gender via ultrasound and experience feelings of disappointment or grief, realise that this is normal and try not to feel guilty about your feelings. The best thing you can do is talk to someone about it who can help, like a social worker or a counsellor at the local hospital. If you are under the care of your midwife, ask to speak to her about how you can handle your feelings and what practical and/or emotional things you may be able to do to feel better about the impending birth and gender of your baby.

Born still: When pregnancy goes wrong

When talking about pregnancy, it is important not to omit 'the bad stuff'. Pregnancies can and do go wrong; most of the time there is absolutely nothing the mother could have done to prevent losing her baby. Losing a baby is almost certainly one of the most traumatic experiences a person can endure. Here we meet Georgia, whose baby was born still. While her loss can never be lessened, it is wonderful for Georgia that she went on to have three healthy children.

Georgia's Story

*I have always wanted to be a mother and thought having a child would be the easiest thing in the world. After years of trying not to have a baby, it took me much longer than expected to fall pregnant as I had **polycystic ovaries**. Thankfully for me and my husband, after a few years of trying and a move to Hong Kong, we found a great doctor and I became pregnant with our first child.*

I was ecstatic but right from the start it wasn't the easiest of pregnancies. While I managed to avoid most of the worst of the morning sickness, appendicitis and a subsequent operation at eight weeks was extraordinarily stressful, especially when away from your family and friends. Thanks to some fabulous doctors, the baby and I both made it through and the pregnancy proceeded as normal for many weeks.

I remember one particular night lying on our lounge room floor, feeling like the luckiest person in the entire world. Here I was living in a fabulous apartment in Hong Kong, with a lovely husband, a healthy baby in my tummy and a relatively new job that I was really enjoying. It was such an overwhelming feeling of gratitude and I was feeling so positive and strong that I can see myself even now, almost as if that night were a vivid dream.

When I was 35 weeks pregnant, my husband went on a business trip to Tokyo—one of his last before I was due to give birth. Everything had been going fine, I was working full time and engrossed in the role; we had our new nursery almost complete and the anticipation of a new life joining us was acute.

One night while he was away, after an extremely long and busy day at work, I was overcome by what I thought at the time was a very bad case of pregnancy blues. I cried for a good couple of hours, for no real reason. I felt absolutely terrible and was so emotionally overcome that I felt physically sick. I went to bed early but didn't sleep very well and, after a terrible night, called in sick to work, hoping to have an easy morning before my regular check-up with my obstetrician that afternoon.

I felt drained but otherwise fine at the appointment, commenting that the baby had been a little quieter than normal that morning. It was my doctor's face while she was giving me a scheduled scan during that appointment that gave away something was wrong. But it wasn't until she said the words that will forever haunt me that I knew it to be the case.

'I can't find a heartbeat', she said. 'I can't find a heartbeat.'

The pain was instant, as if someone had taken every single hope I held for the future in one fell swoop, discarding any happiness I may have possessed, pulling a thick, black curtain down over my life. Absolutely helpless, there was no way I could stop what was the worst imaginable thing I hadn't even allowed myself to imagine could happen to me.

I gave birth to our absolutely beautiful first girl in April 2005, my husband finally by my side. She had a sparkling mass of dark curls, perfect rosebud lips and the most beautiful hands and feet we had ever seen.

Placed on my chest straight after giving birth, Philippa was a perfect baby, except that her perfect little body had been starved of its blood supply. She was always very active in utero and, as we subsequently discovered, a weakened section of umbilical cord had developed an extreme twist only the day before my scheduled appointment, cutting off the blood supply to our first child.

Nothing will ever take away the pain of losing our first child. Nothing prepares you for or can ever take away the pain of losing a child that hasn't been allowed to take its first breath. Nothing prepares you for the size of such a tiny coffin, or saying goodbye to such an important part of you that you were never able to get to know. Nothing prepares you for the years of unhappiness afterwards.

Since losing Philippa, we have been very lucky to have been blessed with three wonderfully happy, very healthy girls. As stressful and as difficult as all my pregnancies now are for me, I am forever grateful for our healthy, happy children and constantly astounded at their perfect hands, perfect bottoms and each new word they are able to express. Every child born safely into this world is a little miracle, a miracle that I am ever so grateful for and appreciate so much more since losing our irreplaceable little Philippa.

Georgia's Wisdom	I will never get over losing Philippa. She was our first-born child and will always be part of our family. There are too many 'hard things' after having a stillborn baby. One of the hardest things to know is when to tell my other children that they had a sister. It is hard to have other people forget Philippa, and hard to know when you should tell a new friend about your loss, and to judge how they will react. It is hard for both people to keep a partnership together after such a loss and often hard on some friendships as well. It is hard to impart wisdom because this is one of the toughest things a mother can endure.
	What I can say is that even though I will never get over Philippa's death, I am learning to live with it, slowly. Put one foot in front of the other. Talk to your partner. Do what you feel is right for you, whether it's talking to a counsellor and friends or being by yourself for a while. What I can tell you is that it doesn't hurt quite so acutely forever. I don't think time heals a loss like this but time smoothes the edges of your pain and helps you to move on with your life. I went on to have three gorgeous, healthy children. You will never be the same, but life does get better.

What is stillbirth and how common is it?

Stillbirth is defined differently around the world (mainly differing in gestational weeks or gestational weight). For example, in Australia, a stillbirth is defined as occurring at or beyond 20 weeks of pregnancy. In England, it is defined as occurring at or beyond 24 weeks. If a baby dies in the womb, it is referred to as an intra-uterine stillbirth. If the baby dies during labour or birth, it is referred to as an intrapartum stillbirth. A neonatal death is one in which the baby dies during the first 28 days of birth.

The difference between a miscarriage and a stillbirth is that a miscarriage is generally defined (depending on the country) as pregnancy loss before 20 weeks' gestation. Simply put, miscarriage is the unplanned end of a pregnancy before the baby can live on its own (and this is defined in terms of time and weight—i.e. 400 grams is used in Australia, if the time of conception is unknown). A recent study by Stanton et al. (2006) estimated the global number of stillbirths to be 3.2 million annually. Their investigation also uncovered the fact that stillbirth rates ranged from five per 1000 in 'rich' countries to 32 per 1000 in south Asia and sub-Saharan Africa. This reflects the tragic disparity between women birthing in OECD countries and their sisters who do so in developing countries.

There has been much research into stillbirth, which has brought hope. For example, in a report by Tveit et al. (2009), 65 000 pregnancies in Norway were followed and a health care plan implemented that stressed the significance of foetal movements. They found that this intervention resulted in a 50 per cent reduction in stillbirth in women with decreased foetal movements.

Stillbirth is an agonising experience and if this has happened to you, or someone you love, there are a few things to keep in mind. According to the International Stillbirth Alliance (ISA), creating memories and spending time with your baby helps to honour your baby's life and existence. You might like to name your baby, touch, feel and hold your baby, give your baby a bath or get some special clothes for your baby. Having footprints and handprints of your baby might also help you to form memories. It is important to recognise that everyone is different and therefore everyone's reaction to the death of a baby is different. Some people may do all of the above, while some people may do none. Everything is normal and you must do things at your own pace, not at the pace of others. This is your baby, your family. There is a lot of support for women and men who have suffered the loss of a baby, whether through miscarriage or stillbirth and you might like to look up the support services on offer in the Resources section if you or your friends or family have been through this.

Losing control: When a car accident leads to miscarriage

Camilla suffered a miscarriage in her first pregnancy; a blow that she will never forget. Here, we read how she coped with it and how it affected her subsequent pregnancies.

Camilla's Story

The first time my partner and I had sex with the intention of starting a family, I fell pregnant. I felt different before my period was due but thought I was perhaps imagining things. All the urine tests I did said 'negative' so when the doctor called me to tell me the blood test had confirmed I was pregnant, it was a wonderful surprise. I can still remember the overwhelming joy that flooded every ounce of me—an uncontainable smile and just wanting to jump in the air. Every morning I woke up, I felt the same feeling of joy and a new sense of purpose. It was a feeling I will treasure forever.

At 11 weeks into the pregnancy, I was sitting at a stop sign in our car and a young driver lost control, smashing into us. A week later I miscarried—a very painful experience, both physically and emotionally. I never had quite the same level of joy with subsequent pregnancies, as they were mixed with a small amount of fear. Saying that, the only thing that healed my feelings of grief was falling pregnant again and then eventually going on to have my beautiful girl.

After the miscarriage, I couldn't help but question why and how this could happen. Even though it happened after our car accident and was in all probability caused by this, there was still the possibility it was something I had done or something wrong with me. I read every possible bit of information I could about miscarriage but felt no comfort or relief that it wouldn't happen again. I did, however, feel the only consolation would be to fall pregnant again and kept telling myself that there must be a good reason for it. Rationally I could tell myself that it was for the best if something was wrong with the baby. Emotionally though, I would cry if I saw newborn babies in the shops or on television—a reminder of our loss.

The second pregnancy happened straight away, and again I was thrilled but it was not like the first time. There were also mixed feelings of joy and anxiety. Every week that went by gave me greater hope and thankfully it was a very busy time so the weeks went quickly. At around nine weeks though, I noticed some spotting and feared the worst. The doctors could find no heartbeat and offered little besides a wait-and-see approach. The first miscarriage had been extremely painful physically; I remember spending hours through the night on the toilet having acute cramps and bleeding, and eventually passing something. The second one was more like a very painful period. Both were heartbreaking.

My doctor explained that investigation into miscarriage is usually only done when a woman has suffered three miscarriages. He said there were differing opinions as to whether you should wait a few months to try and conceive again or try straight away. A big factor to consider was whether you were emotionally ready to try again.

I fell pregnant straight away again and once I was past the first trimester, the anxiety and fear subsided, although I took every precaution I possibly could. I even stopped going to the gym, a probably unnecessary precaution but necessary for me. The doctor I saw was very understanding of my fears and it helped for me to have regular blood tests to see my hormone levels rising. Thankfully the rest of the pregnancy was uneventful and we gave birth to a healthy and delightful baby girl. I look back now and wonder for what purpose we go through such despair. If nothing else, it did make me value what a gift it is to be pregnant.

Camilla's Wisdom

What I have learned from my pregnancies that I would love to share with others going through it is that keeping focused on the wonder of what's going on inside, growing life and creating an individual and special human being is vital to coping with the many discomforts you may experience. Laugh at it, cry at it, joke about it and remember that most of it will change back to normal after the baby is born. Treat it like a nine-month holiday from reality and do whatever you have to do to cope with the changes. Ask for help and give yourself a break whenever you can.

If you suffer from a miscarriage, take it easy on yourself. It's so easy to blame ourselves when something goes wrong, even when it is completely out of our hands. I would discuss your miscarriage with your doctor, particularly if you want to start trying to get pregnant again. And if you're feeling that you just can't cope with the loss or you feel overwhelmed with fear during your new pregnancy, I would talk to people; friends, social workers, your doctor—whatever helps.

How can the loss of a baby affect subsequent pregnancies and birthing decisions?

The experience of pregnancy after previous loss of a baby (during pregnancy, birth or shortly after) has been described using the metaphor, 'one foot in; one foot out' (Côté-Arsenault & Marshall 2000, p. 473). Women often describe going through the motions of their pregnancies (keeping their physical foot in) but constantly remind themselves that pregnancy does not always result in a live baby (keeping their emotional foot out). A study conducted by Côté-Arsenault and Donato (2007) found that pregnant women whose babies had previously died had many issues to grapple with, ranging from uncertainty of the baby's health to waiting for the baby to die (again). Many studies have found increased anxiety and depression in subsequent pregnancies following **perinatal** loss (see Armstrong et al. 2009; DeBackere et al. 2008; Klier et al. 2002; Wright 2005).

Losing a baby can affect decisions surrounding the way in which a woman subsequently chooses to birth, can cause her to seek and form strong attachments to new health providers and can even affect how the birth itself unfolds. If you have suffered baby loss, either through miscarriage, stillbirth or neonatal death, it is important to nurture yourself and take the time you need to heal, at your own pace. You might like to try some of the suggestions listed under Georgia's story and you might like to look up relevant support services in the Resources section for further help.

Pregnancies with health risks

This section is included in the hope that it will persuade every pregnant woman to seek regular **antenatal** care. In doing so, many complications can be detected early and treated appropriately, resulting in both a healthy mother and a healthy baby. Conversely, not seeking antenatal care carries a substantial risk of danger to both mother and baby. These stories are not included to frighten you but to remind you that antenatal care reduces risk to both mother and baby significantly.

Don't panic: Delivery at 34 weeks

Chelsea's pregnancy was a happy time for her. After trying for months to get pregnant, she finally got the positive result that sent her over the moon. However, at 25 weeks, Chelsea experienced a bleed, and, knowing this may be a sign of trouble, went straight to her doctor.

Chelsea's Story

*After trying to conceive for several months, I was diagnosed with **Polycystic Ovarian Syndrome (PCOS)** and I found out I was not ovulating at all. Luckily, after a visit to a fertility specialist and one cycle taking a drug called **clomid** to help me ovulate, I was pregnant. I took a pregnancy test three days before my period was due (at 4 am), as I was too excited to wait until morning. I was absolutely ecstatic when it came up positive.*

I loved being pregnant. I embraced all my symptoms as signs the pregnancy was progressing well and I thought about pregnancy and babies pretty much constantly. I read every book I could find on pregnancy and birth. I bought books and borrowed every book the library had on the subject. I also took my husband along to an 'active birth' workshop. It was very important to me to feel informed. During the pregnancy, I didn't read anything on raising children. Although I knew that at the end of the pregnancy I would end up with a baby, I found it hard to get past the mental hurdle of the birth.

During the first trimester, I had sore boobs, exhaustion and morning sickness. Some people at work guessed I was pregnant because they thought my boobs had gotten bigger. Morning sickness only led to vomiting twice. I was constantly hungry but had trouble finding something I felt like eating. To cope with it, I ate regularly and made sure I didn't do any cooking, as the smell of food cooking seemed to make things worse.

During the second trimester, things got a little easier but I still felt tired all the time and my hips started to hurt a lot too. I saw a physiotherapist who did some manipulations and taught me some exercises to do. I also went to a pregnancy water exercise class which I really enjoyed and which helped my hips somewhat. At night, I slept with four pillows—one under my head, one between my knees, one in front of my chest for me to hug and one behind my back to stop me rolling backwards. Not much room left in bed for my husband! At work, I had to get up and move around regularly because sitting still seemed to make my hip pain worse.

At 25 weeks, I was at work one day when suddenly I felt extremely emotional and exhausted and couldn't stop crying. My boss drove me home from work and I got into bed and had a sleep. Later I woke up and went to the toilet and there was a lot of blood there when I wiped. It took a moment to register that blood was not good and it wasn't simply my period arriving. Thankfully, I could still feel my baby kicking but I was still extremely panicked. I rang my husband and my obstetrician, who told me to go straight to hospital. At hospital, they monitored the foetus and found that everything seemed normal. The bleeding continued for a few hours and I had an ultrasound done. They couldn't find any reason for the bleeding. I stayed in overnight and by the next day, the bleeding had stopped so I was sent home.

I loved being in my third trimester because I so loved feeling my baby move. During the third trimester, the baby was big enough for me to play 'guess the body part' through my tummy and I loved knowing I was patting his bottom or tickling his feet. At 30 weeks, my baby did a somersault and went from being breech to being in the head down position. That was quite painful but I was very happy he was in a good position for birth and hoped he'd stay that way until the delivery.

I had a scan at 32 weeks due to a potential complication found at the 19-week scan. At the 32-week scan we were told the kidneys still looked dilated and they would have to do further investigation once the baby was born; they also told us that the baby appeared to be very large. My obstetrician started talking about inducing my baby early due to its size. I was upset because I wanted a natural birth but little did I know the birth was only two weeks away. My pregnancy ended at 34 weeks with my waters breaking prematurely. I hope I can experience the full third trimester one day!

| **Chelsea's Wisdom** | Try to enjoy the pregnancy as much as you can. Women who can fall pregnant are blessed with an incredible gift. The pregnancy won't continue forever so we have to make the most of every minute—it may end sooner than you expect it to. |

Bleeding in pregnancy

Naturally, women worry when they bleed during pregnancy. You may notice a bit of blood on the toilet paper after you have wiped ('spotting') or your bleeding may be heavier, requiring pads (never use tampons). While frightening, bleeding during the first trimester is quite common. Many women bleed for no particular reason and often the bleeding does not affect the woman or her baby, so if you do experience a bleed, you should try and remain calm.

However, all bleeding in pregnancy should be checked out by your doctor or midwife in order to rule out complications. Bleeding in the first trimester is common, affecting approximately 20 per cent of all pregnancies (Poulose et al. 2006). There are several noted causes: implantation bleeding, post-coital bleeding and bleeding due to vaginal tears, all of which are usually harmless (Smith 2006). However, bleeding in the first trimester may indicate an impending miscarriage or an ectopic pregnancy and this is why it is important to see your doctor to rule these out.

Late bleeding in pregnancy can be more serious and can be due to problems with your placenta or uterus (Harlev et al. 2008; Koifman et al. 2008). For Chelsea, it was associated with a pre-term birth. It is crucial that you go straight to hospital if you experience bleeding in the second half of your pregnancy so that your symptoms can be investigated as soon as possible.

Bleeding in pregnancy is scary but there are things you can do to help your doctor make a diagnosis. The first thing you should do is wear a pad or panty liner so that you can monitor how much blood you are actually losing and what type of bleeding you are experiencing. While in some cases bleeding in pregnancy may be normal, you should never assume it is harmless and you should always call your doctor immediately. If you are in the second half of your pregnancy, go straight to your nearest hospital emergency department. Remember: not all bleeding in the second half of pregnancy results in things going wrong; in fact, it may be your body's way of telling you to seek help.

Shadows on the ultrasound: A subchorionic bleed

Maria also experienced bleeding in pregnancy, which was diagnosed as a **subchorionic bleed**. However, unlike Chelesa, this did not lead to a pre-term delivery but it required close monitoring, regular blood thinning injections and bed rest.

Maria's Story

When I became pregnant for the first time, my husband and I had been married for three years; he was 44 and I was 38. I was a little apprehensive but for the most part, I was just so happy to know our little one was on the way. As soon as my home pregnancy test was positive, I saw my obstetrician and everything was going well. Then, in December, I had some heavy spotting/light bleeding. When I first saw the bleeding, I was scared and worried. I felt fine physically, so why would there be anything wrong with the pregnancy? Did this mean there would be something wrong with the baby? Did this mean I wasn't able to sustain a pregnancy? All kinds of questions went through my mind.

*I immediately called my obstetrician's office. He had performed ultrasounds in his office prior to this and had seen a shadow that he didn't like. When I went to his office that day, the ultrasound showed a larger shadow, and he diagnosed a **subchorionic bleed**, which means there is a mass of blood between the placenta and where it attaches to the uterus. The risk to the pregnancy is if the area of haemorrhage grows and interrupts the connection between the placenta and the uterus—the baby would not survive, as its life-source is cut off. After another ultrasound with the hospital's more sophisticated equipment, he asked that I stay off my feet (although he did not call it 'bed rest') and be restful. He also prescribed blood thinner injections.*

After blanching a bit, I told him and his nurse that being poked in the tummy with something sharp was essentially the biggest fear I'd had as a child, so it would be challenging to confront it head on. I was not able to give myself the shots. The first time at home I'd tried and tried but just couldn't do it. I'd hoped to be all done by the time my husband got home, but instead he found me crying and hyperventilating in the bathroom. From then on, he gave them to me. The injection hurt a bit but we found that icing the area for at least 20 minutes before the shot helped me, although it made the injection site more difficult to puncture. As my pregnancy progressed, and the nice soft gushy areas of my tummy disappeared, finding a good place for the injection became challenging, and I did not want to use my thighs or the backs of my arms instead. I was grateful that these shots would help the pregnancy continue but was not able to find total peace with having to receive them.

For me, the point of 'we're safe now' was when my doctor asked me to discontinue the shots, just a couple of weeks before our baby arrived. It meant that our little one could be born at any time, in good condition. We'd had another ultrasound as well to estimate the baby's size and in that ultrasound we saw a perfect little ear and hair shooting out from the baby's head! We'd decided to keep the baby's gender a mystery but finding out we wouldn't have a bald baby was such a sweet surprise. When the baby was delivered, I asked my husband what we'd had; he told me to look for myself, and when I saw our little boy, pink and yelling for all he was worth, I was incredibly happy that all had gone well.

I've said many times that I'd have another baby in a heartbeat but realise as I recall the details of my pregnancy with Alexander that it was actually a fairly difficult time. Because of our relative ages, it is not very likely my husband and I will decide to have another child. We feel we are very lucky to have gotten through this pregnancy—at the end of it, my health is good, and we have a beautiful, perfect little boy. It is possible the next time we might not be so lucky, so we don't want our 'greed' to colour our judgement.

Maria's Wisdom
I am only now, a few months after my son was born, capable of understanding this. While I was pregnant, it seemed as if it would never end—that how I felt right then was the way it was going to be forever.

Now that my baby is here, I realise that the time I was pregnant was so very short. The precautions and treatments you encounter during your pregnancy may range from inconvenient to really undesirable, but in hindsight, I see they just don't last that long, and my prize at the end was a beautiful, healthy child, which is more than worth the unpleasantness and pain encountered during pregnancy and delivery. Not a bad trade-off, in my opinion!

How do I know what medications are safe to take during pregnancy?

Medicines in pregnancy need to be taken with caution, even over-the-counter medicines. Many women, however, need to take medicine during pregnancy and this should be discussed with your health care provider. There are specialist services in some countries that offer information over the phone about specific medications and their use in pregnancy, birth and lactation. If this is not available to you, you can always speak to your local pharmacist or general practitioner. For more information on support services for drugs in pregnancy, birth and lactation, please see page 245 of the Resources section.

Body image

Body image is a biggie for women and if you have any issues with your body (as most women do), they can be exacerbated or alleviated during pregnancy. Pregnancy has a profound effect on the body; it has to work overtime to ensure the wellbeing of your baby and this can take its toll on even the most patient of women. But what about what's happening on the outside? Obviously your stomach gets bigger but other outward signs can appear as well, such as stretch marks, the development of a **linea nigra** (a brownish vertical line that can appear on your belly) and added weight gain. Some women take to this like ducks to water; some women hate it. Here, we read how a few women felt about their changing bodies.

Strictly exercising: Coming to terms with losing control of your body

Remy had always looked after herself; she ate as healthily as she could and exercised a lot. So when she found out she was pregnant, the idea of 'losing control' of her body completely took her by surprise.

Remy's Story

I have always been proud of having a slim, athletic body—to the extent that in my early 30s I definitely had an undiagnosed eating disorder. I tend to do things to extremes, so when I decided to get fit and lose weight at the end of medical school, I started over-exercising and became very critical of my body shape and size. I was very thin for a few years—mainly as a result of running, but also due to restrictive eating habits—and when I fell pregnant with Jack I had only really been at a normal weight for 18 months. In retrospect, I was using eating and weight as a way of coping with a huge set of life changes that came at me all at once: starting my career, moving interstate, turning 30 and the ending of a long-term relationship. It was a wild time and I definitely coped by focusing on my body and exercise.

By the time I met my now-husband, I was in much better mental and physical shape, but was still pretty careful about keeping my figure in check. I have quite a boyish shape— no real hips or waist, and a modest bust—and I like it that way. When I gain weight I do so kind of all over, not just on my hips and bum like many women, and I don't feel good. So back then I was still very particular about diet and exercise.

The idea of losing control of my weight and gaining the recommended number of kilos while pregnant totally, and I mean totally, freaked me out. My pregnancy was unplanned, partly because I had a secret suspicion that I might have fertility problems after several years of no periods and partly because I don't like taking the pill because it makes me put on one to two kilos at least. So there I suddenly was: pregnant and completely at the mercy of my hormones.

The first thing that happened was that my boobs were suddenly all voluptuous. A very good friend took one look at me when I was about seven weeks and said 'You look really booby—are you pregnant?' I was amazed! Other than that, because I was so fit beforehand, my body did not change a lot. I really didn't start showing properly until about 18 weeks, which allowed me to keep it a bit of a mystery at work. As for feeling sexy, I definitely did, whether it was the hormones or what, I don't know, but my husband certainly enjoyed my pregnancy.

The biggest thing that worried me was stretch marks, but I was lucky not to acquire any. I think that's partly because I didn't gain a lot of weight overall and partly due to genetics. I did get a very prominent **linea nigra** *that took almost 12 months to disappear.*

I was careful not to 'eat for two' and so my diet in pregnancy was pretty much the same as ever, although my sweet tooth disappeared in the first trimester, much to my surprise. I had been a carbohydrate addict and semi-vegetarian, but suddenly my body demanded ham and eggs for breakfast and cheeseburgers for lunch. I was quite relieved when the second trimester hit and I went back to my toast and banana bread fetish. And I did exercise—probably more than people would think wise—but it kept me sane and feeling in control and that was very important in helping me enjoy the pregnancy.

By late pregnancy, I really had that basketball-up-the-shirt look—I was all belly and the rest of me was pretty normal, which was a relief. My husband loved my pregnant belly and in particular wanted to use it as a pillow while lying on the couch—we were both amused when the baby would kick him in the head as a result!

Remy's Wisdom	The biggest thing I learned from being pregnant is that my body is capable of amazing things and that it deserves a break—I am now much

less strict with myself and much less obsessed with diet and exercise. That's not to say that I have let myself go—absolutely not—but I don't worry about a few saggy bits here and there like I would have done before I had babies. I am much more accepting of my body because I spend every day with two wonderful little children whom my body grew, from scratch, and that is pretty awesome.

Is it safe to exercise during pregnancy?

For normal, low-risk pregnancies, the short answer is 'yes', it is safe to exercise in pregnancy. Beginning or continuing regular exercise during pregnancy is safe for both mother and baby (Clapp 2005). In fact, the American Congress of Obstetricians and Gynecologists (ACOG 2003) recommends exercise during pregnancy as a way of reducing backaches, constipation, bloating and swelling. They also say it may help prevent or treat **gestational diabetes**, increase your energy, improve your mood and posture, while promoting greater muscle tone and strength. It is important, however, to discuss with your health care provider what types of exercise are best for you and your pregnancy, as every pregnancy is different.

Not a glower: When pregnancy and smocks clash

Rosetta had no qualms about the changes in her body; she had been comfortable with her body shape for years and saw pregnancy as a natural progression. While she did report problems in the third trimester, these were mainly to do with feeling ungainly and uncomfortable.

Rosetta's Story

Let's just say that I am not a 'glower'. I remember reading about how I would bloom in pregnancy and that I would love every minute of it. I saw the teary moments on television when women rub their belly and smile. I read all the articles in gossip magazines about celebrities who declared their pregnant bodies nothing short of 'wondrous'.

Don't get me wrong—when that stick showed two pink lines, I wept. I was smoking at the time, waiting anxiously for the test results. The lines turned pink, I stubbed out what was to be my last cigarette, I hugged my husband, and I wept. Sure, I was happy—we had been planning this baby for a while and I certainly had wanted this baby for years. But somehow, the moment felt so surreal, like I was watching it in a movie and it wasn't really happening to me.

Slowly, reality sunk in and I began to believe that I was going to have a baby. When we saw the heartbeat on that small black box thump, thump, thumping away, I was completely overwhelmed that I was growing a life inside me. I was actually pregnant. I was going to have a baby!

And then the questions started drowning out all other thoughts. What would my body look like? When would my bump show? How big was it going to get? How the hell was the baby going to get out?

While these thoughts rattled around my brain, I did what I do best when in a quandary—I shopped. Off I went to all the maternity shops I could find and spent ridiculous amounts of money on designer maternity jeans and kaftans. To be honest, I had never had a problem with my body or its shape my entire life and this just seemed to be another natural step in my body's journey and I was going to embrace that with the balance of my credit card.

And it was fine for the first and second trimesters. I did glow. Actually, I rocked. I felt sexy, I felt beautiful and I felt totally at ease with my growing belly. And then I hit 30 weeks. I honestly had no idea how a stomach could get that big. It was huge. Enormous. I no longer fitted into my fabulous maternity jeans, or any pants for that matter. My bump was just too big. So it was smocks—yes smocks—that got me through the last stages of my pregnancy.

I did not glow. I growled. By now my stomach was so big that I actually had to hold my hands underneath it wherever I walked because it was so bloody uncomfortable. My legs hurt, my back ached and I could no longer put on my own shoes. Problems with my body? You bet. And then, at the eleventh hour, the stretch marks appeared. Oh, lovely, purple marks—it was like a map of train lines on my belly! I loved my baby but my body seemed to be giving up on me, joint by painful joint. But out she came, right on her due date and all that I cared about was that she was mine. She was beautiful and she was healthy and she was mine. Oh, and she was big.

After some contemplation, I grew to realise that everyone is different and every pregnancy is different (although unfortunately for me, my babies got bigger with every pregnancy). I realised that my body had been made perfectly to grow and deliver another life. Stretch marks? Yeah, you can still see the silvery lines. Kangaroo pouch? Yep, but nothing shape wear can't fix. I'm pretty sure my back will never be the same but I don't care. My body is amazing; it created, sustained and delivered three human beings and I am incredibly proud of it!

Rosetta's Wisdom

Frankly, I'm tired of the way pregnant women and their bodies are portrayed in the media. It seems that every glossy magazine you pick up, there is another dozen photos of celebrities showing off their bumps (big and small) on the red carpet. And, let's face it, they look hot. That's quite a lot to measure up to. I think there is already enough pressure on women to look perfect. And what about all those celeb bodies that 'bounce' back to pre-baby shape in a matter of weeks? Come on. I don't know one single friend that has bounced back that quickly.

If I were to impart any wisdom at all, I would say this: not everyone is happy with their body and not everyone is happy with their body in pregnancy. If you feel like this, why not try turning that thought on its head? Instead of feeling 'fat' or 'ungainly', why not let loose and revel in the fact that your body—your body—is creating and sustaining life. Now that is something to be proud of.

Embracing change: Enjoying body shape in pregnancy

Mita fits into the 'average' category of women—not delighted with her body but not overly worried about it either. But one thing that sets Mita apart from most women was that she eagerly awaited everything that came with pregnancy—even stretch marks!

Mita's Story

Before becoming pregnant, I wasn't overly proud of my body but I was happy with it. I wouldn't flaunt it in a bikini and there were a few areas I wouldn't mind toning up but generally I was happy. The only things I would change were my breasts. I had an E cup before I became pregnant and always felt they were too large, causing me back pain and making it difficult to find clothes to wear that didn't show too much cleavage.

I wasn't keen on piling on too much weight but my theory was that everything I put into my mouth was for the baby. I was not going to starve my body but neither was I going to pile crap into it at every chance. I did, however, go on a spree of eating a lot of butter, sour cream and high fat milk when the doctors said that my baby was quite small. I also ate chocolate and biscuits a little more than usual. I tried to eat a balanced diet but I never said 'no' to something sweet. I think I ate better than I ever have during the time I was pregnant.

Initially I found my changing shape sexy, although, as I got larger, I was worried about my huge breasts getting bigger. I had a very supportive partner who loved my new belly and breasts. I think that helped me a lot; being desired made me feel more desirable. Funnily enough, I found myself eagerly awaiting body changes like stretch marks and the **linea nigra***. My pregnant girlfriends had both, so I desperately wanted one or both to feel more pregnant. I got what I wanted: the stretch marks appeared at 36 weeks.*

I loved being able to dress to enhance my bump. I loved to wear long-sleeved maternity shirts to work that would frame my belly. I was excited to see my bump growing and others loved to see my progress. The only trouble was most shirts that showed off the belly always showed off my bigger boobs too, which made me feel a bit self-conscious. But every day I got positive comments about my body; how wonderful I looked and how being pregnant really suited me.

Other than eating carefully (as per doctor's orders), I tried to exercise as much as I could. I walked a lot during my pregnancy, as I'm a nurse. But closer to the end of the pregnancy, I started to find it more difficult to walk the dog because I would be tired and aching from my day at work. Occasionally I swam but this was more to relieve the pressure of my ever-growing belly than for exercise.

Another thing that I felt fortunate about in my pregnancy was that most people asked me before touching my belly. I don't mind people I know and am friends with touching my belly, as long as they ask. I loved it when baby kicked and I could say 'Quick, feel this!' I did have a few people try and touch my belly without asking. They were either little children (who don't know better) or people I didn't know very well. I remember reading on a website that if this bothers you, you should try and touch the offender's belly back, and say 'How does this feel!' I tried it, and the lady got quite offended. I simply stated 'Please ask before you touch me. I don't feel we know each other well enough for you to touch without asking.' I was furious. Just because you are pregnant, doesn't mean you don't have personal space!

Other than those space invading incidents, I powered through my pregnancy. I loved my body and the baby growing inside me. I loved everything from feeling a foot poking out from under my ribs, through to the stretch marks.

Mita's Wisdom   I know that some women find their entire pregnancies difficult; I was more fortunate. I loved my body and I loved all the positive comments I received. I did not love people invading my space though! I would say to women who are having a hard time in pregnancy that these changes in your body, in your life, are happening for a reason—you're expecting a child. It is OK to get down sometimes about things changing, but try to stay positive and enjoy what's happening.

Food cravings

Many women have strange food cravings in pregnancy. Perhaps you are eating pickles and ice cream or maybe you can't get enough pineapple chunks (which you've never previously liked). But what if you develop a craving for something that isn't food? Some women develop what is called **pica**, an eating disorder that can present in pregnancy that causes women to eat non-food items. Some of the more common cravings include: clay, charcoal, laundry detergent, soap, hair, toilet paper, pebbles, dirt and even cigarette ashes. While it may seem funny, the consequences of caving in to pica are not; pregnant women can develop serious complications, such as lead poisoning, parasite infections, bowel obstructions and dental injuries. Eating non-food items can also cause harm to the developing baby in utero. A study conducted by Corbett et al. in 2003 investigated 128 women who sought **prenatal** care and discovered a prevalence rate for pica of 38 per cent. (It's important to note that this figure tends to vary according to studies and populations; rates have been found to be as low as 14 per cent and as high as 73 per cent.)

Sex

Sex is different for everyone—pregnancy or no pregnancy. Many books and articles talk about sex after pregnancy but few discuss sex during pregnancy. In this section, we take a look at the sex lives of three women and how pregnancy affected their sex drives, both during and after pregnancy.

Morning sex? No, morning sickness!

Sarah had a very high sex drive pre-pregnancy but discovered that while she was still very much in love with—and attracted to—her partner, she found her pregnant body too uncomfortable to engage in sex. Sarah had always said she would never be 'one of those women who would prefer a cuppa to a romp in the sack' but has had to revise her position somewhat!

Sarah's Story

I took a pregnancy test in private at home one day. I have to say that the moment those two lines appeared was one of sheer wonder and joy. I called Matt in to show him the test and he was so excited he was punching the air and kissing my stomach. We were in a state of suspended belief for a couple of weeks afterwards too. I couldn't wait to start looking pregnant and wanted to shout from the rooftops that I was pregnant and having a baby. I have kept the pregnancy test in my bedroom drawer and each time I see it there, I'm moved with joy and tears well up.

I've always been very highly sexed—up for sex several times every day. But morning sickness really took a toll on my libido in the first half of the pregnancy. I was either exhausted, nauseous or struggling to keep food down, so there wasn't a lot of bedroom action at all in the first months. After the sick feelings faded, it then became an issue of discomfort. I wasn't frightened about the baby becoming injured at all but I did worry about my own back and pelvis as I'd had a lot of pain and problems with those areas. Also, I wasn't feeling particularly sexual—all of my thoughts and feelings seemed to be focussed on the baby and impending motherhood. Sex just didn't come into the picture at all.

I was heavily pregnant when we got married and went on honeymoon. As it was a honeymoon, I felt I had to make more of an effort sexually and put aside all concerns for comfort and 'put out'. I'm glad that I did because it made for some funny and tender moments as my gorgeous new hubby navigated his way around my enormous belly. In the final weeks of the pregnancy, I requested sex quite often too, as I was hoping to go into labour and I had heard frequent sex might trigger that. It didn't, of course. It left some lasting memories of the baby kicking me furiously in the ribs during some awkward moments though.

Straight after we got home from hospital, there was a big spike in libido. I was so desperately in love with my new daughter and with my husband for helping to create her. I was aching, sore, tired and deliriously happy. I couldn't wait to be intimate with Matt, and I think we had sex against doctor's orders the very first night we got home, five days after the birth.

The general lack of libido however has lasted beyond birth and into the whole first year of our daughter's life. It is something I continue to struggle with. I never seem to feel like having spontaneous sex anymore, despite being just as in love with my husband. I've heard various explanations for this ranging from the hormonal (I'm still a breastfeeding mum), to the social (I'm a busy, tired mother of one) to the spiritual (I'm relating to the mother archetype now). I'm also aware that the greater part of the libido issue is that I'm just not comfortable with my post-pregnancy body. My once-fabulous breasts have drooped, my stomach is like a stretched girdle of flesh, and I'm still struggling with extra kilos. I don't look in the mirror and see somebody who wants to get naked and celebrate her body; I see an overstuffed, overstretched mummy mountain instead!

At the end of the day though, sex is the glue which bonds us. It's the special thing we share that nobody else does. So I make what feels like a super-human effort to be sexually available on a reasonable basis for my husband, even though I don't really feel like doing it and would most days much prefer a cup of tea and a nap. I'm convinced that this will change over time so I'm not really worrying about it. It's something that we have talked about a lot as well, as I'd hate for Matt to think that this current state of affairs is anything to do with him. I still enjoy sex vicariously, as I enjoy pleasuring my husband, and the happiness and warmth between us afterwards makes it worthwhile too.

Sarah's Wisdom	Having a baby took a big toll on my entire being. Not a single aspect of my life is left untouched. Before I fell pregnant, I swore on my life that I would never become one of those women who would prefer a cuppa to a romp in the sack. Yet two years later that is exactly the woman I am! My husband and I have learned to be more honest and upfront with each other, and mutual orgasms have been replaced with shared responsibility and mutual respect. It's another form of intimacy which grows out of a shared experience of parenthood, and an all-pervasive exhaustion.
	If you can talk about the changes to your priorities and the ravaging of your libido, it may give your partner a deeper understanding, alleviate some of their frustration, and in turn strengthen your relationship. At the same time don't cop out either—part of a good relationship is shared sexuality and you need to make an effort to step out of your lethargy and become a lover too.

How soon after delivery can I have sex?

The general rule of thumb for when you can first have full intercourse after delivery is after your **postnatal** check up (which is normally six weeks **post-partum**). This is so your treating specialist can check that you are healing well, that any stitches you may have had are healing well (and are not infected), and to make sure your uterus has contracted to its original size (among other things). However, depending on the type of delivery you had, you may be able to resume sex earlier than this. It is important to speak to your health care provider before you resume sex, just to make sure that it is safe to do so.

While you are waiting to speak to or see your health care provider, there are other fun things you can do apart from penetrative sex, such as mutual masturbation and oral sex. However, it is very important that oral sex is only performed on a male, even during pregnancy, as performing oral sex on a woman during pregnancy and soon after she has given birth can be very dangerous, even fatal. Oral sex performed on a woman during these times can introduce infection into the vagina or the womb. More seriously, air can be blown into the vagina, which can very easily get into the damaged blood vessels of the uterus and can cause a fatal illness known as air embolism.

Intercourse is an important part of any relationship but there are always going to be highs and lows. If you are experiencing a lull in your sex life, for any reason, it is important to talk it through with your partner so that he or she understands where you're coming from. And while you're waiting, there's nothing quite like a snuggle in bed to keep you physically bonded.

Why sex in pregnancy? To bring on labour!

For Ilana, pregnancy lessened her libido but increased her sense of connectedness with her partner. Easygoing in nature, Ilana is prepared to go with the flow and is not too worried about the lack of sex she and her partner have.

Ilana's Story

Both of my pregnancies were planned, and I had no trouble conceiving at all, so when I saw those little stripes on the pregnancy test I was absolutely thrilled. In my first pregnancy, I was fairly cautious about sex for the first trimester but had no such worries in my second pregnancy. To tell the truth, it wasn't the pregnancy that made me feel 'unsexy', it was more the tiredness that hindered my libido. As you can imagine, I was far more tired in my second pregnancy. In my experience, it's all normal—sometimes you feel up for it, sometimes not, sometimes in the last few weeks, it's all about ways to bring on labour, not pleasure. But it's all OK; there are no rules on how anyone should feel.

I did feel a deeper sense of connectedness with my partner during the pregnancy ('Look how clever we are, this is a product of our love for one another'). It was a spiritual connectedness, a sense of combining our fates, and creating a world and family of our own, rather than a physical urge. As I said, after a decade or so together, night time can, for some, often be more about sleeping than sex. You get that.

After the births, we waited until all the bleeding had stopped[3] before resuming our sex (or not-that-much-sex) life. Neither of my kids were good sleepers, with the eldest never

---

3 The time it takes for bleeding to cease differs between women. As a general rule, all bleeding should stop by six weeks. Note that your period may take a while to start again, particularly if you are breastfeeding.

sleeping for more than 40 consecutive minutes before needing to be put back to sleep. Yep, baby: one, sex life: zero. As you can imagine, I was asleep almost before I made it into bed. Luckily I have a wonderful, understanding husband who shared the waking up duties and was just as tired.

When we finally got around to it, sex was enjoyable, although after the second birth (and stitches) something just felt a little different. Not bad, or worse, just a bit different. Once again, you get that.

Ilana's Wisdom	I don't have any amazing words of wisdom to impart—it's a journey, and we will all experience different things. Go with the flow, listen to your body (but don't let your fears run away with themselves), hold on and enjoy the ride.

A swinging libido: Sex as usual, thanks

Isobel's libido did not change with either of her pregnancies. She found that she swung from one end of the sexual pendulum to the other for no apparent reason. One minute, she was keen for sex; the next, she wasn't interested at all.

Isobel's Story

I was terrified when I found out I was pregnant with my first baby. My husband and I were living with his parents and saving for a house. We were planning to buy the house, move in and then start trying to get pregnant. I had missed my period, had sore boobs and was starving all the time. I took a pregnancy test (I told myself) to rule out pregnancy. I didn't think I was pregnant but worrying about it was simply delaying my period. I remember sitting on the loo, shaking and willing the little blue line to disappear. It took about a week for this fear to disappear and to become excited about pregnancy. I was still terrified (and remained so, up until after delivery) of giving birth but I was excited to be carrying a child, even if I had the timing a little mucked up.

During pregnancy, I was either overly horny or not remotely interested. And I could never anticipate which way I would swing. Although, as the pregnancy developed, and so did the size of my vagina and the amount of discharge, I found I was more hesitant to have sex. Not less eager, just more embarrassed by my body and what it was doing. To be perfectly honest, I don't think my husband cared one little bit about it.

I felt no greater or lesser intimacy with my husband. We continued having sex as we normally would, right up to the end of each pregnancy. Even when it was uncomfortable, because of my size, we still managed to enjoy ourselves.

With both pregnancies, we didn't have sex for three months after each birth. With the first birth, I had a lot of vaginal damage and the birth was quite traumatic, so I didn't want anything near me. The first time we had sex, my husband went really slowly but I was very anxious. We were able to have sex but it became painful quickly. It took many months after that for the sex to return to normal and for me to lose the fear of pain during sex, although I am entirely sure that this pain was a mental block, rather than a physical one. With the birth of my second child, I was anxious even though the birth was quite easy. I put off having sex for as long as possible due to the fear of it being painful again. With both births, tiredness also was a factor that led to a decrease in sex. It was the last thing on my mind of an evening, especially when I was never sure when the baby would wake up again. All I ever really wanted was sleep. Overall now, we are having just as much sex as we had before but we have to schedule it in around the kids.

Isobel's Wisdom	It is important to remember that your body changes during pregnancy and after birth. You have to trust yourself and be prepared to relax. Men need to remember that sometimes birth can be a fearful experience and that they should be patient. Women should remember that even though they may not feel like having sex straight away, their libido will return and if it doesn't, it might be a good idea to talk to your husband about it, so that you can figure things out together.

Why didn't anyone tell me that …

- For some of us, labour is the easy part.
- I would vomit every day and lose 20 kilos with both pregnancies.
- Pregnancy is only the beginning and there are going to be millions of memorable moments to follow.
- A woman's life changes as soon as the stick turns blue but it takes the man a long time to catch up.
- Pregnancy is awesome!
- Not everyone will get stretch marks or fat ankles and that your body can return to normal.
- It's all so hard.
- Morning sickness sometimes lasts all day.
- I know my body will never be the same but I am so proud of what it has achieved. It has created and sustained life. How wonderful is that?
- It was normal for me to feel grief for the life I left behind, even though I was still happy and excited about the new one to come.
- I would want sex so much—my poor husband was run ragged!
- I would hate pregnancy every single day for nine months.
- I would stand in front of the fridge at 2 am, frantically shoving down cold sausages.
- I would feel like queen of the universe: today, I created eyebrows!

- I would be amazed beyond belief that I could actually feel a foot poking through my tummy and spend hours touching my belly just to say 'hi'.
- That it all goes by so fast and you should cherish it.
- It would never be about me again.
- People would open doors for me and men would always stand up and give me their seat on the bus.

CHAPTER THREE

Birth and post-partum

'Anyone who thinks women are the weaker sex never witnessed childbirth.'

Anonymous

Birth is both a beginning and an end. It is the beginning of a life, the beginning of parenthood, and the beginning of a momentous journey. It is also an end: an end to pregnancy and labour, an end to life without children, and the end (for most) of a personal paradigm. Most of us would agree that birth is a momentous occasion for both women and men, and that the process of giving birth can be as unpredictable as life itself. Bringing a child into the world can be incredibly destabilising but it can also be an experience equal to your hopes and plans. Either way, depending on who you are, birth can bring feelings of joy, elation, fear, exhaustion, boredom, anger, confusion, trauma, love and pain.

We are fortunate enough to live in the Western world, where the rates of maternal and perinatal mortality are at an all-time low. This significant improvement in maternal and perinatal outcomes in recent years—albeit marked by a clear delineation between developing and developed countries—coincides with an increasingly heated focus on the question of *how we give birth*. In some circles, the discussion has been reduced to a mudslinging match. Has birth become so safe, we are now safe to argue about it? As Susan Maushart writes in *The Mask of Motherhood*, 'It is because we can now be so confident about a successful outcome in the form of a healthy baby that we can afford the luxury of examining birth as a process imbued with meaning in its own right' (2000, p. 70). But the intense debate accompanying this luxury has inevitably left many new mothers and fathers feeling confused, disappointed and guilty in the competitive environment surrounding birth.

Indeed, the flip side to the modern luxury of viewing birth as an event in itself is that more than ever, women are judged, or judge themselves, on how they 'perform' on this test of physical endurance and emotional grit. As with so many aspects of becoming a parent, judgement creeps into birth choices in insidious ways. One woman may consider a caesarean section a marvel of modern medicine that she'll gladly benefit from, while another berates her for betraying the power of her body to birth 'naturally'. A woman who chooses a homebirth, wishing to trust her fortitude to birth without the option of drugs, may be admonished by the woman who is shocked at her recklessness for putting herself and baby 'at risk'.

The debate rages in academic circles, among professionals and among parents. Why are there an increasing number of caesareans? Is there such a thing as a '**cascade of intervention**'? Should women be 'allowed' to give birth in their own homes? Should women be discouraged from requesting a caesarean or an **induction**? Is birth becoming dehumanised? Too medicalised? Disenfranchised? The list is endless and the disagreement can be vicious. However, while the debate continues, women right now are birthing in all manner of ways. Controversial or not, for these women, their personal story of giving birth is always incredibly meaningful and significant.

In this chapter, you will read stories that encompass a wide variety of births, from vaginal births at home to emergency caesarean sections in hospital. You will also hear from partners of women who gave birth in different settings. Despite the ongoing discussion and disagreement, the common thread among these stories is that no particular type of birth is necessary to have a positive experience. What seems to matter most to women is that their choices are respected and that they maintain some control over their situation.

Perhaps the best definition of a successful birth is one that leaves the woman feeling treated with dignity and respect—one where her wishes are listened to and support is given in whichever way she chooses to birth, and one in which the safety of mother and baby are paramount.

Vaginal births: Delivery suites in hospitals

There is no doubt that in the developed world most Western women choose to give birth in hospitals (for example, in New South Wales, Australia, the rate is 95.7 per cent) (NSW Department of Health 2009). They choose to give birth in **delivery suites** in hospitals partly because this is the 'done thing', partly for the reassurance of having doctors at hand, and partly because some women want the option of pain relief in the form of **pethidine** or an **epidural**. However, women giving birth in delivery suites can still have significantly different births, as illustrated by the following stories.

Generational baggage: How fear can affect labour

Rachel's story poignantly illustrates a common emotion surrounding childbirth: fear. Many women in Western society fear birth and this can have a detrimental effect on labour and delivery. In fact, it can slow down or even arrest labour. As Rachel discovered, her fear of birth was so intense that she believed it actually heightened her level of pain.

Rachel's Story

I was completely terrified of childbirth. My mother had instilled in me a great fear of the pain that comes with birth. She had never explained the process to me, nor had she given me any emotional input as to how her births had gone. Sex and the body were taboo subjects in our household growing up and because of this, I had emotional baggage that I carried with me into my first experience of labour.

My labour began at the end of a very long day. I was past my due date by a few days and each moment seemed to drag on forever. I went to bed and only slept for an hour before I woke up to a contraction. The contractions were short and uncomfortable in the way indigestion is uncomfortable—annoying but not painful. I sat up and then noticed that I was leaking. My first response was to panic. I remember thinking 'I don't want to be here'. I wasn't at all ready to deliver this baby.

The pains continued and intensified into the night. I have no idea how long it was before they actually became painful, but by that stage, I was a mess. I screamed through each one, not so much because of the intense pain but because I was terrified.

When my husband drove us to the hospital, I was placed into a giant spa bath. It was warm and relaxing and I never, ever wanted to leave it. I was so exhausted that my husband had to hold my face out of the water while I napped between contractions.

*Then **transition** hit. I'd learned that this occurs between the contraction stage of labour and the pushing stage. I wanted to grab my husband by the balls and remove any chance of getting pregnant ever again. It hit like a tidal wave and all of a sudden, I just wanted to get up and walk out. I remember trying to tell my mother-in-law that I was ready to go home. I didn't need to be there anymore—I'd had enough!*

When I started the pushing phase of labour, something amazing happened—I realised that it was almost over. It was truly amazing how much motivation I could muster during this phase. I was no longer quite as exhausted as I first thought. The idea of pushing made everything worth it.

To birth a baby's head is hard to describe. For me, it almost felt like I was being pulled apart. The pressure was so intense but it was not really pain as such. My whole vaginal area seemed to go numb. There was no feeling of flesh tearing (although this is certainly what happened to me), there was just intense pressure. Then there was that final urge to push, which was sweeter than anything in the entire world. That push is what freed my baby from my body; instantly the pain and suffering was over.

Then I got to meet my baby and the feeling was indescribable. Finally, I got to look down upon the face of the being that began from my very own flesh and blood. I got to see her breathe and move independently from my own body. I was so happy to put a face to my daughter. Yet, it was bittersweet too as the cord was cut and my child was now separate and alone in the world. I wanted to cry and laugh and hug my child all in the blink of an eye. I felt an overwhelming sense of joy. And I had survived.

Rachel's Wisdom	My biggest challenge was not dealing with all the emotional baggage that my mum had given me before I conceived. I think my difficult delivery was directly related to my intellectual understanding of childbirth and pain, handed down to me by my mother. I don't think she meant to harm me, but nonetheless, I believe it greatly affected my pain levels during labour.

I can't wait for my daughter to be of an age where I can discuss children and childbirth. I want to help her see that childbirth is wonderful and natural. I never want her to have the fear that permeated my very being with my first pregnancy. Hopefully, I can help her understand that her body is sacred and amazing and perfectly equipped to deal with childbirth.

If I were to have another child, I think I would consider a homebirth without drugs. I would like to experience labour in its entirety. But I would not change any of my other births; they are a part of my life, and they were a wonderful learning experience. I discovered that the power of the mind and the power of the words of others can be a very potent thing.

Can fear affect childbirth?

As Saistao and Halmesmaki (2003) note, fear of childbirth can be 'biological (fear of pain), psychological (related to personality, previous traumatic events or fear of future parenthood), social (lack of support or economic uncertainty) or secondary (originating from previous childbirth experiences)' (p. 202). In extreme cases of fear, a person is said to be '**tokophobic**'. As discovered by Hofberg (2000), women who suffer from tokophobia and who are refused their choice of delivery method suffer higher rates of psychological distress than women who achieve their desired delivery method. The prevalence rate of tokophobia in the community is approximately 6–10 per cent.

Fear of childbirth occurs on a spectrum, ranging from no fear to fear so severe that it causes nightmares, physical complaints and even difficulties in carrying out everyday activities. Recent studies have shown that fear can be present during pregnancy, during delivery and post-partum. Indeed, research has shown that women who suffer greatly from fear of childbirth during pregnancy are 'likely to have the most intense fear during delivery, and also suffer the most from it afterwards' (Wijma 2003, p. 141).

As evidenced in the scientific literature (see Alehagen et al. 2006; Wijma 2003), fear can affect the method of delivery. Fear can be generated by the media, and by friends and/or family who relay 'horror stories' of their own childbirth. While these stories may or may not be exaggerated, many pregnant women take these stories at face value and begin to fear the birthing process. For women who are having second or third babies, fear can be a response to a previous traumatic birth. In any case, studies have shown that intervention in the form of 'talking therapies' such as cognitive therapy and counselling can greatly reduce fear of labour and delivery and also reduce requested caesarean sections (Saistao & Halmesmaki 2003).

If you have a strong fear of childbirth, it is important that you speak to a health professional about your concerns and worries. Fear can be overcome with counselling, education and support from caring birth professionals. If you are overly frightened about giving birth, please look up the support services listed on page 248 of the Resources section.

Bouncy balls aren't very fun: When good intentions fly out the window

Birth is different for everyone and Jaki's story is testament to the unique experience of birth, not only between women but for each birth the woman has herself. It also reflects how quickly birth plans can change.

Jaki's Story

I was 29 when my first daughter was born. I was quite 'herbal' at the time and was right into natural therapies; I thought traditional medicine was all bollocks and so I aimed for a 'natural' birth. I knew that women had been giving birth all over the world leaning under trees for generations and it just made sense to me.

*I did the **perineal massage** in the ninth month and did absolutely everything the so-called expert books said. I took into hospital with me a fit ball, an aromatherapy burner and a tape player. But once my labour actually hit, I was unable to move an inch! I was stuck straddling the back of a chair, frozen every time a contraction hit. Who had time for music, aroma and rocking ... you must be kidding!*

After about nine hours of going absolutely nowhere ('Still only 3 centimetres, dear!'), the midwife suggested I try a warm bath and some gas. But once in the bath, I lost the only thing that was helping me through the contractions—the deep breathing and the back of that blessed chair. Not good. I was nearly crying at this point, looking helplessly at my mum, who suggested (brilliant woman that she is) an **epidural***. Well, decision made. In the anaesthetist came (not soon enough), and the epidural was in, albeit after a few harrowing moments wondering if it was all going to go pear shaped, being naturally reticent about someone about to insert anything into my spine. And thank goodness—relief. God bless whoever invented that thing!*

About an hour later, they said 'Oh look, you're fully dilated—couple of deep breaths honey, one push—there's the head'. Another push and out she came … I swear, only two pushes! I had a couple of stitches but all was fine and good.

My second birth was a terribly practical birth. My daughter, Poppy, was induced two weeks early at my own choice because it worked better for us as a family. I remember arriving on my chosen day at the preordained time (something terribly civilised like 10 am), settling into my own room and being given the **syntocinon** *drip. Seeing the anaesthetist was already there, I decided perhaps it was best to do the epidural at the same time.*

There I was, hooked up to the machine, watching some mild contractions that I couldn't feel, watching television, laughing and joking with Danny and my mum, doing crosswords and generally taking it pretty easy. A few hours later nothing major was going on, so they decided to break my waters to see if that would get things going. Meanwhile, my obstetrician was running late due to the result of some major soccer match causing people to party in the streets, making the traffic shocking. Mum whispered to my belly 'Listen kid, we'll give you till 3.30, alright?'

Needless to say, 3.30 came and went. The contractions were coming thick and fast, I was fully dilated and still couldn't feel a bloody thing—and we were now waiting for the doctor to come, trying to hold off the birth until he could deliver her. He rushed in, Poppy's head already poking out, and voila, one push, two pushes and out she came. I lost a hell of a lot of blood[4]—they were a bit worried and I wasn't to get up for 24 hours, not that I could.

What really sticks in my mind is that my baby looked like a turtle, not a monkey (which is what Jane had looked like to me), and I fell in love a little more quickly. I think that might have been because I knew what to expect and I think that because it was all so much less traumatic, I was more relaxed and nowhere near the same state of physical and mental shock as I was with my previous birth.

Obviously, my mindset completely changed between births. Believe me, I'm the first one to laugh at how different my births were and how funny a 'practical' birth may sound. But even though people may judge me for my choices, I really don't care. Because it's my life, my story, my choice.

Jaki's Wisdom   Do what's right for you. Don't listen to any expert other than your own self. Listen to your body. You are about to embark on the most amazing adventure of your life. Nothing is always as expected. Do your best, that's all you can do, and don't have regrets … just be you.

---

4 See 'What is a post-partum haemorrhage?' on page 89

What are the risks and side effects of epidurals?

Epidurals are often requested by women in labour to alleviate pain and are used when delivering a baby via caesarean section. An epidural is a spinal procedure, whereby anaesthetic drugs are delivered via a tiny catheter inserted into the 'epidural space' in a woman's back. Drugs delivered through this catheter can be controlled during birth.

The risks of epidurals going wrong are rare and most side effects are minor. Common side effects include nausea, itching, shivering, a drop in blood pressure and/or headache. Women may also experience back pain or bruising at the injection site. Around 10 per cent of all epidurals do not provide adequate pain relief (Ravishankar et al. 2005).

There can be more serious side effects of epidurals, however, a recent study published in the *British Journal of Anaesthesia* (Cook et al. 2009) concluded that the estimated risk of permanent harm following a spinal anaesthetic or epidural is less than one in 20 000 and, in many circumstances, is considerably lower.

Since epidurals were introduced in the 1970s as a form of pain relief in labour, controversy has persisted about the possible effects they may have on labour. Epidurals have been linked with longer labours, induction and **augmentation** (where **syntocinon** or **oxytocin** is used to start or speed up labour), instrumental and operative delivery rates (caesareans) and with **maternal pyrexia** (high temperature) and post-partum back pain. However, a number of recent randomised controlled trials have addressed these effects and found that epidurals do not cause higher rates of caesarean sections. They do, however, have a modest effect on labour and augmentation, as well as pyrexia. No consistent differences have been found in **APGAR** scores in babies whose mothers had an epidural. Randomised controlled trials have also identified that epidurals are not associated with an increased incidence of post-partum back pain (McGrady & Litchfield 2004). It is important to note that this is an area of controversy and studies are ongoing.

Jaki's story is not uncommon. Many women enter childbirth hoping for a 'natural' (or intervention-free) process. However, quite a number of those women will opt for pain relief in the form of an epidural—in the United States, that figure is 66 per cent. In Australia, the figure is roughly 27 per cent (Lain et al. 2008), similar to the rate in the United Kingdom (25 per cent) (McGrady & Litchfield 2004).

The best thing you can do if you are at all worried or concerned about having an epidural is to talk it over with an anaesthetist. If you can do so, try to attend a lecture on anaesthesia for birth at your local hospital (if they run such classes) or call your hospital and ask for an appointment with an anaesthetist so that your questions and concerns can be answered. It's great if you can do this before the birth because you will probably 'take in' more information but if you haven't done so and an epidural is imminent, there still might be time to ask those questions!

What will happen to my vagina?

At last count, there were about 200 euphemisms for vaginas. Whatever you or your partner like to call yours, most women (and men) want to know what will happen to it after a vaginal birth. Will sex ever be the same? Will it look different? How much is it going to hurt and for how long?

What will it feel like?

That depends on the type of delivery you've had. Even if you've had no tearing or stitches, your vagina will probably feel swollen, sore and bruised. If you've had tearing (which may need stitches) or an **episiotomy**, which is a cut through the vaginal wall and the **perineum** (which will definitely need stitches), your genital area will feel more tender and sore. Tears are categorised by degrees. A first degree tear involves only the top layer of skin; a second degree tear involves the skin, the underlying tissue and pelvic floor muscles. A third degree tear extends to the opening of the anus and a fourth degree tear extends through to the anus. The chance of a third or fourth degree tear is about 1 in 200.

Will it be stretched?

After you give birth and as the weeks pass, your body gets rid of excess swelling. Things can feel a bit strange—your vagina might feel a bit deflated, stretched, or just plain odd. Every woman is different and so the length of time it takes for things to start feeling normal again will be different for everyone. You can definitely help things along with pelvic floor exercises. These exercises strengthen your pelvic floor muscles (the ones that stretch during childbirth). They are important because they help to increase your pleasure during sex and, when strong, they improve the tone of your bladder so that you are less likely to leak urine in the years following birth. They won't make your vagina smaller but they can make the opening tighter.

How do I do pelvic floor exercises?

- When you pee, clench your muscles to stop the flow for as long as you can. Then start the flow again. This is a good way of figuring out if you're clenching the right muscles.

- Clench your muscles like this as often as you can (if you can do ten clenches for ten seconds each, ten times a day, good stuff!). You can use triggers to remind you, such as stopping at traffic lights, answering the phone, etc.

What will it look like?

That depends on what it looked like before you had a baby! There will be some changes—that is inevitable after having a three-kilo baby (on average) pass through your vagina. It may look swollen immediately after birth and it may also look bruised and quite traumatised. Then again, it may not look so bad. Everyone's body reacts differently to birth. You might like to ask for a hand mirror so you can see for yourself what your post-birth vagina looks like.

What about sex?

Both women and men can have issues about sex after birth. Women often worry that their stitches (if they have them) will open up. They also wonder 'Will it hurt?',

'Will it feel different?', 'Will I even feel like having sex?' Again, the answer is different for everyone. But a rule of thumb is that women who have experienced physical trauma from birth are more likely to experience more painful sex initially.

Is there anything I can do to help after the birth?

Lots! Here are some tried and tested methods for decreasing pain and improving your vagina's health and wellbeing:

- Wear loose clothing and cotton underwear.
- Change your maternity pad often to help reduce the risk of infection.
- Keep your vagina as clean and dry as possible.
- Each time you go to the toilet, wash yourself with plain water and pat your vagina dry with soft toilet paper.
- Drink loads of water to dilute your urine (it reduces acidity and helps reduce stinging).
- If you're pooing, a great tip is to hold a clean pad firmly against the wound and press upward while you bear down.
- You could try ice packs if you've had stitches to help reduce the swelling; lots of women say that witch-hazel pads are helpful too.
- Take pain killers if you think it will help (but go easy on them).

Vaginal births: Birth centres

While the most common choice for giving birth is in a hospital setting, a growing number of women are now choosing to deliver in **birth centres**. Birth centres are usually attached to a main hospital, so that in the event of an emergency, the woman can be quickly transferred. Birth centres are midwife-led and have a more home-like atmosphere. This, combined with the fact that there is minimal intervention in birth centres, attracts women who want to try and give birth in a familiar environment without the use of chemical pain relief. However, as you will see in one of the following stories, some women who intend on birthing their babies in such centres are precluded from doing so.

Meeting baby number two: An unexpected water birth

Nikki has experienced two births; both of them very different. This story is about Nikki's second birth—a water birth.

Nikki's Story

Some memories of the day I gave birth are very strong. One of the most bittersweet moments of that afternoon was watching my first-born walking down our path to my mother's car. I realised in a few hours our lives would change forever. She and I were so very close. We were a little unit, often to the innocent exclusion of her father, and now our relationship would be irrevocably changed; not for the better or worse, just different. I was very sad and a little guilty at what I perceived I was 'doing' to our older daughter by having another baby.

*By 5 pm, the contractions were getting stronger and we knew the baby would be coming soon. I had a **TENS machine** which I used constantly. I'll never know whether it alleviated much of the pain but the psychological aspect of being able to actively manage the contractions was very strong. I felt like I had a lot more control and was more active in my labour; like it was happening 'with' me as opposed to 'to' me.*

*By 7 pm things were happening in earnest. We called the **birth centre** and were told to come in. Walking and the rocking chair became my close friends. The TENS machine was constantly attached and helped enormously.*

At 9 pm, I got in the bath. Being in the water was wonderful; it took a lot of pressure and weight off my back and the heat really helped. By now, the contractions kept coming and coming. The rolling contractions without a break were a surprise to me. I remember banging the side of the bath in agony but at the same time going through each one like it was the first.

*Interestingly, every now and then, the midwife would put a mirror in the bath between my legs to see what was going on. Then I felt the urge to push. With my first labour, I had an **epidural** and was induced, so I had never experienced this. My God, it was powerful. I was squatting in the bath and heard myself yell out 'I'm pushing!' The midwife encouraged me to keep going. I think I pushed twice and at 10.01 pm my baby was born. The midwife scooped her up and put her in my arms. I remember being told to keep her body in the water so she wouldn't get cold. There I was, sitting in a pool of bright red water (no one tells you about that!) holding my beautiful girl. I think she cried a little bit but not much at all.*

I got out of the bath and sat on the side to deliver the placenta. My legs were a bit wobbly from being in the squatting position for so long and I needed support to walk. I had a shower and 15 minutes after she was born, I was feeding her. It was a magical experience.

A few memories have stayed with me, one of the strongest ones being the stitches. What I didn't think about was that because I had no pain relief during my labour, they had to give me an anaesthetic to stitch me up. Well, I can testify that the anaesthetic was more painful than my labour! Hard to believe but it was breathtaking how agonising it was.

Nikki's Wisdom	People are mildly surprised when I tell them I've had a water birth. I think many people think it's a trippy hippy thing to do. They always ask about the pain. I've had two very different births; one with pain relief and one without. There is no doubt the pain was excruciating in and out of the bath. But there is also no doubt that I would have a water birth again in a heartbeat.

What is a TENS machine?

TENS stands for transcutaneous (meaning 'through the skin') electrical nerve stimulation and is a non-pharmacological form of pain relief. A gentle electric current is passed through electrodes that are taped to the skin. The current comes from a small, battery-operated machine that is portable and therefore easy to use for labouring women. One of the major benefits of the **TENS machine** is that it allows women to remain mobile during labour. While it has been established as a safe form of pain relief, you should talk to your health care provider before deciding to use one (for example, you must not use it if you have a pacemaker fitted).

Does the TENS machine work? A study conducted by van der Spank et al. (2000) concluded that women who used the machine during labour reported lower pain scores than the control group (i.e. women who did not use the machine in the study) but that there was no difference between the groups of women on the requested rates of epidural.

Nikki's story highlights the many 'non-invasive' pain relief methods available to birthing women. Aside from the TENS machine, you might also like to try water. Getting into a warm tub creates buoyancy, which can be helpful in **active labour**, as can standing under a shower, especially if you use the nozzle on your lower back and/or belly. Other natural methods that can help relieve pain include **hypnobirthing**, **homeopathics**, massage, aromatherapy and the use of heat packs. You might also like to consider hiring your own **doula**. A doula is someone who can offer physical and emotional support during your pregnancy and labour.

Additionally, you can try to control your environment as much as possible—if certain music calms you down, bring an iPod with some soothing sounds. Some women also find that dimming the lights helps. Everyone is different and you will know best what makes you feel comfortable. If you want to try for a birth using natural pain relief methods, the best thing you can do is research ahead as much as possible. Preparation is the key.

A shock to the system: When plans don't go to plan

Ilka's birth did not go to plan. Wanting to deliver in a birthing centre, she ended up in what she perceived as an unfriendly, medicalised environment.

Ilka's Story

My daughter was a week overdue when my waters broke. Straight away, we noticed that the water was coloured brownish green, so I called the midwife and she told us to come in.

I heaved my mammoth bulk into the shower and thought 'This is probably the last shower I have before I become a mum.'

*At the **birth centre**, the midwife took one look at my pad and said 'Yep. That's **meconium** liquor. You can't stay here, I'm afraid. You'll have to go into the hospital.'*

Immediately I started to feel nervous. I did not want to have the baby in one of those big, unfriendly rooms with lots of medical equipment. Mostly I did not know what to expect. I hadn't met any of the midwives or seen the facilities.

In my birth suite, I tried to set up with my doona and fragrant oils. But really, I was just preoccupied with the strong pains that were starting to grip my bowels. I had to go to the toilet again and again. I was hooked up to a foetal heart monitor, which limited my movement to a radius of about one metre from the hospital bed. The bleeping of the machine and the regular silences which sent my partner and me into a panic became the soundtrack to the day.

The contractions built steadily over the next few hours. I tried to visualise a golden sun and flower petals opening, but it was all too cerebral and the pain I needed to manage was physical. As the intensity of the contractions mounted, I began to lose sight of any positive inner resolve. Each contraction would tear through me; a brutal attack that left me moaning on the floor like an injured animal, terrified that it was about to happen again. I remember my eyes being closed; seeing, hearing and feeling nothing and no one around me except the pain and growing despair.

'I can't, I can't, I can't' became my mantra, and my belief. No one seemed to be arguing with me.

*They offered me **pethidine**, which I took, and with that, my last vestige of mental focus left me. I was stoned and dopey but still in incredible pain. I slept between each screaming contraction. I knew I was not connected to this process. Later, a young, slim, attractive doctor came in on stiletto heels. 'I think your best chance of a vaginal birth,' she told me as I lay sprawled on the floor, 'is if we give you an **epidural**, and hook you up to the **syntocinon** drip to get the contractions a bit stronger.'*

A bit stronger. I knew I could not cope with that. 'Yes,' I said. 'Yes, yes. I'll have the epidural.' All my ideals and politics flew out the window. 'I don't know why I ever thought I could do this', I thought. 'I will never ever do this again. I'll have an elective caesar.' And then the epidural was in. Blessed relief. I lay back to read a magazine, incredulous that my body could be experiencing the same contractions as a few moments ago and yet now I was feeling nothing. Straight away I felt like a failure. I knew I had not coped well with the pain and now it was all over in terms of my involvement—and the baby hadn't even arrived yet.

*The doctor told me to relax for a few hours; she would be back to deliver the baby at 9 o'clock and, as predicted, she was. She needed help with a **ventouse** and I was told to push and push and I did, but there wasn't really much effort in it. I was on my back, with legs raised in stirrups and the pushing I was doing seemed largely theoretical. I couldn't feel it.*

But what I could feel was the love when they placed my little girl on my chest. I will never forget her bright-eyed, inquisitive, exquisitely beautiful face. 'Oh,' I gasped, 'she's absolutely beautiful.' And so she was. And at that moment, my feelings about the birth were left behind and overtaken by something far more important—my child.

Ilka's Wisdom	I learned through my first birth that I needed someone to maintain a very present and intense connection with me throughout the birthing process. I had a very different second birth, which was fantastic for me—much more natural than the first. I had the opportunity to revisit the experience of childbirth and manage it better in my own head and that gave me a lot of confidence. If you decide you want to go ahead with an intervention-free birth, I highly recommend hiring an independent midwife—it made all the difference to me.

Mother guilt in birth

What is mother guilt in birth? According to the book *Mommy Guilt: Learn to worry less, focus on what matters most and raise happier kids*:

> *Mothers sometimes feel guilt over straying from their birth plan. They may have planned to give birth without pain killers, then used them; they may have wanted a home birth, but delivered in the hospital; they may have heard other mothers describe their zero intervention or home deliveries ... and feel a sense of remorse or shame that they didn't hang tough to get that same goal they envisioned for themselves. (Bort et al. 2005, p. 30)*

Unfortunately, many women feel they have 'failed' in childbirth, when their original birth plans fly out the window and they accept an epidural for pain relief. If you are experiencing feelings of guilt surrounding your birth and you are finding these feelings are beginning to interfere with your enjoyment of life, it is important for you to seek help and support. Look up relevant support services in the Resources section or speak with your local health care provider. If your health care provider is unable to help you, they may be able to put you in contact with someone who can. You might also like to try contacting the hospital in which you gave birth (if this was the case). Many large hospitals have social workers who can help you to build networks of support. Most important of all, try not to beat yourself up: childbirth, like many aspects of parenting, can be clumsy and unpredictable.

An important message from Ilka's story (and other birth plans that involve giving birth outside a hospital setting) is to think through all the possibilities and alternatives. For example, if you plan to give birth in a hospital, vaginally, you might be tempted to skip the antenatal class on caesarean sections (because 'that just won't happen to me!'). Don't skip that session. Learn about it, so that in the event you find yourself in a surgical theatre, you will have some knowledge of what is about to happen. Equally, if you are planning to give birth in a birthing centre or at home, you should be open to looking at giving birth in a hospital, because things may not go to plan and you may need emergency medical assistance or intervention. Wherever you're planning on giving birth, learn about where you intend to birth and the process that involves, but pay equal attention to all the alternatives. (You may not plan for an epidural but might end up requiring one, or you may intend to have an epidural but may not be able to obtain one.) This is not a pessimistic message; it's quite the opposite: knowledge is power.

Vaginal births: At home

Until about a century ago, almost all births were homebirths. Now that hospitals have the latest technology, the trend has most definitely swung away from homebirths (apart from The Netherlands, where the homebirth rate is approximately 30 per cent, according to de Jonge et al. 2009). The United States, the United Kingdom, Australia and New Zealand all have similar homebirth rates of approximately 1 per cent.

However, small as the percentage may be, there are women giving birth at home. A recent study by Boucher et al. (2009) sought to ascertain what reasons underpinned women's desire for homebirth. They included: a greater sense of safety, avoidance of unnecessary interventions common in hospital births, previous negative hospital experiences, more control and a comfortable and familiar environment. As you will see in the following story, some women simply prefer to trust their bodies and birth at home, in the same way millions of women did before the arrival of hospitals.

Birthing with friends: A spiritual journey

For Kimberly, birth is spiritual. Kimberly lives in the United States and she hired an independent midwife to help her through her labour and delivery at home. Kimberly is a firm believer in her body and its ability to birth a child but she did create a written birth plan in the case that she needed to go to hospital, so that her wishes might be adhered to.

Kimberly's Story

My journey started on Sarah's due date. I had elected to have a homebirth, as the birth of my first son, Solomon, was an (unplanned) homebirth. His birth was so wonderful and comforting that right then, we decided that if we were to have another child, we were definitely doing it at home. We had learned, hands-on, that we were equipped to give birth unattended.

When my second labor began, I wanted the day to flow as normally as possible, continuing to be active and trying not to give too much attention to going into labor (as challenging as that was). Later, I started feeling 'interesting' sensations; slight contractions that felt more like light menstrual cramps. I was more than able to breathe through the contractions, but later that evening, my husband Kenyatta and I called our midwife, Tolewa, to keep her 'in the know', just in case things escalated overnight.

The next afternoon, I began feeling stronger contractions, more fervent than the contractions from the night before. Each contraction lasted about five minutes, and I thought to myself 'Hmm, this must be the earlier stages of labour, 'cause the contractions are not lasting that long.' With each contraction, the intensity increased, sending me to the 'special birth seat'—the toilet. It's amazing how your muscles instinctively relax when on the throne!

As I returned to the bed, I stared at my living birth plan on the wall. Looking at the plan, I started chanting one of the words from the collage: 'loose, loose, loose.' I also made laughing sounds ('hee, hee, hee') and it definitely soothed the strong sensations. I've always heard that laughing and smiling can chemically alter your body and mood and I'm now a true believer.

When Kenyatta arrived home about 20 minutes later, I was using a birthing ball. Draped over that ball and rocking back and forth was just what I needed to help me though this labour. Each contraction was ten times stronger than the last. I knew that labor was progressing quickly, and I was glad because I was getting a little fatigued.

I asked for help to get on top of the bed and I felt an imminent need to vomit, which I did, seconds later. With contractions rising, I began to chant 'open, open, open.' Tolewa hadn't arrived yet, but immediately, Christy (our Minister) chimed in, simultaneously singing the word as I spoke it, and rubbed my back. I truly wish we had captured this on tape. The moment felt like the physical manifestation of what collective womanhood truly is. For me, it was like being showered with strength, clarity and love from God. When I am giving birth, I truly feel that I am hand in hand with the Creator. I feel connected to a larger consciousness and to my ancestors—it's an overwhelmingly amazing and euphoric space to be in.

At some point, I lay at the top of the bed with Kenyatta behind me, and for some reason, rubbing the stubble on his head became very comforting. I then began to moan, which increased in tone and volume until I was outright howling. In the midst of this, I'm thinking 'Well, something's about to go down because this is the loudest I've ever yelled!' I got on my side, 'the' contraction came, and then my waters broke.

I looked at Kenyatta and asked if he could carry me over to the birth tub and he said 'Baby, I don't think that's gonna work.' So, it was time to do what I knew to do best: I got on all fours just like I did with Solomon's birth, and began to push the baby out. With one push, little Sarah's head came out and I reached down to touch and greet her. With one more push, Sarah entered this realm, right into Christy's hands, who was standing behind me. She later told me that she didn't want Sarah to just fall on the bed and didn't know exactly what to do but to reach out her hands.

The next minutes are oblivious to me; I was in such a euphoric state. I believe Kenyatta and Christy wrapped the baby up in a towel and helped me to the top of the bed again. Next thing I do remember is Tolewa arriving and assisting me in the delivery of the placenta into a bowl (Sarah remained attached to the placenta for about three hours before Kenyatta cut the cord). Family and friends that were on our labor list began arriving in a rhythmic fashion. With each person's entrance, our bedroom grew full of the most beautiful energy, love and joy.

Kimberly's Wisdom	Let your body give birth! Listen to your body and acknowledge your intuition. Do the research for yourself ... learn the benefits and risks of all options. I'll be telling Sarah that she's got everything she needs to give birth.

Are homebirths safe?

Like so many aspects of parenting, giving birth at home is a hotly contested debate, both among women who birth and the medical profession who assist them. Recently, a documentary produced by Rikki Lake (*The Business of Being Born*) re-ignited the controversy in the United States, and homebirth is currently being debated internationally in the public media, medical organisations, within academic circles and among parents.

The guidelines published by the UK's National Institute for Health and Clinical Excellence (NICE 2007) regarding the safety of childbirth state that 'giving birth is generally very safe for both the woman and her baby [and] that among the women who plan to give birth at home or in a midwife-led unit, there is a higher likelihood of a normal birth, with less intervention' (p. 9). They go on to list the information that should be given to all women when planning their place of delivery. The guidelines state that women should consider:

- the locally available services in the case of the need for transfer to a medical facility
- the possible risks to either the woman or her baby relating to planned place of birth
- that if something goes seriously wrong during labour at home or in a midwife-led unit, the outcome for the woman and her baby could be worse than if they were in an obstetric unit
- that if a woman has a pre-existing medical condition or she has experienced a previous complicated birth (that places her at higher risk of developing complications in a subsequent delivery), she is advised to give birth in an obstetric unit.

It is crucial to note that 'freebirth', that is, giving birth on your own without any assistance from a midwife or doctor, is never advised, as it can be extremely dangerous for both mother and baby.

For more information on the homebirth debate, please see page 248 of the Resources section.

Kimberly's living birth plan was a collage on a poster board, filled with words and images of the things she and her partner desired for their birthing experience. This way, anyone who saw it (whether that was friends at home or medical staff in case they had to go to hospital) could understand what they did and did not want for the birth. For Kimberly, the collage was a special prayer of what her heart truly desired. Some of her plan's items read: 'Do Not Speak/Offer Medication!', 'The pain is strong, but you are STRONGER!' and 'Negative energy = Step outside!'

If you are interested in creating a Living Birth Plan, get creative. Think of things you do and don't want for your birthing experience and create a picture or collage of images and words—but the key is to keep it simple.

Vaginal births: After caesareans (VBAC)

Vaginal births after caesareans (**VBACs**) refer to the process of delivering a baby vaginally after a previous caesarean section. VBACs are growing in popularity due to a number of factors. Firstly, newer surgical techniques used in caesarean sections are creating scars that are less likely to rupture in future vaginal deliveries. Secondly, there has been a grassroots push for VBACs to be offered more freely at hospitals. Many women who opt for VBACs do so because they want to experience the feeling of labour and subsequent vaginal delivery. Other women, like Penny in the following story, opt for VBACs because they had a negative experience with a caesarean. Negative experiences range from disappointment at not being 'able' to give birth vaginally (many women feel a deep sense of guilt), to feeling traumatised by their caesarean experience.

Re-defining birth: Uncharted territory

After the disappointment of her first birth not going according to plan, Penny aimed to give birth to her second child vaginally—armed with knowledge and determination.

Penny's Story

*My first baby had been born via caesarean as he was in a **transverse** [horizontal] position. I had been planning to deliver in a **birth centre**, so it was disappointing to find myself in a hospital gown and cap lying on a trolley. I found the whole surgical procedure very scary but it was all over very quickly and I experienced an amazing rush of joy when they showed me my beautiful baby boy.*

Just over two years later, I was pregnant again and this time I really wanted that vaginal birth. I had had no labour with my first pregnancy so I was entering this as a first-timer. I had re-done my birth classes and was as briefed as I felt I could be. But I had no idea just what an individual and unpredictable ride I was in for. And I understood why some mothers maintain there's no point trying to describe labour because it's like nothing else.

After a couple of days of irregular and unpredictable contractions, I started to need Mark for moral support and we tried a few poses during contractions. I needed to breathe through them, groan a little and push against the wall. I was focused inwards. I felt like an animal in my den.

My contractions were getting strong and scary. Scary because they were such indescribable, unfamiliar, internal sensations. Then there was a shift. I got a sense of pushing in my bottom; hard and frightening. I called for Mark and told him to push back. I needed support badly. I didn't like this feeling. It felt wrong, like the baby was coming out and it was too soon. I fought the panic and over the next few contractions, we worked on the best position. I knelt on the couch and Mark pushed hard against my bum. We decided it was time to go to hospital.

The midwife did an internal examination and to my amazement and delight, not to mention relief, I was almost fully dilated. I felt quite elated. She explained that the baby was very low in the pelvis, which explained that dreadful pushing pressure. She kept her hand there for the next contraction, which felt oddly reassuring. It was such a bizarre and practical intimacy.

So with this encouraging progress report, we continued with the work of contractions. Mark offered me sips of water, I rested a bit by dropping my head down like an exhausted horse. I lost track of time. Did I close my eyes for 30 seconds or ten minutes?

At 3 am we decided to break my waters and try the **birthing stool***. Despite being hilariously medieval-looking, the birthing stool was great. 'Imagine you're doing the biggest poo of your life', said the midwife. 'That's the feeling you're going for.'*

I felt the head move down with each push, then maddeningly slip back. It was exactly as she said—a burning, stretching, stinging sensation. It really, really hurt! At first, I was afraid to push. I wanted to avoid the pain. But eventually it just hurt without ceasing and I wanted the baby out. There was no going back; I wanted to push it right out, straight away.

I got onto the bed on my hands and knees. My midwife put down a mirror and I saw a black-haired head crowning. Then, with one final push, at 4.22 am, she slithered out, in one great swoosh—all of her. The relief from pain was instant—brilliant! And there on the bed under me was my baby, crying lustily, bloody and wriggling.

Penny's Wisdom

Birth is amazing. That babies grow inside you and emerge out of your body is incredible, no matter how they arrive. However, for me, giving birth vaginally was an incredible challenge and I felt it redefined me as a woman. I have some insight now as to why people climb mountains or sail solo around the world—it is exhilarating to meet a challenge, come through pain and achieve your goal. But the unequalled bonus of birth is that at the end of the challenge you hold the miracle of a baby in your arms.

VBAC: What are my chances?

Years ago, a caesarean section ended any hope of future vaginal deliveries. But today, thanks largely to advances in surgical techniques, VBACs are possible in many cases. In fact, according to the Mayo Clinic (2008), 60 to 80 per cent of women who attempt VBACs have a successful vaginal delivery.

One of the biggest fears women harbour is having their scar rupture. According to the Mayo Clinic, your chances vary and this is largely dependent on the type of incision you had with your previous caesarean/s. The incision related to the highest success rate in future VBACs is a 'low transverse' incision and fortunately, is the most common type of incision used today when performing caesarean sections. The low transverse incision is a sideways cut across the lower part of your uterus. This type of incision bleeds less and forms stronger scars, which is why it is related to less danger of rupture during subsequent VBAC deliveries (somewhere between a 0.2 to 1.5 per cent chance of rupture).

If, like Penny, you are considering a VBAC, you need to think about what is best for you and your situation. There are some reasons that might preclude you from attempting a VBAC. These include: having a previous classical (or T-shaped) incision, a previous uterine rupture, and/or having two prior uterine scars (American College of Obstetricians and Gynecologists 2004). Your doctor will also take into consideration whether or not you have an obstetric complication and how far you live from a hospital that can perform an emergency caesarean delivery.

A recent study published in the *Australian and New Zealand Journal of Obstetrics and Gynaecology* (Dodd et al. 2004) reported that of the women who had previously had a caesarean section, 41 per cent indicated that they would plan for a vaginal birth in the future. So, if you are planning a VBAC, you are not alone. Refer to page 248 of the Resources section for a list of organisations and websites that can provide you with information, guidance and support. You should also talk through all of the risks and benefits with your health care provider.

Caesarean births: Elective and emergency

Caesarean births have been around longer than you may think. We know, for example, that they stretch at least as far back as 800 BC. Historical accounts reveal a law in Rome dictating that a baby should be delivered via a cut in the mother's womb if it was apparent the mother was going to die before delivery. Caesarean sections were performed for the sake of the child, rather than the mother. One memorable example of this is Robert the Bruce of Scotland, who was born via caesarean section. His mother died during the process. While many believe the origin of the term is from the birth of Julius Caesar, this is unlikely considering his mother Aurelia Cotta lived for many years afterwards.

It was not until major breakthroughs in medicine in the 19th century that mothers were afforded a chance of survival as well. The invention of anaesthesia and penicillin, changes in suturing and incision techniques and the advent of blood transfusions all combined to dramatically improve maternal outcomes. Fortunately, most women living in the developed world have access to excellent facilities, allowing them an alternative to vaginal birth, in the advent of an emergency or other medical reason. Additionally, women are now afforded the choice of requesting a caesarean under special conditions. Caesareans are termed 'elective' when they are decided upon for medical reasons before labour begins and 'emergency' when they are required once the woman has gone into labour.

If you are about to give birth for the first time and you are not planning to have a caesarean, you should at least read a little bit about what happens during a caesarean section, so that you won't be completely unprepared in the event that you need one.

Not what nature intended: Being thankful for modern medicine

Rania's story is a good example of the plans women (and/or their partners) need to make if they live in a remote area, and of how 'emergency' caesareans are not always as scary as they might sound.

Rania's Story

*When I was pregnant with my first baby, I was living 30 kilometres from the nearest town and hospital. I was 'off the beaten track', without any of the mod cons of city living. I was very prepared for my birth—I had even given directions to our farm to the local ambulance officers. I didn't really have a birth plan as such. I didn't have much of a support network or any female friends nearby. I did know that my mum had me via a **forceps delivery** and subsequently had two caesareans. I had an open mind about birth—I certainly had no fear of a vaginal birth (something which bothers me greatly this time—I'm not doing it!). To be honest, as far as birth plans go, I think they are a waste of time. We are all individuals and modern medicine and the science of birth make the whole damn thing so much less of a drama than it has to be.*

*My due date came and went and I was bundled into the car for a check up two and a half weeks after my due date, at which point it was decided that an **induction** at 8.30 pm* *was needed. I went home and collected my bag and merrily headed back into town anticipating a birth that night—how naive!*

I had every form of induction, to no avail. So the next day, they broke my waters with something that will forever remind me of an enormous crochet stick—oh the pain! I was still semi-mobile at this point, with mobile gas, and the only relief I found from the back pain was to sit on the loo, which the midwives were against, so they gave me a bedpan to sit on in bed—by now the glamour was most definitely fading. The contractions seemed apparent from the monitors that were now attached to every part of me but all I felt was severe back ache/pain. All I could think was 'drugs, drugs, give me drugs!' God bless **pethidine***! It was just bliss.*

This went on for the whole evening until at some point after midnight (it had now been about 30 hours since they first started the induction) it was concluded that an emergency caesarean was required. The nurses and the registrar decided I was exhausted; they had trialled my labour to a point where it was obvious I needed assistance, and they thought Mark was stuck under my pelvis. Another hour passed while we waited for the doctors to get out of bed and head to the hospital.

I was prepped for surgery. The last bit all happened so quickly that I just remember the **epidural***, being lifted from the theatre bed and then having a beautiful bundle of 'Mark' being shown to me as I was asking if it was a girl or a boy. I was wheeled into recovery and anxious to see my new bub. I remember just staring at him in awe and pestering him, wanting to see every nook and cranny of what I'd made.*

My recovery was swift and I had no complications. In fact, I had such a good and speedy recovery that I was walking outside the hospital the day after the birth.

With this pregnancy, I have **placenta praevia***, so I am having an elective caesarean (I have ten weeks to go). I have no desire to prove to myself that I can deliver vaginally. I quite obviously didn't fit into any part of 'natural' last time round. Birth, for me, is to enable a child's entry into the world in the most safe and non-stressful way possible. I thank God for modern medicine and the advances that have been made, as I am one of the women who could quite possibly die during childbirth without it.*

Rania's Wisdom	I would tell people to be flexible and open to everything and anything. I think that doctors and midwives are the experts and they do know best. All your plans and wishes can end up causing pain and disappointment if you're fixed in your thinking. We are very lucky to be birthing in this century. Imagine being set on a vaginal birth and ending up dead due to lack of technology or assistance.

Are caesarean sections safe?

According to the UK's National Institute for Clinical Excellence guide on caesareans (2004) and the US National Institutes of Health's statement on caesarean delivery on maternal request (2006), the following are more likely to occur after a caesarean:

pain in the abdomen, bladder injury, injury to the tube that connects the kidney and bladder (ureter) needing further surgery, hysterectomy (in repeated caesareans), admission to an intensive care unit, developing a blood clot, having a longer hospital stay, returning to hospital afterwards and/or having **placenta praevia** (where the placenta covers the entrance to the womb) in a future pregnancy. It is important to note that some of these risks are very rare.

The guidelines go on to state that there is less likelihood of having pain in the perineum (the area between the vagina and anus), urinary incontinence three months after birth and prolapse (sagging of the womb) through the vaginal wall after a caesarean.

If you wind up having an emergency caesarean section, you should not be frightened. However, like everything in life, individuals have different reactions to emergency caesarean sections. Some, like Rania, take it with a grain of salt but on the other end of the spectrum, many women feel traumatised, emotionally and physically shocked, as well as feeling guilty and/or 'let down' by the system (or indeed their own body). These feelings can occur even when a baby is not delivered by emergency caesarean. A study conducted by La Trobe University in Melbourne concluded that 'physical and emotional health problems are common after childbirth, and are frequently not reported to health professionals despite the fact that many women would like more advice and assistance in dealing with them' (Brown & Lumley 1998, p. 156).

If you feel traumatised, either emotionally or physically, after you give birth, it is important that you seek help and support. Talk to supportive friends and family, your midwife, early childhood nurse, GP or obstetrician. You can also try phoning the local hospital and finding out whether they have any supports or services, such as social workers or support groups that you can access. Also, look at the Resources section at the end of this book for a list of services that might be helpful. Remember, we all need help sometimes; maybe now is the time to tap into your networks.

Not according to plan: When pre-eclampsia leads to a caesarean

Emilia's tale is another example of just how unpredictable pregnancy and birth can be. Although she had visions of a straightforward vaginal birth, Emilia wound up having an elective caesarean section.

Emilia's Story

I never expected that I would arrive at hospital ready to birth my son with my perfectly straightened hair and neatly packed overnight bags in a calm, unhurried manner and announce to the person at the reception desk 'I am Prof's 3 pm caesar.' I always imagined a dramatic trip to the hospital, a panicky husband speeding through red lights and me in slight discomfort but reciting mantras and calmly reassuring panicky husband that all would be fine. For some reason I had even pictured my waters breaking in the middle of the kitchen floor. I would have been in the throes of cooking something delicious and nourishing. The reality of Nathan's birth is quite different to how I imagined it to be, though.

*I was 31 weeks pregnant and had a standard **antenatal** appointment at which it was discovered my blood pressure had suddenly shot up and my baby was in the **breech position**. I left the hospital that day five hours later. Pregnancy so far had been an absolute breeze and suddenly after one little blood pressure reading, everything seemed to have changed. I was to report to the hospital twice a week for monitoring and was encouraged to investigate natural ways of getting the baby to turn.*

*At 38 weeks, my blood pressure was 190 over 110. This is dangerously high. The obstetrician decided that the baby was coming out and as he was refusing to get into the right position or was unable to, he would have to be removed manually. Thus two days later, during which I could not sleep, concentrate or indeed focus on anything but the fact that I would shortly be meeting my precious new baby, I turned up at the hospital with freshly blow dried hair (I thought it would be important to look nice for the baby in the photographs afterwards) and my suitcases. I was so excited about it all being over shortly and so fed up with the constant monitoring of the **pre-eclampsia** that I hardly had the opportunity to feel nervous about the caesarean. As the anaesthetist was sticking a needle the size of a knitting needle into my spine, I had a few moments of panic but then felt quite relaxed (probably due to the drugs).*

In the theatre, I remember looking up into the lights that were made from very shiny stainless steel and I could see a hazy reflection of myself lying on the table, Ross (my husband) and the anaesthetist sitting at my head and the obstetrician and his assistant on the other side of the curtain bent over my body. Ross stood up and looked over the curtain (I still have no idea why he did this) and as he sat back down I thought he might have been about to pass out. Afterwards he told me that he now understands why they put the curtain up and that is all he had to say about what he saw.

*After what felt like an age, they managed to evict Nathan from the womb. He was immediately held up for me to see and the obstetrician announced 'You have a son'. 'I knew he was a boy', I shouted and then burst into tears. The midwife wiped all the **vernix** off him, wrapped him up snugly in a blanket, and then carried him over to me. She held him close to my face so that I could see him properly. He was perfect; I truly thought that he was the most beautiful baby that I had ever seen. I was then told that it was time for me to go to recovery and that Nathan needed to be checked over by the paediatrician. As they wheeled me out of the theatre, I shouted back at Ross 'Do not let him out of your sight!'*

After a stint in recovery, I was wheeled up to the ward and as they pushed me along the corridor, I was wheeled straight past Ross who was sitting outside the nurses' station.

He was holding Nathan and there were tears streaming down his face. It was a magical moment for me.

Emelia's Wisdom	For me, birth wasn't something I could plan too much for. I think it is best to be open-minded about what might happen and to expect the unexpected. Also, there are so many people around to help—the obstetricians, midwives, **doulas**, your partner (if you have one) and family and friends—so use them while you have them!

What is pre-eclampsia?

Pre-eclampsia affects roughly 10 out of every 100 pregnancies. It is an illness that only occurs in pregnancy and can affect both the mother and her baby. It usually develops after 20 weeks (although developing the illness at such an early stage is considered rare) and is most common in first pregnancies.

In the mother, it can cause problems such as leakage of protein into the urine, high blood pressure, thinning of the blood and liver dysfunction. Because the illness is usually asymptomatic, it is essential that you have regular antenatal checks. Among other things, your health care provider will test your urine for protein levels and monitor your blood pressure for possible signs of pre-eclampsia.

If left untreated, pre-eclampsia can lead to very serious complications. Some of the advanced symptoms include severe swelling, bad headaches, vomiting and/or visual disturbances and/or abdominal pain just below the ribs. Try not to panic if you experience any of these symptoms but make sure you call your doctor or midwife immediately to rule out pre-eclampsia.

Pre-eclampsia cannot be predicted, but researchers point to several factors that may increase your chance of developing the illness. For example, if this is your first pregnancy, you are at higher risk. Additionally, if you have pre-existing high blood pressure, a family history of the condition or you are diabetic, your risk is increased (Bhattacharya et al. 2009; Hernández-Díaz et al. 2009).

Symptoms in the early stages of the illness can sometimes be controlled with certain medications but if the illness is advanced, the only cure is delivery of the baby (Haddad & Sibai 2009). If you have pre-eclampsia or want to find out more about the condition, please look up the support organisations on page 245 of the Resources section.

Emilia's story stresses the importance of seeing your health care provider regularly throughout your pregnancy. Most pregnancies and births are uncomplicated but it's best to make sure that you and your baby are doing well. If a complication is detected, it can usually be treated. While Emilia's delivery was radically different to what she had intended, she was fortunate enough to be living in a country where modern facilities were available and surgeons were on standby in the case of emergency. This is in stark contrast to developing countries, where maternal and infant mortality rates are much higher.

Sheer terror: When past trauma leads to a general anaesthetic

Zahra had her third baby under general anaesthesia. While epidurals are internationally recommended over general anaesthesia due to its higher risk, some women, like Zahra, are left with no other option.

Zahra's Story

*My first baby was delivered via caesarean section. At 38 weeks, I was leaking **amniotic fluid** and in light of my weight gain (I had put on 50 kilograms) and the fact that I was extremely tired, my very patient doctor decided that the best thing to do would be to induce me. After two days of **induction**, however, nothing happened. My baby went into distress and I ended up with an emergency caesarean.*

*I had really hoped to have a **VBAC** with my second daughter Keira. Little did I know how far from reality that would turn out to be. I bled intensely for the first three months[5] and was told to go home and wait to miscarry, as they couldn't find a heartbeat. At three months, they found a heartbeat but at no time did I ever think I would deliver a healthy baby. I'd previously had a miscarriage at three months due to a Down/Turner syndrome baby girl, for which we'd had **genetic counselling**. So I was pretty prepared for something to happen again.[6] I figured I was just lucky we had Tressa. Even at the end of my pregnancy with Keira, I still didn't think I'd have a live baby. But I did, even though her birth was one of the most traumatic experiences of my life. It was decided that I did in fact need another caesarean, so when the time came for my **epidural**, my anaesthetist turned up and that's when all the drama began. It took hours to get the epidural in. He poked and prodded; basically he tore my back open. My blood pressure dropped, everything was pretty awful and they wouldn't let Ron in to see me, so we were both panicking. After three very long and painful hours, he managed to get the needle in.*

The day after Keira was born, I had visitors from all over the hospital wanting to see what he'd done to my back—insurance people (apparently they thought I might seek legal action), psychiatrists, doctors, nurses—everyone! I looked like a victim of war crime and to be honest, I felt like a freak show.[7] Even the anaesthetist came to check on me. He blamed it on my weight, although my obstetrician disagreed. The anaesthetist was such an arsehole—I hated his attitude. He made it seem as though I was the reason he couldn't get

5 See 'Bleeding in pregnancy' on page 45
6 See 'How can the loss of a baby affect subsequent pregnancies and birthing decisions?' on page 42
7 See 'What are the risks and side effects of epidurals?' on page 65

it right—that it was my weight that was the issue. There are many, many people who are much bigger than I am who have had successful epidurals. And he had the hide to charge me for all of the three hours he fucked up.

Then I became pregnant with Shaun. Again, I was booked in for a caesarean—there was definitely no chance of a VBAC after two caesareans and a **low-lying placenta***. Also, Shaun was in a* **transverse** *position. Knowing that I needed a caesarean, I asked the obstetrician to ensure I had a different anaesthetist. I just couldn't bear the thought of having the whole thing happen again. He assured me he would book in another guy and the day before I went in, the office called me to confirm who was booked in for my birth.*

There have been a lot of twists and turns in all of my pregnancies and births but none so unforeseen as what happened on the day I gave birth to Shaun. Twenty months later, I was sitting in the theatre and in walks … the same anaesthetist. To this day, I have no idea what went wrong; why he turned up instead of the other person we had specifically booked. When I saw him, I froze. But then I gathered my wits enough to ask for the other anaesthetist.

When the new anaesthetist arrived, I just remember wanting so badly for everything to go according to plan. I desperately wanted a different experience. Then I started completely freaking out. I'm pretty sure that even Ron could hear my heart beating outside. I had a massive panic attack and I couldn't control my breathing. I remember trying to calm down but it wasn't working. I started crying, asking if it was going to work and getting very angry with everyone.

My obstetrician told me that he thought I should have my baby under a general anaesthetic given the circumstances. I can't remember his exact words but they were along the lines of 'We gave it a go, we've tried inserting the epidural, but it's not going to work out for you'. He's a great doctor. At that point, I just wanted it over. I just wanted Shaun out! So I agreed and the next thing I remember was waking up to the sounds of someone talking about Shaun and I figured that they must be talking about my baby because that's what I was going to call him. I was pretty out of it and it took them two hours to take me back to see him.

I had never seen a more beautiful creature (well, besides Tressa and Keira). And my recovery went really well—it felt no different to my previous two caesareans. And for that, I am grateful.

Zahra's Wisdom   I believe it doesn't matter how your children come into this world, as long as they come out screaming! You need to assert yourself and feel confident in your own decisions. Remember, you will never ever experience anything in your life that will even remotely resemble birth, so try to enjoy it, love it and remember it as long as you can. My last baby was born under general anaesthetic but in the end, that's not what's important. What is important is that he was healthy. And he was coming home with me.

Caesarean births: Requested

This topic may be one of the most hotly contested in the birthing community. If you look at birth on a spectrum, you would find a natural homebirth on one end and a requested caesarean on the other. While they may seem extremely different, there is a central similarity: choice. Both types of birth have been chosen by the mother. Just like their homebirthing sisters, women who choose to have a caesarean section without medical reason have made a conscious decision to do so.

There are a variety of reasons why women choose to have caesarean sections, ranging from fear of vaginal birth through to convenience or simply a preference for a controlled, medical environment.

Civilised and calm: Preferring a medical environment

Factors influencing Therese's decision to opt for a requested caesarean included fear of childbirth and having a strong background working in the medical field, thus making her feel more comfortable in a surgical setting. Therese thoroughly researched all of her options and, like many women who request caesareans, did not enter into the decision lightly.

Therese's Story

*I am terrified of vaginal births.[8] I remember coming home from an **antenatal** class once, crying, and feeling even more terrified and helpless than before. I had already seen several births, as I had worked in a maternity unit as a young nurse, and I had hated it and begged to leave.*

*In the years leading up to my pregnancy, I had severe **endometriosis**, which entailed pain to the extent of passing out. I had two very huge surgeries for that and I guess I was at a point in my life where I was just 'over' having pain. That was one of the reasons I elected to have a caesarean. I also chose it for convenience. My husband worked 40 minutes away and travelled to and from work by bus.*

The lead up to the big day was so exciting! I was not at all concerned about complications. I knew my doctor was an excellent surgeon. He came highly recommended and had a very good reputation. Driving in that day was terribly exciting and wonderful—I remember it like yesterday.

We got out of bed at a good hour, took some pictures of my belly, and drove into town. I felt I was almost in labour anyway (I had had diarrhoea and felt 'odd' for the past 24 hours). Anyway, we chatted as we drove in and I can remember saying to Michael 'I just know we

---

8 See 'Can fear affect childbirth?' on page 62

are going to have a blonde-haired, blue-eyed girl that looks just like you.' (I was absolutely correct about that!)

*We turned up and were taken to the **delivery suite**. They did the standard checklists, changed me into a gown and I went into the pre-op room. My obstetrician came in with the anaesthetist. I was worrying about how long the surgery would take, when the doctor said 'There's the head!' I hadn't even realised they'd started!*

I recall they sort of described what they were doing—'Just getting bub out now, you'll feel some tugging and pressing on your upper tummy which might be uncomfortable … but we'll be as quick as we can'—that sort of thing. Then they held her up.

They let me have a quick cuddle and then asked if they could check her. It was really only about a minute that she was out of sight, as she was perfectly fine. While they sewed me up, they brought her over to me and Michael and I held her easily. I remember thinking it took a while to sew me up, but I later found out that it was because my doctor saw some endometriosis that had been missed, so he cut it out for me. Saved me another surgery!

Overall, I felt the experience was just amazing, fantastic, relaxing, calm and 'civilised' for me. Mind you, I always knew that if I did have to give birth, by myself, on the side of the road, I could do it. I never doubted that my body would do what it needed to do if it needed to. I had gone to my local hospital midwife clinic, been assessed and had a chart created just in case I had to deliver there.

I think women have to think about all these sorts of things. Overall, it's about one's attitude to one's body and to risk. I felt that an uncomplicated surgery, in the best possible scenario (best surgeon, best team and best hospital) in a healthy woman, was low risk for me. There is no right or wrong—I am just very glad I had the choice.

Therese's Wisdom

Parenting is so much more than just the birth. I find that some women are the same with birthing as they are with the wedding. They focus so much on that one day and get it out of perspective in the context of a lifetime. I wonder if much of the angst felt by some women about their birth experience is simply because they built it up to be such a massive 'event' … what could live up to that sort of expectation? Some women seem to think their whole being is going to change after giving birth. Maybe it does for some. But for me—I'm the same person I was before—I just now have two kids to raise as well.

I knew my obstetrician; I trusted him and knew that he was experienced and very good at surgery. Another thing to consider is how many children you want. I knew I only wanted one to three (maximum). The stats I saw showed that most of the catastrophic issues with caesareans rise dramatically after three caesareans.

I think you do have to think a lot about how you will feel about not giving birth vaginally. I knew I might feel disappointed at not experiencing labour and I guess, from time to time, I still do. But for me, the pros outweighed the cons.

Does the number of caesareans you have increase your risk of danger?

The simple answer is 'yes'. The Royal Australian and New Zealand College of Obstetricians and Gynaecologists (2008) say that when weighing up the pros and cons of repeat caesarean sections, you need to be aware that the risk of scar rupture, placenta praevia and **placenta accreta** increases with each caesarean. They go on to state that women who are good candidates for requested caesareans are those who are older, and/or those planning only one child (or perhaps two). If you are a young person and are planning a large family, that advice is reversed.

If you are thinking of requesting a caesarean or you are considering one based on medical grounds, you are strongly encouraged to research all of your options. A good starting point for research is the Resources section at the end of this book. While caesareans are generally considered safe, they are (like any surgical procedure) not without risk. And as Therese pointed out, an important factor to think about is how many children you want to have, as well as how you might feel about not experiencing a vaginal birth.

Use the Resources, where you will find a list of support services and websites dedicated solely to caesarean births. Also, make sure you talk with your obstetrician about any concerns you may have; they will be able to assess your health and talk you through any risks that are involved in the procedure that relate specifically to you as an individual. Lastly, if you make a decision to have a caesarean birth and you have researched your options and spoken to professionals, be prepared to stand by your choice—because it is your choice and no one else's.

Partners' perspectives

It's easy to forget about the birthing woman's partner. After all, she is the one going through the process of labour and birth, and so all attention is focused on her. However, partners are just as involved in the process of birth. They witness their partner in labour, and they often act as a support person and advocate. But how the partner feels about the birthing process is often overlooked.

A frightened dad: Complications after delivery

Here, Matt tells of the birth of his first child and the intense fear and shock he felt when his wife had a **post-partum haemorrhage**. Left alone, literally holding the baby, Matt sobbed for the first time in 20 years.

Matt's Story

The majority of people that talked to me about childbirth before the birth of our first baby told us what a 'beautiful experience' it was. To me, the phrase 'beautiful experience' conjures up images such as a balloon ride at dawn over the Serengeti. Although I wouldn't describe it as a 'beautiful experience', the birth of our second child was not too bad. But the birth of our first had some complications.

Like many, my wife was unlucky enough to go into labour late one evening. We hadn't had much sleep the night before. This meant my wife was awake and labouring all night, rapidly running out of the physical energy to push and the emotional energy to cope with the pain. I managed to catch a guilty hour or so of sleep on a chair beside her hospital bed at some stage during the night.

The next day, our baby was born. Unfortunately, there were complications delivering the placenta—it wouldn't all come out, meaning the womb wouldn't contract and wouldn't stop bleeding. There are various things that can be tried for this. All of them seemed quite painful and none of them worked. Due to the blood loss, my wife's blood pressure was all over the place. At one stage, it was 40 over 20 [normal blood pressure is 120 over 80]. I noticed that although doctors and nurses kept reassuring us, there were some very worried looks passing between them.

My wife was very weak and almost delirious at this stage; certainly in no condition to care for the baby more than a quick hug. Eventually they carted my wife away for surgery under a general anaesthetic.

I spent a few anxious and exhausted hours in the delivery room, waiting for news of any sort. I was by myself, except for my new baby girl, who I was desperately trying to comfort. You can imagine what goes through your mind after seeing the anxious looks between doctors, seeing a blood pressure level that I didn't know was physically possible and not hearing anything.

At some stage during these hours, my brother-in-law popped in to visit the hospital. His first reaction was a smile for his new niece but his first question was to ask how his sister was. For the first time in about 20 years—the first time in my adult life—I broke down into a blubbering mess.

Eventually someone came to tell me that my wife was OK and led me to her. She was in bad shape, having had so little sleep, been through such an experience and lost so much blood. The first few weeks were a real struggle as she tried to recuperate while looking after what was a very 'high maintenance' baby.

In the end, there is nothing that we could have done differently and since we all came through the experience and our baby has grown in to a healthy, happy and loving little girl we are lucky.

Matt's Wisdom	For the birthing process, you have to be there. I think men have realised this and nowadays things are different to when we were born, when the men would wait at the pub with their mates for the news. It's not OK to sit out in the waiting room. If, God forbid, something awful happens, you're not going to want to live with yourself if you missed the whole thing because you were sitting in a room reading a *National Geographic* at the time. Your presence can help your partner and, considering what she has to go through, it's not too much to ask for the man to 'suck it up' and stick with her.

Expect the unexpected. Whether your expectations are forged through reading a million books or listening to a million people, however you imagine it's going to be, the chances are, it's not going to be that way. This doesn't just apply to your first child either—your first child will have forged an expectation that the second could be the same—it won't. If things don't match your expectations, don't despair—roll with it.

Speak up. While you should listen to the doctor, nurses and midwives, you should also stand up for yourselves so that you get what you want. Hospitals can be intimidating places and you might be tempted not to be 'rude' and not to ruffle feathers. Don't be. You'll probably never see these people again. Don't feel bad about ruffling someone's feathers by asking for a second pillow or whatever for the second time in five minutes. This is the time to stick up for your partner. If she wants something, or says something's not right, believe her and pester someone to do something until she's happy. She mightn't have the energy to do it herself.

What is a post-partum haemorrhage?

Post-partum haemorrhage (or PPH) is excessive bleeding after the birth of a baby. Primary PPH is when the blood loss occurs within 24 hours of delivery and secondary PPH occurs between 24 hours and six weeks after delivery. It is normal for blood loss to occur during childbirth (the 'average' amount is 350 mL). If blood loss exceeds 500 mL (1000 mL for caesareans), it is regarded as pathological and given the name 'post-partum haemorrhage'. The main reasons for excessive blood loss are: **uterine atony** (the inability of the uterus to contract after the placenta has been delivered), genital tract trauma (for example, tears or an episiotomy), retention of tissue (from the placenta, as in Matt's story) or the presence of a bleeding disorder.

While PPH may sound scary, the good news is that it is treatable. In fact, some women who are diagnosed with PPH don't need any treatment at all. All women are different and therefore some women can tolerate more blood loss than others without deleterious effects. However, if the blood loss is causing problems, there are several things doctors can do. You may be given medicine (to stimulate uterine contractions), your uterus may be massaged (again, to try and stimulate contractions), and/or genital tract injuries may be repaired. If the haemorrhage is more serious, a blood transfusion and/or surgery may be required. The emergency bell might be called and many people may come into the delivery room to help, which can feel quite overwhelming and scary. The midwife or doctor will try to deliver the placenta if it is not out.

Again, it is very important to remember that PPH is treatable. If you are concerned about PPH, you should talk to your health care provider. In some instances (particularly where there is a history of PPH), you may be given preventive treatment during the third stage of your labour. For more information on PPH, talk to your doctor or look up page 248 of the Resources section.

A walk in the park? Born breech in the hallway

Alex knew that his wife Clara was probably in labour, as she was experiencing light contractions. Although he wanted to go to hospital, the midwives had advised Clara to stay at home for as long as possible, so instead they went for a stroll around their local park. Soon afterwards, Clara delivered her baby on their front porch, with the assistance of the paramedics, a neighbour and one very freaked out husband.

Alex's Story

The day my wife, Clara, gave birth to our second child was a Monday, which of course is a work day. She had felt light contractions the previous night and we decided it would be OK for me to go into work, so off I went. I kept in touch with her throughout the whole morning. People were telling me I was crazy and that I should go home but Clara kept on reassuring me that everything was fine. But by about 1 pm, I knew from what she was telling me that the contractions were coming closer together and I just couldn't bear to be at work any longer.

I got home about one hour later. She'd been in touch with the midwives and they told her to stay home as long as possible. She was being a cool cucumber and suggested we go for a walk. So we went for a walk around the local football oval and by this stage, the contractions were about four minutes apart. I can still picture her hunching over trying to handle each contraction. It was just crazy.

By the time we got home, the contractions were still about four minutes apart. I encouraged Clara to think about going to the hospital but she wanted to wait a while, as the midwife had said to her 'No point coming in and sitting around waiting'. Silly twit of a midwife.

Clara finally decided to leave for the hospital when the contractions were about two minutes apart, when she suddenly ran to the toilet, saying 'I have to poo!' That's when I knew we were in trouble. Her **mucous plug** had come away, she had to poo and, quite frankly, so did I!

She asked me to turn the shower on for pain relief. So I helped her in, ran down to the car and left it running in the middle of the road while I ran back up to get her. I must have been in a state of denial, thinking we could make it to the hospital in time. I think she was as well—when you're in severe pain and looking for relief, you don't tend to think straight, especially when you're in a situation as strange as that. Looking back on it now, I think we both realised we'd left it too late.

Luckily for us, we live next door to a nurse who had heard Clara screaming and knew exactly what was going on, so she raced over and got to her at the same time as I did. Thank God she did, because just as we got to her, the baby was crowning. I was completely freaking out but our neighbour was such a calming influence. She called the ambulance crew who arrived within about five minutes. When they arrived, they first tried to carry Clara outside but realised it was too late. So we placed her on the floor near the front door. It was the tiniest space you can imagine! There was me, Clara, our neighbour and the two ambos, plus all our shoes and the cat!

Clara was on her back with our neighbour cradling her head. One of the ambos was ready to catch and I was freaking out. Clara started to push and the baby started coming out. I remember turning to him and saying 'What's wrong with its head?' At which point, as he had a better view, he yelled at his colleague 'Shit, it's a breech. Call for backup!' The other ambo was running around trying to call base but there was no reception. It was too late for help anyway.

So Clara gave an almighty push and our daughter was coming out bum first, as if she was touching her toes, with her back up against Clara's stomach. But she stopped halfway—her bum and a bit of her back and legs were out and the rest was still in. I thought Clara was going to split in half. I didn't know that the circumference at this point was still smaller than the head. The next contraction came and the baby's legs flopped out, but her head was still in. Me and the main ambo were freaking out and I was yelling 'Pull it out, it's stuck!' Thank God he didn't because with the next contraction, her head popped out. In the end, it turned out to be a textbook breech labour and birth.

Obviously, I was completely relieved that everyone was OK but I do remember feeling a lot of anger towards Clara. Maybe it was a natural reaction when placed in a life and death situation. I was shitty at her for putting us in this situation and I really felt we should have gone to the hospital as soon as I came home—it would have saved all of this from happening.

I was quite frightened when it was all happening but I could see that Clara was OK. My biggest fear was due to the fact that our baby was breech and was being delivered by two ambos who had not delivered a baby before—let alone a breech. Most doctors aren't even trained for that.

After the delivery, we were bundled into the ambulance and they injected Clara with **oxytocin** to help the placenta come out. Clara reckoned the pain of delivering that was almost as bad as the birth itself.

Actually, the story became a bit legendary because friends who birthed at the same hospital a few weeks later were told our story by the midwives!

Alex's Wisdom

It takes a while to fall in love with your kids; really in love. So many people say 'Oh my God, I loved it from the first moment' but I think everyone's different.

The midwives and obstetricians tell you to stay away from the hospital until the contractions are thick and fast. I guess most people have a low pain threshold but not my wife ... that's how she tolerates me! I guess partners have to ask themselves this question: 'Would you prefer to sit around bored in a hospital with all the amenities at your disposal or take a punt and wait till the last minute at home?' Sometimes it's different for subsequent births because they have a tendency to come out quicker, but still, I think I'd rather hang about at the hospital!

Birth and recovery: Tips and tricks from those in the know

- I recommend bringing a bag of jelly beans—they were great for throwing in my mouth between contractions for a bit of extra energy, plus the midwives enjoyed eating them too!

- I got out of bed as soon as I could. I had a caesarean birth and asked the nurses to help me shower 18 hours after my operation and I took a shuffle around the ward afterwards. Not only did it help me to get back on my feet psychologically, it also helped to disperse the fluid I had retained.

- Keep mobile, keep hydrated and keep focused.

- Stress balls were my best friend in labour.

- I had a caesarean birth and I found that the waist of my trousers irritated my wound, so I simply put on a 'bump band' underneath.

- If you have back pains with your contractions, have someone put pressure on the pain site with their hands—kind of like CPR for your back.

- It helped me to remember that the pain was purposeful, to try to re-frame it more positively and to remember that each contraction does end. Oh and breathe, breathe, breathe!

- Drink Ural in labour—it takes all the acid out of your urine so that your first pee doesn't hurt so bad.

- If you ever have to go through something traumatic with your pregnancy or birth, it may well be helpful to seek out a professional to chat to, even if it's your midwife or health nurse; it may help sort out things in your mind and hopefully help to ease some of the emotional trauma.

- Go with the flow. Your body is in control and knows what to do, so go with it. Maintain a focus on the goal, which is to have a healthy baby and mum, and all the rest will fall into place.

- I found that music really helped me. I knew I was going to have as many drugs as possible but I was still frightened of giving birth. I borrowed my husband's iPod and created a playlist of all my favourite songs. They were all upbeat songs— songs that I would normally have listened to pre-children to get ready for a party. I found them brilliantly distracting. I could almost pretend it wasn't happening— almost!

- Be calm. Remember the pain won't last forever. It is just one day of your life.

CHAPTER FOUR

Babies

'If your baby is beautiful and perfect, never cries or fusses, sleeps on schedule and burps on demand, an angel all the time, you're the grandma.'

Theresa Bloomingdale (Kids 2008)

There is no doubt that parenthood is one of the toughest jobs in the world. While conception and pregnancy can be difficult and laden with emotion, bringing home a new baby can be one of the most overwhelming experiences of your life. For starters, this tiny being has taken nine months to create (on average) and in many cases, has been longed for and dreamt about for much longer. So when your baby eventually arrives, the moment can seem surreal, beautiful, scary, perfect and anxiety-laden all at once. Especially as babies, as the saying goes, don't come with instruction manuals. You are now on your own; to ensure that this baby not only survives but also thrives.

Parenting is an area of intense scrutiny, particularly when new babies are involved. How babies are fed, how they sleep and how parents cope with the challenges inherent in these issues have become matters for public consumption and dissection, parental debate and academic scrutiny.

This chapter focuses on families' experiences of feeding, sleeping and coping with a new baby. The first stories that follow talk about breastfeeding and bottle-feeding and the judgement that many parents can face regardless of which method they use to feed their baby. It is apparent that women are experiencing heightening pressure to breastfeed, and often end up feeling like failures if this method of feeding is unsuccessful for them. Many women also feel judgement when they cease breastfeeding, or choose not to breastfeed from the outset.

Judgement is also cast upon parents when deciding how to help their babies sleep. Whichever method the parents who tell their stories here chose to use, they felt judged because of it. It is significant, however, that although they were judged by others for using different sleeping techniques with their babies, the parents who used them were all happy with the choices they made for their family. Perhaps this illustrates that so long as your baby is brought up in a loving and stimulating environment, one in which your baby feels safe and cared for, it doesn't really matter what method you choose to help your baby to sleep.

In this chapter, we also look at coping—without support, with sleep deprivation and with babies who are sick or premature. These stories are included to show you some of the issues that may arise when you bring your baby home and how you might deal with them, should they happen to you.

A note on **controlled crying**: This term is used interchangeably throughout the literature (and the stories in this chapter) with **comfort settling** and teaching to sleep. While I have not changed the terminology in the stories, I have used the term comfort settling throughout my commentary and within the information boxes to avoid confusion.

Feeding: Breast and bottle

In recent years, there has been an increasing international push for breastfeeding due to an ever-expanding research base providing evidence that breast milk is superior to formula; as a consequence, breastfeeding is on the increase in many OECD countries. However, many women still choose to bottle-feed and many women begin breastfeeding and cease due to a vast array of problems.

The stories that follow are from women who had very positive experiences of breastfeeding, and also from some who experienced great difficulties with breastfeeding, resulting in feelings of desperation and grief. You will also hear from a woman who chose from the outset to formula-feed and the judgement she felt because of this decision.

Breastfeeding success: A premature baby thrives on expressed milk

Cathie's story of breastfeeding is a positive one. Although her son was born prematurely under general anaesthetic, Cathie was able to express her milk and went on to have a hugely satisfying experience for over two years. This she attributes to her 'stubborn' persistence and the wonderful support she received both from her workplace and from her family, who respected her choice to feed her son exclusively on breast milk.

Cathie's Story

*My son was born after a difficult pregnancy, via an emergency caesarean under general anaesthetic. The first time I saw him, he was in a **humidicrib** and I was drugged out of my mind. The next couple of days were (and still are) hazy, so I only have snapshots of memories. I remember the paediatrician asking if there were any allergies in the family and wanting to use soy formula. I told him 'no', I was breastfeeding. I remember the really empty feeling of waking up and not having my baby with me—I was no longer pregnant and he was in the special care nursery. However, I do have a really strong memory of the first time I breastfed him. It was more than 24 hours after he was born that we breastfed for the first time, as he had been on a drip after the delivery.*

The nurse said that because he was premature, he might be too small and weak to breastfeed. Someone obviously forgot to tell John that. He knew exactly what to do. I remember seeing his little head suckling, and thinking 'Wow, his head is smaller than my breast—he must be tiny, because my breasts are not all that big!' That was the moment I fell completely and utterly in love with him.

*John did tire easily, so it was decided to alternate a breastfeed with a tube feed. I was determined that he would only have breast milk, so I asked a midwife if I could express for him. She had some doubts, because she didn't think my milk had yet come in, but after a quick go at hand expressing, she got me an electric pump. I had plenty of **colostrum**. Once my milk came in properly, I had loads of it. My only regret is that there were no facilities for me to donate my milk to other babies whose mothers couldn't feed them— I had more than enough to go around.*

John came home after a week because he had put on so much weight during his first week. He absolutely thrived on breast milk. We followed a feed-on-demand routine. John wanted to feed every three hours, for about one hour each time. Although this was draining, I knew he was just trying to gain the weight he didn't have at birth, so we persisted. I knew the most important job in the world was nurturing this precious baby and I felt breastfeeding was the best way to do it.

John and I both loved breastfeeding from the first moment—we fed whenever and wherever. I went back to work part-time when John was eight months old and made the decision to express milk. My workplace was very supportive and I had two 'lactation' breaks a day to express. Initially, the main problem was that John refused to take a bottle, so for the first two weeks he starved all day, then fed all night to make up for it. Pretty exhausting! I persisted, probably because I am really stubborn, and eventually he took the expressed milk from a bottle. I am so thankful that my father-in-law, who was minding John, was incredibly patient and respected my wishes to breastfeed.

We breastfed until John was just over two years old and stopped then because I was pregnant and didn't want him to think the new baby was 'stealing' his milk. He actually gave up quite happily, which I was surprised (and a bit sad) about.

Cathie's Wisdom   My main advice is to do what works for you and your family—if you want to breastfeed until your child is two, don't let other people tell you that is wrong. Likewise, if you want to sleep with your baby in your bed for more convenient feeding, that is OK too—as long as it works for you, your partner and your baby. Just make sure you know what the guidelines are for **co-sleeping**, so that you are all safe and happy.[9]

What are breastfeeding rates in developed countries?

Breastfeeding rates vary greatly from country to country. In under-developed countries, breastfeeding rates are, in general, consistently higher than those of their developed counterparts.

One paper (Cattaneo et al. 2005) attempts to unravel the reasons behind the consistently lower rates of breastfeeding in Europe and why they do not meet the international standards set by the World Health Organization's (2003) *Global Strategy on Infant and Young Child Feeding*. The findings suggest that health care professionals' pre-service training on breastfeeding is inadequate and in-service training achieves only low to minimum coverage. Additionally, the **Baby-Friendly Hospital Initiative (BFHI)** is well developed in only three countries. While legislation for working mothers meets, on average, the International Labour Organization's (2005) standards, it covers women under full employment only. Other factors include a lack of volunteer mother-to-mother support groups and a lack of trained peer counsellors. While Norway seems to be the 'holy grail' of breastfeeding, with initial rates at 99 per cent and a six month (non-exclusive) rate of 80 per cent, Cattaneo et al. point out that even Norway's exclusive breastfeeding rates are substandard at six months.

So how does the rest of the world compare? This is difficult to answer accurately, as there is no standard methodology in place for data collection. However, we can approximate that 73.9 per cent of babies born in the United States are breastfed at some point but that rate drops to 13.6 per cent at six months. Canada's initial breastfeeding rate is 87 per cent (comparable to Australia's at 83 per cent), however this rate drops to 14.2 per cent at six months, compared with Australia's six-month rate of 48 per cent. It should be strongly noted that these rates are calculated

9   See 'Co-sleeping safely' on page 124

differently (some countries use 'ever breastfed', some use 'exclusively breastfed', and some 'initially breastfed'). Clearly, a standardised methodology for data collection needs to be devised and implemented on an international level if we are to gain an accurate insight into the real breastfeeding rates around the world.

No support in sight: The grief of discontinuing breastfeeding

The beginning of Aisha's breastfeeding relationship was a good one, however, when Aisha moved countries, things took a turn for the worse.

Aisha's Story

Let me start by saying that before pregnancy, I thought the idea of breastfeeding was pretty weird. I could not imagine how having a baby sucking on my nipple would feel or that I would think it normal—it seemed somehow so raw and animalistic. But when I got pregnant, suddenly I realised: these boobs must be for the baby; I mean, they're enormous and I certainly don't need them to be that way! So there was never any question that I would breastfeed. None. Of course I would.

When Joshua was born, they put him to my breast immediately, but I had a caesarean so there was not much room to feed and it was more of a token gesture than anything else. I felt kind of spaced-out at the time, so I don't even really remember it.

When I got back from recovery, though, it was a different experience. My husband was sitting in an armchair in my room, holding Joshua, who had his whole fist in his mouth and was sucking furiously. He knew exactly what he wanted and where he wanted to get it from! It felt very normal to offer him my breast and he was very good at latching on and was sucking almost straightaway. I did get very sore nipples and my milk took a long time to come in, which was a source of much stress to me at the time but we went home as planned on day five and everything was fine. I had seen a lactation consultant who was helpful and the midwives were also great, so we were off to a flying start.

*When Joshua was five weeks old, we moved to the United Kingdom, due to my husband's work. That was tough, but breastfeeding went well for the first four months at least. Then I started to have a problem. My **let-down reflex** inexplicably became very slow at times. Joshua began to get frustrated and would pull off and scream. This made me tense up and thus began the downward spiral that eventually saw me finish breastfeeding him at five months of age; much sooner than I wanted.*

I believe I was definitely affected by a lack of resources in Scotland—there was no such thing as a lactation consultant and the only helpline I could find was constantly engaged. I tried to increase my milk supply by taking brewer's yeast and all kinds of herbs. I tried warm baths and compresses, expressing, relaxing (not so easy when all you can think to yourself is 'Relax, damn it, relax!') and everything else that I could find on the internet. I posted pleas for help on pregnancy website boards but to no avail. I could not cope with Joshua's impatience and it was easier to satisfy him with a bottle of whatever was available—at first expressed breast milk and later, formula—than to listen to him wail with frustration. Sometimes preparing a bottle would mean that my milk would let down normally and it would not be necessary but as my milk failed to flow, so did my supply begin to fail.

Initially, I was devastated when it became apparent that Joshua much preferred the ease of a bottle to the unpredictability of my breast. I felt that since I was now not working, my main job in life was to nurture my son and that not breastfeeding meant I was failing at this task.[10] It took a lot of agonising and obsessing until I was comfortable with what happened. I even tried to call my Australian lactation consultant but couldn't get through. My online friends were supportive and it did help that at least two of them also had to stop before they were ready (due to various personal and medical issues) but it was so hard.

Aisha's Wisdom	Breastfeeding is one of the most emotion-laden experiences you can ever have as a woman and everyone has an opinion on what you should do but you can only do your best. The grief over having to stop breastfeeding Joshua prematurely was something that stayed with me for a long time. It was only really soothed by the successful and longer breastfeeding relationship I subsequently had with my daughter, who never took a bottle and was patient enough to weather the slow let-down, which happened again but was overcome with our persistence.

However, I think through my experience with Joshua I learned that a mother nurtures, loves and provides for her baby no matter how she feeds it, whether breast or bottle or whatever. Joshua is a well-adjusted, strong and happy little boy, and no one would ever know that he was only breastfed for five months. |

How to find breastfeeding support

If you plan to breastfeed your baby, the best time to learn about it and seek support is before your baby is born. This way, you can take your time; it is a much different game trying to come to grips with breastfeeding when your baby is howling at three in the morning and you are tired and desperate for help but don't know where to start looking.

The first place to try is the hospital in which you intend to give birth. Many hospitals run antenatal classes that include a discussion on breastfeeding but often this is not enough. You might like to find out if your hospital has dedicated lactation consultants who are available for consultation before your baby is born. This way, if you have difficulties feeding your baby when he or she arrives, you have already established a relationship with a health professional that can provide you with support and assistance.

---

10 See 'Breastfeeding is "natural", so it must always be easy, right?' on page 102

If you don't intend to birth in a hospital, you can always consider hiring a lactation consultant privately. Alternatively, your attending midwife can provide much support and advice throughout your pregnancy, as well as a list of resources. Remember, midwives don't just 'catch the baby'—they are responsible for prenatal and post-partum care (up until six weeks after birth).

However, midwives and lactation consultants are not your only options. Many countries have national help lines, as well as online support. There are also some excellent websites containing helpful information, as well as online communities where you can chat to other mums in similar situations. For a full list of helpful organisations and resources, please see page 250 of the Resources section.

Lastly, never underestimate the power of your local network. Find out who runs your local breastfeeding support branch, join local mothers' groups and even playgroups. You never know who you will meet; many people go through similar experiences and may have found a solution that might just work for you.

Discharged too early? Failure to latch causes thoughts of failure

Cassie never gave breastfeeding a second thought; it was, for her, the only path to take. However, when Cassie faced difficulties with breastfeeding, she was also met with a lack of external support in her US home town.

Cassie's Story

I knew without a doubt that I wanted to breastfeed my baby. I never gave it a second thought. I wanted to breastfeed because it can provide a wonderful bonding experience between mom and baby and it provides perfect, natural and free nutrition for baby. So, I did everything I thought I was supposed to do to prepare for breastfeeding. I read the books, I attended the classes. I even listened to the difficulties that my best friend was having breastfeeding her newborn. I was six months pregnant at the time. But, as I did all this, I was thinking to myself 'How hard can this be? Animals in nature don't do all this preparation and they still manage to feed their babies without difficulty the vast majority of the time.' Well, my breastfeeding experience went nothing like I had envisioned.

I went into labor at 39 weeks and 5 days. When my daughter was born, she was placed on my chest. My daughter then began to scream, and she screamed solidly for four hours. I tried to put her to the breast repeatedly but there was no soothing her. Eventually, she calmed down and slept for several hours. When she woke, the first couple of times she was put to my breast, she latched on, which was a huge relief.

It was not until the second day that we experienced problems. That day, she just could not seem to latch on correctly. The nurses were wonderful and spent hours at a time trying to assist us. Finally, we called in the hospital lactation consultant. She was unable to get her to latch on either. So her suggestion was to express, since it had been 18 hours since my daughter had successfully nursed. I felt in my gut that this was not the right thing to do but this was my first baby and I was not confident in my abilities to mother at this time, so I did as she suggested. I pumped and fed the breast milk to her in a bottle. Supply was not an issue; I pumped more than she could drink.

Each time I tried to feed her, I would attempt to get her to latch on without success. I was encouraged to keep trying; told that she would eventually get the hang of nursing. We were discharged from the hospital on the third day. At this point, we still had not managed a successful latch since day one. This was over a weekend, so there was no lactation support in the hospital. I was not given any advice about who to contact if the breastfeeding did not get any easier in the next couple of days.[11]

Once we got home, things did not improve. I sat up in bed all night long and attempted to get her to latch on. I was desperate for this to work. I re-read all my books and tried all the suggestions they had to offer. I cried for hours on end because I could not do what should have been 'natural' for a mom and baby. I just could not understand why she couldn't latch on. I was frustrated, sleep deprived, feeling like a failure and in major pain from cracked, split nipples. It was a rough 48 hours.

On our third day home from the hospital, my husband told me that it was not so much what we fed our baby that mattered but that she was fed and loved. He was supportive of my decision either way. He pointed out that we were both formula babies and had turned out happy and healthy. So, I made the decision to give up my attempts at breastfeeding.

I did pump breast milk; my daughter was exclusively fed breast milk for eight weeks. This was a struggle also. I felt like I was totally chained to my breast pump. I pumped every two hours during the day and every four hours at night. Outings took some major planning around my pumping sessions. But at least I felt like I was feeding my baby breast milk.

My family lived an hour away at the time of my daughter's birth. I had no close friends nearby who had small children or who had breastfed. I felt alone in my struggles. My best friend eventually ended up with a successful breastfeeding relationship, however, she was two hours away. My husband was as supportive as he could be but knew nothing about breastfeeding. I really wish that I was given information at the hospital about who to contact for help. I didn't know at the time that there was help out there, so I didn't know to ask for it.

Cassie's Wisdom

Would having had access to external help have changed things? I will never know. I later found out that my daughter has a very tight upper **frenulum**, so she may not have been able to position her lips to get a good latch. With my second child, I was told that I have flat nipples and should have been wearing a nipple shield in order to correct this. But, I do know one thing: I did bond with my daughter, even though she was fed from a bottle and not the breast.[12] I always snuggled close to her and talked to her while she drank. So I have to agree with my husband: it is not so much what the baby is fed but that they are fed and loved

---

11 See 'How to find breastfeeding support' on page 99
12 See 'Breastfeeding, formula-feeding and bonding' on page 105

completely. If you are not successful at your attempts to breastfeed, you can still have that strong, loving bond with your baby.

Breastfeeding is 'natural', so it must always be easy, right?

As noted by McCarter-Spaulding (2008):

> Breastfeeding ... is an interaction between a mother and an infant, which at its most basic physiological level is a form of providing nourishment to the infant. If breastfeeding were only that simple however, there would be no need for the plethora of lay and professional literature available to provide guidance and instruction to women who are breastfeeding and to the people who are responsible for supporting them. (p. 206)

Many studies have concluded that the provision of information, education and support to women who choose to breastfeed improves women's ability to establish and maintain breastfeeding. This evidence is counter-intuitive to the notion that because breastfeeding is 'natural', it is therefore easy.

It is certainly clear that 'breast is best', due to the unique qualities in human breast milk. For example, there is evidence that breastfeeding protects babies from all kinds of maladies, ranging from eczema to **SIDS**, as well as providing 'buffers' against breast and ovarian cancers in breastfeeding mothers. However, while many mothers initiate breastfeeding (see 'What are breastfeeding rates in developed countries?' on page 97), many also end up weaning due to a number of factors. Some of these are physical (e.g. breast refusal, poor milk supply, breast and nipple pain), obstetric-related (e.g. caesarean births, premature infants), postnatal experience (e.g. conflicting advice), poor support and/or return to work.

As Crossley (2009) points out, the strong rhetoric of 'the natural' that surrounds childbirth and breastfeeding practices can lead to women feeling as though they have somehow 'failed' as mothers when breastfeeding is not successful for them. Wilkinson and Scherl (2006) examined studies in which mothers expressed feelings of disappointment, guilt and failure, and that

> they were ... 'bad mother[s]' when they weaned the[ir] baby from the breast to the bottle. They were ashamed of their weaning and actively hid their change to formula from friends and professionals in their community. (p. 6)

If you are one of the many women who have difficulties establishing and/or maintaining a breastfeeding relationship with your baby, don't despair: you are not a failure as a mother and you certainly should not feel ashamed. You are not alone. Breastfeeding, for many, is a learned experience and one that is not always successful. For more information on seeking out support, see 'How to find breastfeeding support' on page 99.

Sticking to her guns: Formula-feeding by choice

Mothers may choose to formula-feed for many different reasons, ranging from medical issues to personal preference. Devyn is one of the 13 per cent of new Canadian mothers who choose not to breastfeed.

Devyn's Story

Throughout my long and difficult pregnancy with my daughter, the thought of how I was going to feed her never really crossed my mind, to be quite honest. I knew breastfeeding was not for me, and that was all. There was no dwelling, no weighing the pros and cons, no spending countless hours researching and trying to make a decision … it was just like common sense for me: I was going to bottle-feed.

When my daughter was born, once again, I felt no stress about it at all. I had a caesarean and saw the most perfect pink bundle wrapped up before me—she seemed too perfect to be real. I reached out and touched her petal soft skin; it was like silk. As with all caesarean babies, they needed to take her away for a bit and monitor her as I was being taken care of. We were to meet again in the recovery room when she was ready.

Immediately upon being reunited with my perfect angel baby, my nurse moved my blanket, lifted up my gown and literally grabbed my breast. She squeezed it so hard and shoved it into my daughter's mouth before I could even gather my thoughts. I could not believe it. All I remember was lying there in awe, my husband by my side looking equally as shocked and watching what seemed like someone else taking control of my body, my private and sacred body part, and manipulating it like it was putty. Then I saw my daughter's perfect little face pushed into my breast so hard as her mouth started sucking away. Ouch! I was in agony! And hey, drugs or no drugs, I was starting to get my bearings and was realizing that this was not what I wanted to do.

After about five face plants to my breast, our new family went into our private room. There were nurses all around trying to get me comfortable, reassuring me like they do every new mom I am sure, and once I was settled into my bed, we noticed my daughter seemed to be fussing. Once again, she was seized and before I knew it, my gown was pulled up and the same thing was done. Why were they doing this? Is this what they do to all new moms? And why wasn't I saying anything? The nurses were making me contort my body to try and get my breast properly in my daughter's mouth, putting pressure on my newly stitched up incision from the c-section when I finally regained control. 'Nurse,' I began, 'please get me a bottle!' The nurse looked stunned, like I had just done something unfathomable. I repeated myself: 'Nurse … get me a bottle … please.' All she said was 'Are you sure?'

The rest of our hospital stay was filled with visitors coming to see us and quite a bit of flak coming from my mother about why I was not even trying to breastfeed. I didn't get it. What was the big deal? I didn't want to, this was my child, end of story. Once again, I did not make a big deal about it. I was in love with my baby girl, in complete awe of this perfection that we made, and that I had carried for nine long months. I didn't want to focus on what other people wanted of me. I was happy with my choice and people would just have to deal with it. Little did I know, I was in for a very big surprise.

When I got out into the mom world, my feelings, emotions, personal beliefs, everything went out the window. I am a very confident person by nature and a very opinionated person as well but the kind of treatment I had got for—gasp—choosing to formula-feed, shook me to the core. I loved my daughter more than anything and here I was, thinking that as long as I was feeding her, that was enough. But suddenly it wasn't … it really wasn't at all. I wasn't doing a good job. I was failing somehow because she was not receiving breast milk, not being protected by my antibodies, not being given the perfect food made for human babies. Everyone who I met questioned, badgered and belittled me in some way for choosing to formula-feed my daughter. How could I be so selfish? Why didn't I at least try? This happened so much that when my daughter was two months old, I panicked. I contacted a lactation consultant and considered a process called re-lactation, which is the rebuilding of one's milk supply weeks or even months after lactation has stopped.

As my daughter got older, I began to meet other formula-feeding moms who supported and encouraged me.[13] It was a breath of fresh air, a feeling of not being alone, or being a bad mom, or like I did not measure up. I also did my research on both sides of the fence. I began to regain my confidence and realize that the decision I had made, to formula-feed my daughter, was a wonderful one for us. My daughter was thriving, our bond was everlasting and had nothing to do with me breastfeeding her or not. I knew I did the best thing for my daughter and our family. My daughter is healthy, my daughter is smart and my daughter is the reason I breathe. Formula-feeding was the best choice for us and one I do not regret. I have living proof that I don't need to anymore.

Devyn's Wisdom

If I had one wish for all moms and moms-to-be who choose to formula-feed (or had to formula-feed), it would be to stop feeling bad. It's not worth the struggle or the personal torment when formula-fed babies can be just as healthy and, most importantly, just as loved as their breastfed counterparts. Formula-feeding can promote wonderful bonding and is a wonderful option for women to turn to whatever the reason. It's time we focus our time and energy elsewhere and be confident in our decisions. I'm sure our kids will thank us.

---

13 For a list of formula-feeding support organisations and websites, see page 250 of the Resources section

Breastfeeding, formula-feeding and bonding

There have been some studies to suggest that while breastfeeding is wonderful for bonding, bottle-feeding can be equally so. For example, a study conducted by Britton et al. (2006) concluded that it was the quality of the mother–baby bond at six months, rather than the type of feeding (that is, breast or bottle), that predicted stronger attachment (see also Wilkinson & Scherl 2006).

It is important to remember that bonding with your baby is facilitated by many factors, not just by feeding. Singing to your baby, cuddling your baby often (skin-to-skin contact is great for bonding), wearing your baby, laughing with your baby, bath time and baby massage all contribute to secure attachment. Think about it this way: if breastfeeding were the only way to bond with your baby, how would fathers be able to bond?

You can ensure that your baby feels secure when feeding from a bottle, just as you would do if you were breastfeeding, by holding your baby snugly in your arms and looking into their eyes. Your baby will feel safe and comforted and this will likely be a wonderful time of bonding for both of you.

If you have chosen to formula-feed, you may like to seek advice and support. Look up page 250 of the Resources section. If you don't have a support group nearby, you can try online forums or you could even try starting up a support group in your area (see Appendix B: How to start a support group, on page 225 for further information).

Sleeping and settling

There is a plethora of books and resources online and in bookshops on getting babies to sleep. According to Balter (2000), parents lose around 350 hours of sleep in baby's first year. It is little wonder, then, that there is so much information available on how to get more sleep, for both you and your baby. The stories that follow come from parents who have tried varying techniques with varying success, from comfort settling to co-sleeping.

Jumping for joey: When 'kangaroo nursing' brings joy to both mum and baby

Cho read all about settling crying babies while pregnant with her first baby and immediately warmed to the 'kangaroo nursing' method, a term used by her paediatrician for constant holding, soothing and comforting of newborns.

Cho's Story

When I was pregnant with my first baby, I was extremely fortunate to stumble across a wonderful book about settling crying babies. I honestly had no idea what to expect and since I did not attend antenatal classes (waste of time when you know you have no option other than a caesarean delivery) I certainly didn't learn anything there. I had of course heard some horror stories about baby behaviour—mainly from my mother, because she did not know she was having twins (my brother and me) until she was in the delivery room, so I think the shock of suddenly having two babies instead of one made the whole of our infancy a kind of horror movie for her.

The book taught me some very valuable lessons. It talked about crying as occurring on a spectrum, with **colic** at one extreme and normal baby 'fussiness' at the other; the lesson being that all babies fuss and cry and that it is normal for them to do this, even to the point of being inconsolable, especially in the first 12 weeks of life. These weeks are, according to this book, like 'the missing fourth trimester', when it is theorised that babies want to be back in the snug warm environment of the womb. So, the settling techniques this book teach are centred around re-creating that environment: swaddling, rocking, patting, 'shushing', offering things to suck on and generally the things that we all naturally do with babies, but doing them simultaneously and in a certain way.

As a result, I felt that while I was heading into very unfamiliar territory in becoming a mother, at least I had a few tricks up my sleeve to deal with whatever I might find there. I had also read about **controlled crying** and regarded it as a kind of magic silver bullet, to be used when all else had failed. It would supposedly work reasonably quickly. I had not thought about how it would feel to listen to hours of crying.

Unfortunately, I quickly discovered that I absolutely could not bear to hear my little son cry. The look of bewildered grief on his face as he would lie in his cot, crying for me to come to him, was enough for me to resolve never to leave him to cry it out.[14] Believe me, at times during the seven months that he was waking at night, I was sorely tempted to let him just cry! But I never did.

My baby was very unsettled in the early weeks of his life and I spent a lot of time holding him, patting his bum, walking with him in the sling—whatever worked. I remember staggering along the boardwalk at the beach near my mother's house one evening at about 9 pm, horribly sleep deprived, just willing him to finally conk out and let me go home to sleep! I did **co-sleep** with him and had to deal with some negative comments from people about this—I dealt with them mainly by ignoring them—but I never felt pressured not to comfort him as much as he needed. The paediatrician who saw my baby and me in hospital was very much in favour of kangaroo nursing, his term for constant holding, soothing and comforting of newborns. I found that a good match for my own situation.

Cho's Wisdom	There are so many schools of thought as to what you should and shouldn't do to settle a crying baby—let them cry, don't let them cry, pick them up, don't pick them up, sleep with them, don't sleep with them … it goes on forever. I realised that I could only follow my own

---

14 See 'What is comfort settling?' on page 112

instincts and ignore all the other advice that didn't fit with what I felt was right for me and my baby.

There are two other things I would tell all new parents to remember. Firstly, if your baby cries and you cannot make them stop, it's OK.[15] They are safe and cared for, and you are doing your best. Secondly, there is light at the end of the tunnel! When you make it to the end of the 'fourth' trimester, things will get a lot better. Which is always a good thing to remind yourself of when it feels like they have been screaming forever.

Commonly used methods for helping your baby to sleep

There are many techniques used by practitioners and parents alike to help their infants and babies to sleep. Comfort settling is discussed in 'What is comfort settling?' on page 112.

You might like to settle your baby in your arms until they fall asleep and then put them in their cot. This can be useful when your baby is very young. As your baby gets older, however, this might become more difficult because your baby will be bigger and therefore heavier.

'**Hands-on settling**' is commonly used for babies under six months. This is where you put your baby into their cot and stay with them. You can gently 'pat' your baby, rock the cot (if possible), stroke your baby and try using 'ssshhh' sounds. Not all babies will fall asleep this way, but if yours does, you can leave the room and have a break!

Being in the same room with your baby, otherwise known as the '**camping out' method,** works for some babies and parents and has proved most helpful with babies aged between 6 and 24 months. Essentially, you put your baby in their cot and lie down (or sit down) in the same room and close your eyes. This method can be a great choice for parents who don't want to use the comfort settling technique.

Another commonly used method is '**co-sleeping**'. Co-sleeping is an umbrella term used for different variations on a similar technique; that is, sleeping with your baby. Your baby can sleep with you in your bed (which is great if you are breastfeeding) or you might like to have your baby's cot in the same room as you. Another idea is to have a cot with a side that slides right down, so that you can push it right up next to your bed. If you decide that co-sleeping is something you would like to try, please see 'Co-sleeping safely' on page 124.

Other methods include: taking your baby for a walk in the pram, carrying your baby in a pouch, or letting your baby fall asleep at the breast or bottle before putting them to bed.

---

15 If your baby cries persistently (that is, three or more hours a day for at least three days a week), you should visit your doctor to rule out **colic**, reflux or any other illness/condition.

There are many different methods from which to choose (and there are more than are listed here). Try to ignore judgement from other parents or health professionals. Rocking or soothing your baby will not 'spoil' them; comfort settling will not 'damage' them and co-sleeping with your baby will not mean you will have a teenager in your bed in the years to come. Talk to other parents, friends and family; seek out and speak to midwives, health care nurses and doctors, all of whom will have different ideas and suggestions. Which methods you try are entirely up to you. And bear in mind, you may need to use different techniques for different children in the family.

Tears at bedtime: Teaching baby to sleep brings heartbreak for mum

Trina tried everything to get her baby to sleep, including the comfort settling method. Interestingly, Trina's choice to use methods such as 'wearing' and rocking were met with the harshest judgement, over and above her use of the comfort settling method, showing that many parents are judged whatever they decide to do.

Trina's Story

Before having kids, I thought the phrase 'sleeping like a baby' meant long, deep, peaceful sleep. I now think it means just the opposite.

Nobody told me that babies need to be taught to sleep and that my baby's sleep was going to consume my every waking (and sleeping!) thought; that every conversation with other mums was going to be about sleep and just how little sleep I was getting. All I could think about was sleep!

*Sleep was not covered in any of my **antenatal** classes. All I was shown was how to wrap (swaddle) my bub and told to always put him on his back. So I did this and all was great; he slept for three to four hours at a time. Then my blissful bubble of ignorance burst and those days of long sleeps were a thing of the past.*

As soon as my little boy hit six weeks, he would only sleep for about 45 minutes at a time, if that. I would have to rock him to sleep every time and often have to start all over again when he woke up as I lay him down. If I really wanted him to have a decent sleep, I would have to lie down with him and we would both sleep for two to three hours. Left alone to his 45 minute catnaps, he would become so tired and miserable by the time his next feed was due that he would fall asleep, not feed properly, and then suddenly wake again. And so it would go all day until the sun went down, at which time he would happily sleep five to six hours at a stretch.

I tried to read just about everything I could get my hands on. I was desperately needing one of those babies who just puts themself to sleep and I had no idea that there were so many different 'schools' to help my baby do this.

At first, the rocking didn't bother me so much and I did, over time, accept that my guy was a catnapper but by the time he was six months, he was so much bigger and heavier, and I was starting to feel that I was setting up a pattern that needed to change for me and for my son.

*I tried the **comfort settling** method first.[16] I would stay with my baby and pat and shush, pat and shush for up to 45 minutes at a time. I tried and failed three times. It simply broke my heart to see him cry with such distress and feel that I was the reason for it. I went back to rocking him to sleep, telling myself that he slept well at night, so I should just accept it.*

We went out a lot and did lots of walking (he would never sleep in the pram either) and soon after he was eating solids well and crawling around a bit, sleep just happened for him—he would have long day sleeps and he was happy to put himself to sleep.

*Interestingly, it was the gentler style of comforting that I was most criticised for. Rocking my baby was met with comments such as 'You will spoil him', 'You'll do your back in', and more commonly 'Just let him cry'. It was like **controlled crying** was being forced upon me as if it was the only way to get him to sleep. I often felt like I was being a bad mother for not wanting to let my baby cry. I would get a lot of criticism for 'wearing' my baby too. I was once told to 'Get rid of this thing [my sling] and let the kid breathe' by a woman with a baby of similar age to mine. I just smiled and said how much happier my baby was when he was with me or laughed and said 'Yes, I am a marsupial mum'.*

I find other mothers are sometimes the quickest to judge, which is sad because I think we should be supportive of each other's choices.

Trina's Wisdom	I don't think there is a right or wrong way to settle a baby, just do what works and feels right for you and your baby. Just because leaving my baby to cry didn't sit well with me doesn't mean I would judge a person for doing it and likewise for baby wearing—it works for me.

How much sleep does my baby need?

According to the Raising Children Network (2010), babies aged between three and six months need about two or three sleeps during the day of up to two hours each. Babies who are seven to twelve months need about two to three hours in total (usually taken as a morning or afternoon sleep). It's important to note, however, that every baby is unique and therefore will have different sleeping needs.

---

16 See 'What is comfort settling?' on page 112

Regaining control: When teaching baby to sleep brings a flood of relief

Lucja tried everything to get her daughter to sleep. Desperate to get into some sort of routine, she contacted a parent helpline and was 'talked through' the method of controlled crying.

Lucja's Story

I'll never forget that day. Lucy was about seven months old; she was in her cot screaming her head off while I stood over her watching. I was on the phone with a nurse from an Australian helpline for new parents. I was desperate. She was seven months old and had not slept by herself once during the day up until that point.

She needed her sleep—if she didn't get it, she would be cranky and irritable all day. Our 'witching hour' as they call it, lasted all day, not the usual, quaint period between 6 pm and 7 pm. So, in order to stave off her unhappiness (let's face it, who wants to scream and cry all day?), I would watch for tired signs and either quickly grab my baby pouch and wear her for two hours while I got some housework done or I would lie down with her on the bed until she fell asleep. And there I would lie, pinned down with her head in the crook of my arm, until she woke. In the early weeks, I wasn't bothered by this much. She was little and light and I didn't mind the rest when we lay down together, as I was exhausted both from her birth and the long, sleepless nights. Besides, I loved being so close to her.

But seven weeks turn into seven months very quickly. My back could no longer sustain 'wearing' her for hours on end and if I chose the alternative, nothing could be done with the day. I couldn't do the most basic of things (such as the laundry) let alone indulge in some 'me' time. An hour would have done it. Just to sit and read a book or pick up the phone and chat to a friend or even to have a hot bath. Any of these 'indulgences' would have been a wonderful re-charger for me. But as it stood, I was literally attached to my beautiful daughter all day.

I tried everything. Everything. I tried rocking her to sleep and putting her in her cot. But she knew—just knew—the minute she was out of my arms, that something was amiss and would howl until I picked her up. I tried going for walks in the pram, I tried driving her around in the car—anything to get her to sleep. But nothing worked. I felt hopeless and at my wits' end. If something didn't change—and soon—I knew my hopelessness would spiral.

So luckily for me that day, the nurse who picked up the phone calmed me down. With tears streaming down my face, I put Lucy in the cot and went to look for pen and paper as instructed.

*'Now,' said the nurse, 'I want you to write this down.' She then gave me detailed instructions on how to get Lucy to sleep by herself. She sounded so comforting and so confident that I immediately began to feel hopeful. She explained the **controlled crying** method to me. In a nutshell, it was a method that revolved around the principle of leaving Lucy in her cot for lengthening periods of time. While this aspect of the technique was crucial, there were other elements that were equally important, such as establishing a*

sleeping routine and learning to understand the difference in her cries. I'm ashamed to say that I didn't even know there was a difference in Lucy's cries. But this blessed woman actually stayed with me on the phone while I tried controlled crying for the first time. She could hear Lucy through the phone and together, we learned which of her cries were 'whinge' cries (most of them were) and which were 'comfort me right now' cries. Unless Lucy's cries were 'comfort me right now' cries (when I would go in and do so straight away), I was to leave her firstly for one minute, then three, then five, then seven minutes and so forth. They recommended that I stick to a maximum upper time limit of 15 minutes.

I decided to wait until the weekend when my husband could help me. We talked it over and concluded it was the right choice for us. We also set an upper time limit of ten minutes—it was a time frame that we were both comfortable with. And so the weekend came. We steeled ourselves; we just knew it had to be done. Unbelievably, it worked. Lucy learned to sleep. And it had flow on effects—she was much happier during the day, as was I. And when bedtime came, we would read her a story, she would smile at us and cuddle her teddy as we whispered good night, and nod off to sleep.

But then I made a big mistake. Huge. In my newfound spare time, I visited an internet forum to find out more about this technique and how other parents had used it. I was completely unprepared for the viciousness that came from other women. I can't describe to you how awful I felt that I had control-cried my baby. 'Don't you realise that she needs to be picked up and cuddled? That's your job as a mother!' 'Why did you bother even having children if you can't be bothered looking after them properly?'

God, I felt like I'd been stabbed in the heart. What had I done to my baby? When I recovered from the shock, I remembered something crucial: these people were not Lucy's mother. They had no idea what we had been through and did not know me as a person or as a mother. So I decided to stop feeling guilty and stick to my guns. And I did some research while I was at it. As it turns out, my instincts were right. I waded through all the research that so many had pointed to in their heated discussions on controlled crying (having a strong background in scientific research myself helped, I was experienced and confident enough to interpret scientific papers) and I was comforted and reassured by what I found.

My daughter was (and still is) a very happy child who knows that she is loved to bits. And me? Well, I went on to have two more children and there was no second-guessing on my part anymore—once they hit the six-month mark, they were taught to sleep. And we are all the happier and saner for it.

Lucja's Wisdom

Women can be so competitive when it comes to mothering. I don't know why. I have heard parents refer to the controlled crying method as the 'abandonment' technique and the women who use these methods as 'baby torturers'. Not only are these labels completely inaccurate (and very unkind), they are also very unhelpful when you're a new mother looking for reassurance. There are many reasons for mother guilt and I firmly believe that one of those reasons is the way in which women can denigrate each other's parenting practices.

You need to find out what's right for your family, not what's right for other people's families. Maybe you desperately want to carry your baby until he or she is two years old. Maybe you want to co-sleep. Maybe you want to teach your baby to sleep. Whichever method you choose, don't let anyone else make you feel guilty for your choice. It's your family, your choice.

What is comfort settling?

There is much confusion about the term 'comfort settling', partly because there are so many variations of the technique, and partly because it is often used interchangeably with the terms 'controlled comforting', 'teaching to sleep' and 'controlled crying'. One very important distinction to note, however, is that comfort settling is not the same thing as the 'cry it out' method. The 'cry it out' method is not widely recommended, as it entails leaving a baby to literally cry it out until they fall asleep from exhaustion without any comfort. This method has come under some scrutiny—most notably from Sunderland (2006) who theorises that leaving babies to cry it out may cause the stress hormone cortisol to rise, which, she asserts, is not good for baby, in the short or long term.

Within this book, the term 'comfort settling' is used when referring to controlled crying, as it is increasingly becoming the term of choice. Cooke (2003, p. 217) describes comfort settling as 'a structured way of getting … babies to sleep without parents'. While the technique used can vary slightly, it remains true to the following central tenets: learning about your baby's cries and 'cues', making sure your baby is not hungry, has a clean nappy and is comfortable, and implementing a 'pre-sleep' routine (for example, reading stories, singing calm songs—basically winding down in general).

Babies' cries can mean many things, for example: 'I'm bored', 'I'm hungry', 'I want a cuddle' or 'I'm tired'. With practise (or with the help of an experienced professional), you can learn the difference between your baby's cries. Distress can be indicated by an increase in the intensity, loudness or tone of your baby's cry, whereas tiredness is usually a quieter, grizzly tone. The first step in the comfort settling technique is to watch out for your baby's tired signs (or cues/cries).

Once you have noticed that your baby is tired, make sure their nappy is clean and they are fed and comfortable, and put your baby in their cot. You might say something like 'Night night, sleep tight'. It doesn't really matter what you say, so long as it is reassuring and said in a calm tone. You then leave the room for a short period to give your baby a chance to settle on their own.

The next step is to leave your baby to settle themselves for increasing periods of time. For example, you may start with 30 seconds before you return to your baby and then increase this interval by one or two minutes at a time, until you reach your maximum time interval (this might be five minutes, ten minutes, fifteen minutes—it's entirely an individual choice). Green's (2001, p. 126) method illustrates this well: 'Leave them crying for 5 minutes if you are average, 10 minutes if you are tough, 2 minutes if you are delicate and 1 minute if you are very fragile'. If, however, your baby's cries become distressed, you should go in to them and provide comfort, no matter how long they have been crying.

There are a few things to note with this method. Firstly, some babies like to be picked up and cuddled when you return to comfort them. However, this seems to make some babies more distressed when you leave the room. If this is the case with your baby, instead of cuddling them, you could pat them softly on their bottom and reassure them with your voice, for example 'Ssshhh, it's alright, mummy/daddy is here'. Secondly, you need to be calm, confident and consistent. Lastly, you need to be persistent. This method has a high success rate, but only if you persist with it.

There are, of course, many techniques for helping your baby get to sleep; this is just one of them. For more information on some other techniques, see 'Commonly used methods for helping your baby to sleep' on page 107.

The catnapper: When comfort settling lengthens sleep and strengthens mum

Sleep was a big problem for Nerralea when her baby was born, as he only ever slept for 45 minutes at a time.

Nerralea's Story

After my first son Ivan was born, I honestly thought this parenting thing would be fairly easy. What a shock. My baby came home from hospital not really knowing what sleep was. In the beginning, he would sleep every two hours, but his sleep progressively worsened until he was on a 45 minute routine, day and night. He woke up every 45 minutes around the clock. The strain it put on my marriage was incredible. We were both exhausted. Neither of us functioned properly; we just walked around like zombies.

We tried rocking him to sleep in our arms but as soon as we put him in the cot, he'd wake up and begin crying again. We tried patting him in his cot, but again, as soon as we tried to sneak out of the room he'd wake up. We tried playing music in his room … everything, including a visit with both our doctor and our paediatrician who both said there was nothing wrong with him.

*We got to a point where we were so desperate we'd try anything and **controlled crying** was an option we started to think about. Of course, as a new mother, I was anxious about letting my baby cry. I reached out for help but felt judged by other parents and even health care professionals. I'd more often than not hear 'They're babies for such little time—why would you want to allow them to cry? Just hold them', or 'Why not try **co-sleeping** or just keep offering the breast in order to get them to sleep?' All these ideas were well and good but we had tried them—repeatedly—and they just weren't working for us.*

Some of the judgement was really harsh. Once, I got hit with 'How could you let your little baby cry? Your son will think you don't love him'. It made me feel awful—like such a failure as a mother that I would even consider going down the path of controlled crying. But I could no longer maintain the status quo. Things had become so unbearable that I ended up with **postnatal depression**.[17]

Having postnatal depression is the worst thing I've ever had to deal with. I was constantly crying. I didn't want to have anything to do with my son. Every time he cried, I would feel so angry. I wondered every single day what I was doing, having a child. The lack of sleep was horrific; the strain it put on my marriage unbearable. What was meant to be one of the happiest times in our lives was one of the most difficult to endure. I didn't want to cry anymore. I would just hold Ivan, not even wanting to look at him, while he and I both cried. We were a mess. It was time to do something.

So we ended up going to a parenting **live-in service**. *In all honesty, while I was nervous about how much they'd allow Ivan to cry, I was relieved that I was going to get some help and guidance and hopefully bring home a 'new' baby.*

We discovered that the controlled crying technique required us to listen to his cries. I was relieved it wasn't about leaving him for hours to scream. We were taught to listen to what our baby was needing. If his cry was quite high pitched, then he was wanting some comfort. We would go straight into him and pat him in the cot. Once he was calm, we would walk out of the room again.

What we found was, more often than not, his cry wasn't high pitched and he had more of a 'whinging' cry. Once we allowed him to have a little cry, we could hear that he was settling in between and even having periods of no crying. It was such a relief when he first went to sleep. I felt like we might finally be getting somewhere. Finally, we had a glimmer of hope in what had been a very dark world of constant crying and no sleep.

After four days, the change in Ivan was unbelievable. He was still waking every now and then but he was also having periods of two to three hours' sleep. So once we returned home, we continued listening to his cries. We were more confident as parents, knowing that we weren't in any way harming our child by allowing him to have a cry. Within two weeks of returning home, he was sleeping 100 per cent better. Even his stretches between night feeds lengthened and we were managing to get some sleep. I could actually look at my son again and think how much I loved him.

The controlled crying technique was like a breath of fresh air for us. I can't even begin to tell you the difference it made once Ivan started sleeping. My moods changed and I was better able to deal with the postnatal depression. Our marriage became stronger and we started to enjoy what was the most exciting time in our lives.

Nerralea's Wisdom	What would I say to those who are about to become first time parents? Never say 'never'. Don't judge others about their parenting choices. It's all good and easy to say 'I'd never do that to my child' but unfortunately, our babies don't always fit into the mould we have for them. And when that happens, the higher your expectations are of yourself and your baby, the more difficult you will make it on yourself.

17 See 'Is there a link between poor infant sleep and postnatal depression?' on page 115

I know there are people out there that think that by using the controlled crying technique I have in some way harmed my child. But I can say with absolute certainty that we as a family are much happier because of it. My boys get the sleep they need and we as parents are far less stressed than we were during those early days.

Parenting and motherhood is absolutely one of the most difficult things I've ever done but also the most satisfying. If women could just support each other through this process without passing judgement, it would make it so much easier.

Is there a link between poor infant sleep and postnatal depression?

Martin et al. (2007) state that postnatal depression (PND or post-partum depression) affects 15 per cent of Australian women, a figure similar to other developed countries. The prevalence of depression in fathers during the post-partum period can be as high as 50 per cent when their partners have PND.

Hiscock et al. (2008) note that maternal depression and anxiety are consistently associated with infant sleep problems (for example, baby sleeps poorly, wakes often at night and stays awake), even after controlling for known depression risk factors. Such factors include a history of depression, having a depressed partner, reduced support from partner and other social networks, marital conflict and recent negative life events.

Postnatal depression affects a parent's mood, cognition and ability to conduct daily tasks. Additionally, as noted by Hiscock et al. (2008, p. 622), both maternal and paternal depression are associated with: 'relationship breakdown, insecure mother–child attachment, child cognitive, child behaviour and emotional problems, and (in rare cases) child abuse'. These negative impacts on children have been reported in many clinical studies (see Barr 2006; Boyce & Stubbs 1994; Buist 1998; Murray & Cooper 1997; Paris et al. 2009; Wisner et al. 2006).

In 2008, Hiscock et al. conducted a cluster-randomised controlled trial that measured the effects of implementing brief behaviour modification programs designed to improve infant sleep. The behaviour modification program consisted of training sessions conducted by nurses (who were trained by Dr Hiscock, a paediatrician and Dr Bayer, a clinical psychologist). These training sessions were conducted with 114 parents who were taught how to help their baby to sleep using the comfort settling method and the 'camping out' method (parents stay in the same room as their babies). Parents were given a choice as to which method they used, as Hiscock's clinical experience suggested that different families prefer different sleep management approaches. The study found that mothers in the intervention group reported significantly lower depressive symptoms (59 per cent) relative to the control group.

Hiscock's findings confirm other studies that demonstrate significant improvement in maternal mood and depression due to modification of problematic infant sleep behaviour (see Armstrong et al. 1998; Bayer et al. 2007; Dennis & Ross 2005; Fisher 2009; Morgan 2009).

Postnatal depression is a serious problem, for both parent and child. If you find it difficult to get your baby to sleep (and to stay asleep), you may well benefit from using either the comfort settling method or the 'camping out' method described above. For more information on these methods, see 'What is comfort settling?' on page 112 and 'Commonly used methods for helping your baby to sleep' on page 107. However, it's important to remember that teaching your baby to sleep is not a panacea for postnatal depression. If you are experiencing any signs of depression (see 'Postnatal depression' on page 154 for a list of symptoms), you should go straight to your doctor so that a treatment plan can be implemented as soon as possible.

Coping without support

Rearing babies and children takes an enormous amount of effort. There is truth in the adage 'it takes a village to raise a child'. Parents who are isolated— whether they are far away from family and friends, are single parents or have partners who work long hours—often struggle to cope with the day-to-day tasks of raising a baby, as well as the sheer loneliness that can accompany scant adult interaction.

Relocation and dislocation: When moving leaves you without support

Marcella relocated hundreds of kilometres away from her family because of her husband's job, and sought to meet other women through playgroups and reduce her sense of isolation.

Marcella's Story

My family lived about 200 kilometres from us when I fell pregnant, so I got support over the phone from them but as far as practical support goes, my friends from work were the most helpful. I was relieved of some of the more physical parts of my job and was often excused from after-hours meetings and activities. My assistant kept the pantry stocked with Italian sponge finger biscuits and peppermint tea. My husband had never really had much to do with pregnant women, so he didn't really know what to expect. I don't think he completely understood how utterly exhausting pregnancy is. Bless him though, he never complained about holding my hair out of my face as I held onto the toilet bowl.

When our daughter was 12 weeks old, we were transferred to Melbourne for my husband's work. It was quite difficult having all of our family and friends on the other side of the country. I only knew one other person in Melbourne; thankfully she had a daughter the same age as ours but she was also a first-time parent and new to Melbourne, so it really was a case of the blind leading the blind. Those first few weeks were really difficult. I didn't even know where the supermarket was, much less have someone around who could babysit while I went to the hairdresser or out for dinner.

The awful Black Saturday bushfires happened a few weeks after we moved. Thankfully, the fires didn't reach our area but they were close by. My husband was heavily involved in coordinating the relief effort and was away from home for almost four weeks. I was in a new state with a young baby on my own. I found myself going to the shopping centre just to talk with other adults. I would chat with anyone who stood still for long enough. I also spent a lot of time on the phone with my mum in Perth.

Around the same time, I started looking for a playgroup to join. Obviously with my daughter being only 12 weeks old, it was more for me than her. I found several playgroups in our area, but they were all for much older children and often there were a few siblings of each family attending. This wasn't really what I was looking for—as a first-time parent, I wanted to share my experience with other novices. I eventually found a playgroup that was full of new parents and all our babies were born only a few months apart … I haven't looked back. These women have become my closest friends. We experienced the same milestones at the same times and were able to share these wonderful experiences together.

Marcella's Wisdom

I think the most important advice I could give anyone would be to make the effort to develop your own support crew. You really need to put yourself out there and meet people. Join a playgroup or some sort of activity you can do with your child and with other parents. Then talk to people—get to know them and make friends. There are people out there who are going through similar experiences and who will help you get through the tough times. The only other advice would be to accept offers of help. It's OK to ask a friend to watch your child just to take a nap or go to the hairdresser or just give you some time to yourself. There is a lot of support out there if you look for it.

Where can I find extra support?

Support is vital for first-time parents and maybe even more so for second, third and fourth time parents. Without support, parents can quickly feel isolated, which can lead to loneliness and even depression (Hiscock et al. 2008). It is vital that you seek out and develop networks if you have none in place. Aside from the resources listed at the end of this book, you can try a number of avenues. If you live in a highly populated area, seek out your local child health nurse or community health centre, as they will have long lists of groups you might like to join, such as playgroups and mothers' and/or fathers' groups. If you live in a rural or remote area, you could think about starting up your own parents' group or playgroup (see Appendix B: How to start a support group on page 225), or you could make use of the internet to join online community groups.

Coping with sick or premature babies

Coping with sick or premature babies is probably not foremost in parents' minds during pregnancy or when waiting for a baby to arrive (such as through adoption or surrogacy). The stories that follow are must-reads, because they may help prepare you in the event that you have a sick baby.

From despair to hope: When a diagnosis of acid reflux brings relief

Tamara had an exhausting and confusing time with her son who was finally diagnosed with, and treated for, **acid reflux**.

Tamara's Story

Alexander was a beautiful, calm baby while we were in the hospital and for the first few days we were at home. My husband and I both fell in love with him immediately. I remember being in the hospital, holding Alexander in a rare moment when no one else was in the room, and feeling so lucky in every aspect of my life—my marriage, my family, and this new little life.

Around the second or third week, Alexander began crying for extended periods, without any hope of consolation. As new parents, my husband and I weren't sure why this was happening—did we just not know how to calm a crying baby yet? Was he just supposed to be crying? He would simply start crying from a very peaceful state and this would continue for hours. He'd pull his legs up into his tummy, then arch his back, and absolutely scream.

I tried every comforting technique I could think of—swaddling, cuddling, feeding, singing, walking, swinging, rocking, car seat on the clothes dryer. None of these worked for more than a few minutes. I felt like I had failed as a parent, especially as a mother, because I could not calm this poor little guy. At one of the lowest points, my husband came home from work to find both Alexander and I crying on the floor. I'd laid him down and wrapped myself around him, and we were both entirely distraught. My doctor was watching me closely for post-partum depression,[18] *as being around endless crying and not being able to help stop it was making me feel hopeless, not to mention depleting my energy and strength that were already at very low levels.*

Around the third week, my mom had been able to be around Alexander long enough to see a number of crying spells. She said that yes, all babies cry, but babies shouldn't cry like this. With her support, I was able to gather some strength to take him to the paediatrician. Initially, he was diagnosed with gas, and sent home with drops and the advice that they may or may not work. We tried this for a week, and then went back when no change was found. Finally, he was diagnosed with acid reflux.

I was so relieved to know that he had something else impacting his ability to be soothed—that it wasn't my ineptitude. But I was frustrated that he'd had to go through four or five weeks of misery and that he hadn't been diagnosed at our first visit. I felt the paediatrician (and my husband) thought I was an alarmist mom, and that I should just deal with his crying.

My mom was the only other person to be around to see my boy's behavior and total inconsolability. My husband knew it happened but said he could not really understand what it would be like to be around it all day, and also couldn't judge how realistic my stories were—maybe I was exaggerating based on my own stress or fatigue. Mom is the only reason I've kept pushing the doctors to get different treatment for my son and is the person who found out about the different medications to begin with.

I find that because I endured so many days of non-stop crying, my own reactions when he starts crying now (when his reflux is managed a bit better) are that the crying is not going to stop. Depending on how hard he cries (even if it's just because he's very upset with his current situation), I will start sweating profusely, I cannot think properly, and ultimately I will start crying myself. Sadly, I've had a bit of conditioning based on his first two months of life, and I am learning to 'detune' my response to the more normal crying that occurs today. My mom has been helpful in giving me the mental, emotional and physical breaks I have needed to get back to a more balanced place. By watching her with my baby, I've learned a number of techniques that work to help a little one to sleep, to calm them down, or to distract them from the beginnings of a fuss, and I use these tricks daily!

Tamara's Wisdom

This experience has taught me that being a mom can be very lonely, even when you have great support. Being a mom of a baby with health issues can be absolutely isolating. Keep looking for options and alternatives for your little one. You're the only one who can advocate for them, which can be an incredible burden as you second-guess your efforts, or lack thereof, to help. Keep trying, and realize that if you've done your best for that day, that is enough. Don't settle for the complacent 'this will pass with time'. That may be true, but you're going through that hell today, tomorrow and the next day. You deserve to be and feel well too and that can only happen if your little one is properly cared for by all involved.

---

18 See 'Is there a link between poor infant sleep and postnatal depression?' on page 115

How to cope with persistent crying

Persistent crying can be a very distressing experience for both parent and baby. Parents who are desperate to soothe a baby who won't stop crying can end up feeling desperate, frustrated, hopeless and angry. While it is important to try to soothe your baby, you should also be aware of your own feelings. If they appear to be escalating to anger (or even rage), you need to take immediate action. Ideally, ring a friend or family member who can come and help you. Maybe they can take over for a while so you can recharge. If this is not possible, put your baby safely into their cot and walk away. Breathe deeply and take a few minutes to calm down. If you feel that your anger is getting out of control, you need to call a helpline immediately (see page 256 of the Resources section for a list of organisations in your country). It is vital that you do this, as these types of incidents (that is, persistent, inconsolable crying) have led to Shaken Baby Syndrome, which can result in severe brain trauma and death.

The importance of learning first aid: When baby stops breathing

Kristen's son was born prematurely and stopped breathing, necessitating CPR and an emergency stay in hospital.

Kristen's Story

My son was definitely impatient—he came six weeks before his due date, to be precise. I remember distinctly the day labour started. I had back pains, which I put down to too much exercise the day before. I was in a work meeting about lunchtime and needed to go to the loo and when I did, I had some spotting (not very much). That night, I thought I should drop into the birthing centre to make sure that Ollie was OK. When I got there, I was sent to the labour ward. I was still in denial, but Ollie was born at about 10 pm that night.

A few days after Ollie was discharged, I was holding him just after a feed and he was asleep in my arms. I was looking down at his face (as you tend to do a lot with a newborn) and noticed that it was going blue (at this stage, time is all over the place—going very fast and very slow all at once).

I called to Michael, who was in the same room, that Ollie had gone blue. Michael came over, immediately took Ollie from my lap, put him on the floor and started doing CPR. While Michael was resuscitating Ollie, I called the ambulance—as expected, the despatch operator was wonderful, talked us through what we should be doing (which Michael was doing). Ollie was alternating between breathing and not—Michael would get him started, he'd gasp or have a cry, then he'd stop again. This happened a couple of times before he started breathing properly again, just before the ambulances arrived.

Two ambulances, from different areas, were despatched ensuring that one got there within a few minutes. As Ollie appeared OK at that stage, the paramedic asked if we wanted to be taken to hospital (glad we said yes). Ollie and I went in the ambulance and the paramedic was taking down the details 'How long did he stop breathing for? Ten seconds? Twenty seconds?' It seemed like an eternity and you don't really think to count while it's happening.

Oliver was taken into the children's emergency department immediately. He was put into a cot and hooked up to a monitor—anyone who has experienced their child ill in hospital will have memories of the 'beeping' monitors. At first you jolt at each alarm, scared that something is wrong with your child. You look round and see the nurses going about what they are doing, wondering why they aren't responding, then a nurse comes over and says 'Nothing to worry about … these things go off all the time'. At which point, your heart starts beating again.

Ollie was being monitored and was breathing fine and having no issues, but the head doctor in the children's department insisted on getting a 'line' into him in case they needed to administer anything quickly. A doctor and a nurse attempted to get the needle into Ollie's arm (remember that Ollie was still three weeks premmie and weighed under 2.5 kg). After several unsuccessful attempts (and me having to leave the room—no point them having me fall on the floor) they called for the head doctor. The head doctor came and had a go, but still no luck. Finally, a doctor from the neonatal unit was asked to come down and assist. Success! The line was in.

Ollie was admitted just after lunch and by early evening, no repeat events had occurred. He was hungry so the nurse said I could give him a feed. Given that the last incident happened just after a feed, you can imagine that I was feeling a little bit nervous about feeding him again. We went through the changing, feeding, burping routine without a problem. Until, a short time later, Ollie went blue and the alarms started going off …

Within seconds, there were five or six doctors and nurses around his cot, bagging him and trying to pump drugs into him. What was panicking me was that Ollie wasn't making a sound. I expected to hear him cry out but he didn't. Ollie was wheeled to the resuscitation unit with Michael and me following. We sat there, dazed, watching the doctors and nurses working on Ollie. We hadn't seen any sign of life but they were still working on him.

Each resuscitation room opens onto a corridor that passes all rooms. Michael and I were sitting on chairs in the corridor watching Ollie in the room in front of us. It was at that moment when a paramedic came over to us and said 'I'm so sorry. Your son is dead'. It was the most surreal moment I have ever experienced. Michael and I looked at him, then back to where Ollie was still being worked on. We were both thinking 'But if he's dead why are they still working on him?' It turned out that the paramedic had the wrong family; lucky for us—unimaginable for the other family whose baby had died. Ours was still fighting on.

Once Ollie was stabilised, which took quite some time, he was transported to a specialist children's hospital. Over the next two weeks, Ollie progressed from the isolation unit, to intensive care, to high dependency (which he moved through within a day—I think he was too noisy!), through to special care and finally, back home. It wasn't smooth sailing—Ollie did need a blood transfusion at one point—but our road was a lot easier than many others with premature babies. During this time, a number of specialists checked everything that could be checked with Ollie. He had heart scans, brain scans, bloods checked for everything—not a thing was found.

*The final diagnosis, made on the basis that they couldn't find anything else, was **reflux apnoea** associated with him being premature. That certainly didn't make it easy taking him home. How were we going to watch him 24/7 to make sure it didn't happen again? A small device made that possible. You tape a small tube (which connects to a monitor) to the baby's tummy and the monitor alarms if the baby stops breathing. The baby wears it all day and night … peace of mind. We had the monitor on Ollie for three months and of course, there was not one emergency.*

Looking back, if I had put Ollie to bed after his feed he would simply be a cot death statistic. For a short period, we thought we had lost Ollie. We then had a period where we didn't know if Ollie had sustained any brain damage or other problems associated with not breathing, let alone any issues associated with him being premature. Luckily, to this day, Ollie hasn't shown any signs other than normal development.

Kristen's Wisdom

Having a premature baby can be scary—especially if things go wrong. My strongest advice to every new parent is to find a local first aid course for babies and children and learn how to cope with emergencies. If Michael had not known how to conduct CPR on babies, there would be no Oliver.

If you have had similar problems with your baby, such as breathing problems, I urge you to seek out a sound and motion monitor. We didn't get one before Ollie was born but we certainly got one after his incident. We joked about using it through Oliver's teenage years but we did use it until Ollie moved into his bed when he was three.

First aid for babies and children

One of the most important things you can do for your new baby is to take a first aid course for babies and children. In Australia, these are offered through the St John Ambulance Service (www.stjohn.org.au) and sometimes parents' groups organise in-house training sessions. As clearly illustrated in Kristen's story, had her partner Michael not known how to perform infant CPR, Oliver would likely have died while waiting for an ambulance. For a list of organisations that provide infant first aid courses in your country, please refer to page 254 of the Resources section.

While you are strongly urged to participate in a first aid course for babies and children, if you choose not to do so, at the very least, you ought to purchase—and read—a first aid guide book (specifically for babies), buy a fully equipped first aid kit and have emergency numbers pinned somewhere easily accessible. You can also purchase instructional DVDs from many organisations worldwide. For a list of such organisations, refer to page 254 of the Resources section.

Coping with sleep deprivation

Sleep, sleep, sleep! Sleep, or lack thereof, is a prominent aspect of new parenthood. As illustrated in the following stories, sleep deprivation can lead parents to the brink of despair. However, many parents have devised cunning strategies to deal with sleep deprivation.

Where's the off switch? Finding out that babies don't have one

Savannah was unprepared for the total lack of sleep that is part and parcel of being a new parent, especially as she thought that the long and irregular shifts she had worked for the majority of her career would help her to adjust smoothly to irregular sleep.

Savannah's Story

I naively thought, while pregnant with my first child, that my work would have equipped me well to deal with sleepless nights with a newborn. I was used to working up to 26 hours without a break or any sleep and to being woken at ungodly hours while on call. 'Bring it on,' I thought, 'it'll be a piece of cake.'

Wrong, wrong, wrong.

The thing that wears you down when dealing with a newborn is the sheer relentlessness of it all. Before, there was always an end to the shift, an end to the on-call when I could switch off the phone, throw my pager in the bin and dive into the arms of my welcoming doona. No matter how bad it was when I was on, there was always going to be a time when I was off.

My baby had no concept of 'off'. He declared himself early, on the third night in hospital, when he decided he did not like sleeping alone in that big hard old bassinette. He preferred to be held, thanks very much. Or breastfed. Preferably both at once, actually. Every time I put him down, his eyes would pop open and I would hear that sound that I soon came to dread more than the chirp of my now-retired pager: that 'uh uh uh uh …' which precedes the inevitable 'WAAAAAAAAHHH!', which roughly translates as 'PICK ME UP RIGHT NOW!'

*That third night was awful. I got no real sleep at all. I did not know what to do and was quite teary the next day, which everyone put down to the normal **baby blues**. The next night I was tense with anxiety about what would happen. I put him down—he opened his eyes—and so I did something I thought was terribly naughty, but I had to do it: I pulled the side rails of the hospital bed up and brought him in to bed with me.*

It worked an absolute treat and we slept one solid stretch of four whole hours together. I even fed him while lying down and mostly asleep myself. But I was wracked with guilt. I mean, isn't that how babies get smothered and die? I felt like I had done something wrong for sure.

*I was saved by our paediatrician, a wonderful man who is a firm believer in **co-sleeping** if it is what it takes for the mother—and baby—to get enough rest. He reassured me that unless I was morbidly obese, drunk or on drugs, I would never smother my baby by accident, since co-sleeping mothers and babies sleep more lightly but longer (this has been shown in sleep studies on the subject) and the mothers tend to be very aware of where the baby is, even when asleep.*

So for the first six weeks of his life, my son and I snuggled in together every night and he slept curled up cosily in the crook of my arm. If we had a good night, I might patch together six or even seven hours of sleep. If we had a bad one, it might be much less but it meant I did not spend the whole night trying—and failing—to get him to stay asleep in the bassinette. I was still pretty sleep-deprived overall but it was much better than it could have been.

Sleep deprivation makes me tense and ever-so-slightly insane. I get to a point where I am so tired that I can't fall asleep, which would be funny if it wasn't so completely awful. I cry at the drop of a hat. I sit hopelessly on the edge of the bed and sob and refuse to be comforted. I am no fun for anyone and this is certainly what I would have been like much more often if I had been spending my nights trying to get my baby to sleep on his own.

People say that you should just sleep when the baby sleeps but I am a terrible daytime napper and find it hard to fall asleep at the best of times. When you are already sleep-deprived and wound-up because you just know they are going to wake up again soon and the whole cycle is going to repeat itself, it is not the best of times!

I also had people shake their heads and tut-tut when I confessed that my baby was sleeping in my bed and say 'Oh you mustn't do that, he'll still be there when he's three.' I wanted to scream 'But he's only two weeks old! He doesn't know!'

Savannah's Wisdom	When you have a newborn to care for, and even more so when you also have a toddler to amuse all day, you need all the sleep you can get. My wisdom is that it's OK to do whatever you need to do in order to maximise the amount of sleep you are getting. Even if other people think it's wrong. Because sleep-deprivation is far worse than any number of disapproving comments, really!

Co-sleeping safely

Co-sleeping (also known as 'bed sharing' or 'sleeping close by') is an umbrella term that includes baby sleeping in the same room as the parents and/or in the parental bed. There have been many positive reports of co-sleeping, particularly with regard to facilitating breastfeeding and the enhancement of mother–infant bonding.

However, there are instances in which bed sharing can be dangerous. For example, infants should not be brought into bed when parents are excessively tired or if they are using medications (even over-the-counter medications such as cold and flu tablets can be hazardous). Parents should not be under the influence of drugs (street drugs or prescription medication that makes you tired) or alcohol. Additionally, if you smoke, you should not bed share, as this is associated with an increased risk of Sudden Infant Death Syndrome (SIDS).

You also need to be careful about what type of surface you and your baby are sleeping on. For example, it is never recommended that you sleep with your baby on a couch, a waterbed, a recliner, or any other type of surface in which your baby could become wedged between the surface and you. If your baby is premature, of low birth weight, has a temperature or you are overweight (being overweight/ obese is a risk factor for bed sharing and is not recommended), you should speak to your doctor before considering sharing a bed with your baby. Lastly, don't let other children sleep with your baby, as they are not as aware of the infant in the bed as parents are.

The information given above does sound a bit scary. However, if you heed the safety guidelines (and better still, talk through any possible safety concerns with your doctor), you and your baby could have a great bonding relationship and you may even get more sleep. For more information on co-sleeping, see <www.attachmentparenting.org> or read the American Academy of Pediatrics' policy on SIDS <www.aap.org>. And remember, if for some reason you cannot bed share, you can still co-sleep by sharing your room with your baby (bearing in mind that smoking increases the risk for SIDS, both with bed sharing and with room sharing). For further information and support, see page 252 of the Resources section.

On autopilot: When lack of sleep leads to forgetfulness

Yasmin talks about how her husband's depression, combined with the lack of help she received with her two small children, led her to feel like a zombie from lack of sleep.

Yasmin's Story

I can honestly say that I haven't slept well for close to five years. By the time Poppy had learned to sleep through, I was already pregnant with my second daughter, Saffron, and couldn't sleep for myriad reasons.

Just thinking about all that lost sleep makes me feel exhausted but, like anything else, you learn to deal with it. I have adjusted and have even gotten used to walking around like a zombie and functioning on minimal sleep. I have become accustomed to constantly losing my keys and forgetting where I parked my car. Sometimes I find that my sentences don't quite make sense; I often feel shocked by my struggle to find words appropriate for the occasion.

And it's not just the lack of actual sleep; it's the bad quality sleep that is a bigger problem. Because of my husband's depression[19] and inability to cope with our newborn, I was forced to sleep on the sofa with my baby so that my husband could have the bedroom to himself. She was waking every two to four hours to feed or just to be settled back to sleep. We were squashed on the sofa together, so we were waking each other up. And it was January in Australia, so we were practically cooking in each other's sweat.

It wasn't like I could rest during the day either. There was a depressed husband and an energetic three-year-old to care for, a household to maintain, plus, I was going back to work very soon, to a new and very grown-up job. I was so tired that I felt nauseous. The worst of it was at midday, when I would think 'This is it, I am going to die. I simply can't get up again.'

I didn't have the luxury to sit and think about being sad or depressed or how hard my particular situation was. But physically, it had a big impact. I lost all my baby weight dangerously quickly because I didn't have the energy to eat properly. I cooked for the family but I remember thinking that I simply didn't have the energy to chew. I lost my usual enthusiasm for exercise and stopped going for long walks with the kids. Soon, I just got used to the lack of sleep and simply got on with it.

My sleep deprivation was the cause of an incident that I still think about every day. Saffron was only about eight weeks old and I had to see my accountant. I remember putting her in the baby seat and driving to the accountant's office. I did my business and came out of the accountant's office and got back in my car. I was gone for about 20 minutes. It was only when I got back in the car and started the engine that I realised I had left my sleeping baby in the car (in the heat of the March afternoon sun). I was startled enough by my unforgiveable absent mindedness but then a homeless, toothless woman kept knocking on my car window and screaming that she was about to call the authorities and that I didn't deserve to have a baby. All I could say to her was 'I am sorry, I am sorry; I am having a bad day.' I drove off with tears streaming down my face. I was ashamed and horrified at my exhausted state. The hideous possibilities of what could have happened to my daughter never cease to escape me. I had completely forgotten about my baby's existence for the entire time I was at the accountant's office—that's probably the very definition of exhaustion for you.

I can count on one hand the number of times my husband got up to help with Saffron in the middle of the night. He put in earplugs and slept through. It was my fault too; I allowed him to become lazier by the day and not share the load. I made excuses for him—he was depressed, he had to get up for work. All of this sleep deprivation did cause me to have some very bad moments, like when I picked up my hungry baby and aggressively told her to 'Shut the fuck up!' But those moments would pass and I would feel bad for my anger. I never beat myself up about it though, as I knew Saffron would forgive me.

---

19 See 'Can men get postnatal depression?' on page 34

Yasmin's Wisdom	Life phases change and kids' patterns change and even the bad times will be missed and maybe even remembered fondly. I know I will miss the warm little bodies of my kids cuddled next to me in the middle of the night, even when I am so tired that I can't speak or open my eyes properly.
	Kids will sleep eventually. I have made a rule for my team at work—nobody is allowed to talk about how tired they are, because nobody is more tired than me!

Bonding with baby: How fast does it happen?

- It was a wonderful welling of joy when I first met her. We bonded immediately. I was just so elated at meeting this beautiful little person.

- I looked at him and thought 'Oh, it's you! Hello!' There was no huge rush of emotion or maternal feeling (I don't describe myself as particularly maternal, more logical and practical than emotional, I guess) but it was just a fact: there he was, and I was his mother. OK. What now?

- When I first met my baby, it was after a caesarean section and she was put on my chest while they were still stitching me up. I felt in awe of her with these big eyes looking at my husband and me and it hit me what a huge responsibility it was to have this baby. It took a while before I was able to be alone with her again and the bonding then started.

- When I met my first baby, I was just overwhelmed. Not a good type of overwhelmed, more like a shock. She was screaming her head off; the noise was incredible. I felt out of my body and not part of any of it. I can't remember when I bonded with her but it certainly took a while. And it was an up and down type of thing.

- I was overwhelmed. My labour was 22 hours and by the end of it, I think I had forgotten that a baby was the end result. Sasha was put on my chest straight away and I remember looking at her like she was an alien. I did not bond with her immediately. I was in shock. My body felt like it had been through a war and my mind was trying to make sense of what had just happened. I did feel a sense of awe that this little baby had come out of my body but I felt that I didn't know her at all.

- I cried when she was placed on my chest. It was a relief after such a long labour. I didn't bond with her straight away but I didn't worry about it for a second. I had done enough reading to know that it often doesn't happen immediately and I actually think it's unrealistic to think that's the case. This is a whole new person you've just met. No one becomes your best friend the first time you meet them. It took us about three weeks and then I just looked at her and had a bit of a eureka moment. Kind of like 'Of course, it's you. Couldn't be anyone else.'

- I bonded with my second baby straight away, but not the first. I had postnatal depression the first time, which really affected our relationship. It took me a long time to bond with her in a way I'm happy with (and the birth of my second child has totally cemented our relationship now, and it's more wonderful than I ever imagined). I feel really sad that I missed out on her first year, all those cuddles I could have enjoyed!

- I was emotionally shocked by how much love I had for both kids when they were born. You think you know love until you have a baby.

- We are certainly 'attached' and 'bonded' as well as I could ever have hoped. It annoys the crap out of me when people infer that children born by elective caesarean section are traumatised and don't 'bond'. I am as wonderful a mother as I could ever hoped to have been and am as close to my children as anyone.

CHAPTER FIVE

Motherhood

'The next time you read about Sarah Jessica Parker's perfect marriage and motherhood, don't sigh and say "Oh, I wish that was my life". Instead, say "Give me a break."'

Susan Douglas and Meredith Michaels (2004)

The term 'transition' is used in social science literature when describing a period of significant change, either positive or negative, in a person's life. For example, if you get married, move house or experience the death of a loved one, you will experience strong emotions and will naturally undergo a period whereby you adjust to your new life. Perhaps one of the most common (and significant) transitions for women is the move to motherhood. Making the decision to become a mother, being pregnant and bringing a life into the world is an emotionally charged experience. For some, this is a process to be embraced and happily incorporated into the new identity of 'mother'; for others, the ride is not so smooth.

Perhaps one of the strongest influencing factors for women during their transition to motherhood is the way in which mothers are portrayed in the media. Gossip magazines sell pictures of impeccably groomed celebrities looking slim and gorgeous, effortlessly juggling their movie star careers with children. Stars themselves often gush about how motherhood is more important than their careers and that becoming a mother has forever changed their lives for the better. Yet the reality of motherhood is quite different to the idealised existence portrayed by magazines. Without the entourage of helpers available to public figures, real women cannot hope to live up to the slim, well-rested images of 'perfection' they are constantly confronted with. Sadly, not only do women judge themselves against this false premise, they also judge each other.

Women are judged on countless issues regarding motherhood, as many of the stories in this book make evident. But most of these judgements can be boiled down to arguments about 'good' and 'bad' mothers. According to the standards set by society, 'good' mothers are always happy, never upset or angry, and always put themselves last. 'Good' mothers look fantastic while juggling careers with home life. 'Bad' mothers let their babies cry, don't breastfeed and go back to work straight after having their babies. Fortunately, there are voices of reason counteracting these unhelpful stereotypes. Books like *The Mommy Myth, The Mask of Motherhood* and *I Was a Really Good Mom Before I Had Kids* challenge the new cultural ideal of the 'supermum'.

The accounts from real women in this chapter also help set the record straight. Bodies do not 'bounce back' within four weeks of birth, motherhood is not always mentally stimulating, and women struggle daily with their parenting decisions. Every mother who tells their story in this chapter loves her children unconditionally—there is no doubt about that. But this does not mean that their lives are perfect and it certainly doesn't mean they are perfect mothers, for there is no such creature.

In this chapter, you will hear from women who discuss their feelings on the transition to motherhood and how becoming a mother forced them to re-think who they were and how the new role of 'mother' fitted into their lives. You will also read about the challenges facing women regarding work and family life—to stay at home and be the primary carer or go back to work? You will hear from women who experienced postnatal depression and how they managed their illness, as well as stories about 'mother guilt', the common leveller of many mothers. What unites these women is not the structure of their family lives or the way they parent; it is the pressure to be the 'perfect' mother, to always 'get it right'.

Learning about real motherhood is inspirational: far from the Vaseline-smeared image of motherhood, you will see that today's mothers are incredibly resourceful; they think deeply about every aspect of parenting and love their children fiercely, even on bad days. They face major challenges and still manage to come out on top, without the assistance of 'staff'.

It is hoped that you read the stories of these women and take comfort in the fact that everyone finds motherhood a tough gig at times. That doesn't make you a 'bad' mother, it just makes you a real one.

Identity

Women's concept of self is multidimensional and complex. Often, a woman's identity is shaped by her social roles, such as worker, daughter, partner and friend. Given that becoming a mother is such a life-changing event, it is not surprising that this new role can play havoc with a woman's sense of identity. It can leave her reeling in shock ('What the hell is happening to me?'), fear ('I can't do this') and even grief ('I want my life back, please'). Women respond to motherhood in many different ways; some find the transition a smooth one, while others find the ride bumpy and emotional. Your identity will always be a work in progress, and figuring out who you are once you become a mother is also a matter of time and patience.

Give me The Cure: Learning how to remember who you are in the midst of motherhood

Rebecca has three children and has learned that she didn't need to lose all sense of her old 'self' to be a good mother.

Rebecca's Story

Before I had children, I was on the way up. I had completed two university degrees and had worked in several countries establishing my career; a career that I loved and was passionate about. During this time, I also met the love of my life. The moment I saw his long hair and his worn-out leather jacket, I was sunk. We spent our years travelling—we trekked around Nepal, we breakfasted in Austria and we spent a year living in Ireland together. In between our travelling bouts, we lazed around our Bondi flat or graced the local café with our presence when we eventually climbed out of bed. If we were feeling particularly energetic, we visited mates or drank at our favourite pub. Life of leisure? You bet.

But when I hit 30, I started hankering for a family. Before I knew it, having a baby was all I could think about. He wasn't so sure; he wasn't ready. I was. Very. I remember crying a lot because, at the ripe old age of 30, I truly believed that time was running out for me. And so it went until one day, back in Australia, Gordon asked me to marry him. Not so long after that night, we were standing at the kitchen sink, smoking furiously while we waited to see if the pregnancy test I had bought turned positive. It did. We were stunned (seriously, we couldn't believe that sex had actually led to pregnancy). I put out my cigarette.

When the shock wore off, I was so excited about the prospect of becoming a mother. And when my gorgeous Sarah was born, I threw myself into the mothering role. I had given up my job and my career for this. I had also given up daily showers, washing my hair and, apparently, any sense of Rebecca. In my desperate bid to take care of Sarah, I just assumed that all of my needs should come last, if at all. So what if my daily attire was a pair of daggy tracksuit pants, no make-up and hair combed back so no one could see how dirty it was? This was my job now. I lost all sense of moderation. Had I not received intervention from my husband, I might well have made it past the 'no-showers' stage but then quite blindly moved on to the 'perfect mum' stage with that same, dogged determination that left my own needs at the bottom of the pile.

But around the three-month mark, Gordon cottoned on to what was happening and booted me out of the house, despite my protests ('But I have to feed her in a few hours!', 'But what if she wakes up and wants me?') Reluctantly, I showered, washed my hair, put on some make-up and decent clothes, and went for a drive. I remember turning up The Cure as loudly as possible. It felt good, evocative. A man pulled up next to me at the lights and evidently liked what he saw. Pre-Sarah, I would have ignored him but this look, this glance of approval, was like a flicker of light; it reminded me that I was not just a milk machine. I was not the sum total of the nappies I changed. I was, somewhere in there, still Rebecca.

That was the first time I realised that maybe I didn't have to throw out the baby with the bath water. I could be Rebecca the mother and Rebecca the Cure-loving, lipstick-wearing, conservative-loathing, armchair polemicist. Only problem? I wasn't sure how that was possible. I wasn't even sure if it was possible. Was it possible to wear miniskirts, say the 'f' word a lot, feel like a 20-year-old and be a responsible mother as well? Wasn't I meant to bake cakes and sing nursery rhymes, preferably in a twin set and pearls? Of course it is possible to be yourself and be a mum at the same time. But it was a hard lesson for me to learn and it was a long one in the making.

I am now mother, not only to my graceful and loving Sarah, but also to my fairy-loving, angel-haired Zoë and to my Ollie Wobble Bliss Bomb. Without undermining myself or my capabilities as a mother, I have managed to embrace my role as mother and retain a sense of self. I guess there are certain, obvious things that help me integrate my new and old self. An example that springs to mind is the dance parties I have with my kids. Just the other day, I put on Dee-Lite's 'Groove is in the Heart' and let loose. It's not a nightclub and I'm not drinking shots but I get to do my thing while deriving the unbelievable pleasure of watching all three of my kids (aged four and under) dance around like lunatics.

Instead of always cooking from scratch (OK, I never cook from scratch anymore), I often enjoy freshly re-heated pizzas with my kids and have great fun mucking around in the sand with them. I may not know many nursery rhymes, but I know every lyric George Michael ever sang and, believe it or not, my babies never seemed to mind the difference. So in this way, I've managed to have fun with my children while staying stay true to myself.

That said, it is equally important for me to have my own moments; moments where I don't integrate my new and old self—moments when I can just be me. These moments are rare but they are precious to me. Like when I dress up and go to a restaurant with my husband and all talk of children is banned after the first five minutes of conversation. Like when I go shopping, on my own, try on ridiculously priced dresses, and then buy them. Or when I spend one hour by myself, browsing through a bookstore, unhindered by nappies that need changing and babies who need feeding.

I have learned to turn situations with my kids to everyone's advantage and I have learned to take time to nurture myself. Both of these things I do to retain a sense of self (and sanity). But I have also learned (as most mothers will tell you) that it is not all about me. Just as I need my own space and my own moments, I need to create moments and space that are just for the kids. So you will hear me singing Twinkle Twinkle for the umpteenth *time on any given day. You will see me colouring in endless fairies and butterflies (always in the same colours, for fairies only ever come in pink and gold, according to Zoë) and you will see me on my hands and knees picking up bits of playdough after an especially enthusiastic session. And yes, you will probably see me in my pyjamas on many a day. But most importantly, you'll see a mum who has learned that when it comes to identity, you can have your cupcake and eat it too.*

Rebecca's Wisdom

It's easy to allow motherhood to gobble you up and spit you back out as a Stepford Wife if you let it. But if you're in any way like me and want to retain part of your old self, as well as honouring and valuing your new role as 'mother', then you need to be conscious of the process that is taking place. For me, that process was acknowledging my life as being distinctly different pre- and post-children.

I think that our identity, our sense of self, is made up of many different things. It's important to remember that taking on a new role doesn't necessarily mean your whole identity needs to be different. Roles are fluid and change over time and with events; each new role that we take on (or have thrust upon us), needs to be integrated into our sense of identity.

My roles (mother, wife, friend, author) do not define who I am as a person. Much as I may love a particular role (and 'mother' is right up there with 'author'), I try to remember that I am not just the cookies I bake or the books I churn out. I am Rebecca.

Excuse me, is your sense of identity changing? Finding peace with motherhood

Heidi thinks of herself as a mother first and foremost, but has learned to balance this role with other parts of her identity.

Heidi's Story

I started to feel a change in my sense of identity a few weeks after the shock of having a newborn had worn off. But I was very surprised to feel the exact same effect after I had my second baby. Why would it happen again, when I'd already been through such a deep change? For me, it must be more than just in my head, maybe a primitive, instinctual change; like the fabric of my being was being re-woven to incorporate a new life.

I thought about it a lot. I wasn't especially happy about it. It was an all-consuming transformation that I wasn't in control of. I definitely struggled to adjust to the whole thing but didn't really express it. I felt like I was the only one going through this experience. And no-one really talks about it. You can't just walk up to another mum in the parents' room and say 'So, is your sense of identity changing?' I felt lost. Both my babies slept and ate well, and were generally 'good'. I could cope with them. But I had trouble coping with what was going on inside my head. I began to think that going to work was the answer, where I would be normal. But when I had my first baby I was forced back to work very early and it was definitely the wrong place for me. I was quite depressed but didn't admit it. By the second time, I knew that I just had to ride through the transformation until it was complete.

I felt that everything had changed for me, especially my relationship with my husband. I couldn't even go to the toilet when I wanted to, whereas my husband was still able to do whatever he wanted all the time. I'll never forget one day when I was at home alone when my first baby was only a few weeks old. I had been counting the hours until my husband came home. He came straight home from work and promptly told me that he was going out. I burst into tears because I couldn't ever leave. He still went. He doesn't remember it now at all but it was such an obvious demonstration of where both our lives were. To me, he seemed to be so free. I was jealous but couldn't change my position.

With my second baby, I was better able to express what I was going through and could put together the words that my identity was changing. I tried to explain to my husband that all I had room for in my head was the children and that I simply didn't have much space for him right now. He didn't feel a change in identity at all; he simply went about his usual day. I feel some resentment against him for this, that he sometimes acts like he doesn't have kids. I could never act like that because they are part of me.

Although I fought against the change in the beginning, now I think that it's made me a better parent. I'm very strongly attached and bonded to my children. I have now embraced my role. I'm a mum first and foremost but am also able to balance that with other identity-defining activities, such as part-time work (that I love), spending time with my husband and time for me to read (which is how I relax). I think it's important to find that balance between being a mum and being me, which takes some figuring out.

Heidi's Wisdom	I don't think there's really any way to fully prepare for having a baby. If you think you know what to expect, you're probably wrong. Read and talk to others as much as you can but everyone's experience is different.

Missing me: How will I ever get my life back?

Silvana is in the early stages of her motherhood journey. Wary of jumping into motherhood in the first place, Silvana has fought feelings of anger and grief for the loss of her old self. She wonders how she can ever get her old life back and feels cheated that her friends didn't warn her of the journey she was about to embark upon.

Silvana's Story

One of the main reasons it took me so long to want to have a baby was because I was nervous about losing my 'self'. I had an amazing career, had conquered past weight issues and was happy with my own identity; an identity that I felt did not need to include motherhood. My husband has a great job in the music industry that is not very family-friendly and I was worried about being the wife at home while he was out partying. I needed a lot of assurances from him that this would not be the case before I felt confident enough to be pregnant and still be me.

I started to feel a change in my sense of identity when I was pregnant. I hated what pregnancy did to my body and this really affected my sense of identity and self. I was used to being in control of my life and that included my body and my weight. When Carla was born, however, I found that my sense of self changed even more. I felt lost and depressed. I felt overwhelmed that I was stuck with this baby forever. I know this sounds terrible but that is the truth. It didn't mean I didn't love my daughter, but I was not prepared for how the responsibility of having a child would make me feel so trapped. I felt like running away.

I was now a mother and that was it. I felt I could not marry the two roles of mother and career woman together. I had lots of people, including family and health professionals, telling me what to do in the first couple of weeks and while some of it was helpful, I also felt overwhelmed and lost.

I found this change very hard. I grieved for my old self and I continue to grieve for my old self. But the older that Carla gets, the easier it is to connect my old self with my new self. I do believe the older you are when you have a baby, the harder the issue of identity becomes. You have been this person your whole life and then you have a baby and your life is totally changed. My partner was extremely supportive but I do think he was a little shocked in those first few weeks when he saw how badly I felt about my new role and how I was coping with it. I was very worried about him seeing me differently. I wanted him to still see me as the sexy and confident woman he married; not as this depressed, bloated, sobbing woman. I had unrealistic expectations of how I should look and feel post-birth and this only made me feel worse. My partner did everything right in trying to make me feel good and it's only now (12 weeks post-birth) that I believe him.

I miss everything every day. I am hoping this fades over time. It is still too recent for me to have forgotten my old life and the 'old' me. I really miss sleep but I also miss time for me and time for us. At the moment, I don't see how I will be able to find time for me ever again. But I know it should get better. Both my partner and I struggle with parenthood. There have been moments when we have both thought we might have made a mistake. How will this baby fit into our lives? But then we look at Carla and fall in love again.

Silvana's Wisdom	I think it's important for people to tell the truth about what parenthood is really like. After Carla was born, I gave some of my friends a hard time for not telling me the truth about how difficult it is. I think I would have been better prepared emotionally if I had known how tough the first couple of months are; how you are struggling with parenthood while your body is still recovering from labour. I think people don't tell the truth as they don't want to scare people off parenthood but I think it's better to know than not.

Is it normal to feel so overwhelmed?

Yes. Many studies investigating how mothers cope with motherhood have been carried out. Nyström and Öhrling (2004) conducted a literature review in order to reveal some of the feelings expressed by new mothers. They discovered that the underlying theme in all the literature they reviewed was that parents were 'living in a new and overwhelming world' (p. 319). The authors found that while mothers expressed feelings of satisfaction and love, they also expressed many negative emotions. For example, mothers often felt powerless and inadequate, and expressed feelings of loss, anger, guilt and exhaustion. Women often felt unprepared for what it would be like to be a mother and reported feeling disappointed, lonely and isolated. Mothers also stated that they felt 'tied up' and more restricted since the birth of their baby.

Some people reading Silvana's story may feel shocked to read that she felt 'stuck with this baby forever'. However, Silvana should be applauded for her candour, as many women feel exactly the same way. In the same literature review noted above, Nyström and Öhrling also found that women expressed awareness that 'life had changed and there was no turning back' (p. 326). If you are feeling like Silvana, take heart in the fact that many women feel like this at some point. But also remember that becoming a mother is a process and a journey; it is not an instant transition. There will come a time when you figure out what being a mother means to you.

If you become so overwhelmed that you feel you cannot look after yourself or your baby, you should seek outside help, in the form of a counsellor, psychologist or social worker. You may be experiencing symptoms of postnatal depression and it is important to ensure that if this is the case, it is detected and treated early. For a list of organisations and information, please see page 258 of the Resources section.

Working mums and stay-at-home mums

Whether a mother decides to stay at home with her children or return to work should be a simple matter of choice. Unfortunately, it almost never is. Like many of the issues discussed in this book, the question of mothers in (or out of) the workplace has become a topic of media debate and judgement, to the extent that it has been dubbed 'the mommy wars'. The mommy wars dispute, put simply, asks: 'Who is the better mommy, the stay-at-home mom or the working mom?' (Zimmerman et al. 2008, p. 204). Described as 'facile' by Stone and Lovejoy (2004, p. 64) and a 'convenient way to divert the dialogue away from real issues' by Zimmerman et al. (2008, p. 204), the mommy wars are essentially a falsely reductionist argument. As Zimmerman notes, the discussion neglects issues such as 'affordable health care, quality childcare, gender and racial equality, fathers' roles in parenting, media effects, fair wages and benefits, and family-friendly work arrangements' (p. 204), and pits working mothers against those who stay at home.

The question of going back to work is a complex one, often involving difficult emotional and financial issues. The stories in this section reflect the challenges faced by many mums. Roshini decided, after much agonising, to stay at home to look after her child while her partner stayed at work. Mei felt she was forced back to work too early and experienced a great deal of distress as a result. Celia couldn't wait to get back to work so she could reclaim some adult interaction and sanity. All of these women made choices that involved emotional or financial hardship of some kind, and none of their choices were as straightforward as the mommy wars make them out to be.

A feminist act: Exercising the choice to be a stay-at-home mum

Roshini initially grappled with the idea of staying at home because she felt she was letting the feminist team down. However, after reading more on the subject, she realised this wasn't the case.

Roshini's Story

I have always wanted to be a mother. I enjoyed being pregnant and started maternity leave four weeks before our baby was due. We had planned for me to take 12 months off work but were open to the idea that this might change, although I didn't know how long we could afford to live on one income.

As time passed, the need to make a decision became larger in my mind. At that stage, I could not imagine placing my son in day care. Sam had only been cared for by his grandparents once or twice, for a few hours at a time with me close by. He was still breastfeeding regularly and he needed my help to go to sleep. I couldn't imagine how a day carer could look after five babies like him at once—I found it hard to meet all his needs and I only had him! So we agreed that we would not enrol him in formal day care until he was at least two years old.

I considered going back to work part-time, but after paying for childcare, we would only be $100 or so in front. My work hours could be long and unpredictable, which would make juggling childcare pickups, dinner and bedtime hard. Initially, I felt I was letting the feminist team down by giving up my career. But after reading more from the perspective of maternal feminism, I now strongly feel that being a stay-at-home mother can be a feminist act too. I don't think the solution for women's liberation is for all kids to be in day care from when they are young. Longer term maternity leave, more men taking time off work to look after kids and financial support for stay-at-home parents are all ways to support women's needs as well as children's needs.

I had to think of what it meant for me to not have a career (for a while), which is a big part of many people's identity. I was a high-achiever at school and university, and prior to having my son, I'd worked in social work—which a lot of people thought was enough of a step down, when I had the marks to be a lawyer! Dropping out to be a stay-at-home mum seemed unthinkable. People sometimes said things to me along the lines of, 'It's OK for mothers who have no other option to do this, but you could do anything—it's such a waste.' I find this attitude insulting, as it implies looking after children is not hard or important work. In fact, I think it is one of the hardest things you can do, especially if you want to do it well.

There are still days when I feel guilty or worry that I am being lazy or a cop-out, thinking that because I don't have a paid job maybe I am just a layabout not contributing anything to society. But when I look back at my day, there's not much time when I am sitting on my arse doing nothing! Just because my work is not paid, it does not render it worthless. For many of our middle class friends and family, a career is supposed to bring you happiness, however the reality is that for many people, work is just a job. My partner feels differently— she would still rock up every day if she won the lotto, and sees her work as a vocation. I think she is very lucky to be working in a career she is passionate about. I have come to realise that for me, motherhood is my vocation—I enjoy it, it's something I am passionate about and that I would like to do every day for the rest of my life.

Roshini's Wisdom

Sam is now 16 months old and a lot has changed in the last few months in terms of him being ready to be apart from me—he is much more outgoing during the day and has happily spent a whole day with extended family. I think giving him that time and not rushing him has helped. However, I still know that I am the best carer for him. No one else knows him inside out the way I do. The attention and love that comes from being his parent could not be matched by anyone else—from the silly games and cuddles we have, through to analysing the contents of his nappies. Just by being his mum, I feel I am giving him the best care possible.

How much money is a stay-at-home mum worth?

According to a report published by Salary.com (Hanrahan 2008), a stay-at-home mum (SAHM) was worth approximately US$116 805 (that's approximately €92 000 or A$134 000) per year. To calculate this figure, Salary.com looked at ten jobs that most SAHMs do each day: housekeeper, childcare centre teacher, cook, computer operator, laundry machine operator, janitor, facilities manager, van driver, CEO and psychologist. In calculating a mother's wages, they also considered the overtime that would be put in by mums: a whopping 52 hours each week.

If you want to find out what you're worth as a SAHM today (in US dollars), you can use the personal calculator on their website: <www.mom.salary.com>. The next time someone asks you 'What do you *do* all day?', hand them the list of jobs as well as your estimated worth—that should give them food for thought!

Not happy: Going back to paid work when the timing isn't right

Although Mei was officially back at work when her daughter was six months old, she found that work intruded on her daily life before this, probably because her place of work is the family business.

Mei's Story

Grace was six months old when I went back to work. I didn't necessarily decide to go back to work. My work was the family business. I supported my husband in his career, and ran his practice. For that very reason, he insisted I return to work, as he wasn't coping with me not being there to help. I really felt as though I was guilted back into returning to work earlier than I wanted or felt ready to. This was incredibly distressing for me, as I really did not want to leave Grace in care. I was worried, like any mother, I guess, that the carers wouldn't look after her like I could; that she might fret for me, or worse I'd fret for her and not be able to concentrate on my work. I was very angry with Rick for putting me in a situation that I didn't want to be in. I was even angrier with myself for not having the balls to stand by my intention of not returning to work until Grace was at least a year old.

We went to two different childcare centres that had available spaces (most places we rang were full), and the centre we went for was very friendly and had a great attitude towards the children. They were helpful and encouraging and made it easy for me to leave her there on workdays without any anxiety. Grace has been at the same centre for two and a half years. From there, she'll be going to primary school, hopefully with well established friendships. She loves the carers and can't wait to see them on her childcare days. That speaks volumes for me.

Balancing work and family life was a 'two steps forwards, one step back' situation for a very long time. I felt that I was always working or looking after Grace or running after the stepchildren. Work often came home with us—I received numerous phone calls at home and there were many times in the first six months that I was in the office on my days off because instruments weren't found, machines weren't working and help was needed.

I often felt guilty both at work and at home. While I was at work, I was often thinking of Grace and wondering if she was OK. I was also exhausted from lack of sleep, so I knew work was no longer getting all of my attention and dedication. I also felt guilty when at home, because I wasn't at work, or I was wishing I was at work if Grace and I weren't having a good day together.

At some point, I finally said 'enough is enough' and managed to close the office doors at the end of the day, walk away and say 'That's it, that's all I can do for now'. While I'm a great planner—scheduling in and working by the family calendar—emotionally I was stuffed. I was running on empty and would have meltdowns every couple of months. I often have difficulty asking for help, so that's been a big lesson in achieving balance. Get help, don't be shy and definitely don't be embarrassed about asking for help.

Mei's Wisdom

Family for me is the ultimate. Work will (generally) always be there. Jobs can be completed by others. Precious moments lost with your family can never be regained. Relax the rules and remember to take time out. So what if dinner is on the table ten minutes late? Be with the ones you love and love the moment you are in.

Loving motherhood, loving work: The decision to return to work

Celia couldn't wait to return to work outside the home. While she thoroughly enjoys being a mother, Celia also enjoys the company of adults and found that returning to work helped her to be a happier mother.

Celia's Story

I went back to full-time work when my son was 13 weeks old. Part of it was financial—we were saving for a house and losing one income meant losing about 35–40 per cent of our joint earnings. The other part was emotional. While I am not in love with my job, I enjoy working. The three months I spent at home with Alex drove me nuts. I need adult interaction, which I found sorely lacking while on maternity leave. By the time I got to the end of my maternity leave, I found myself checking my work emails and looking forward to picking up where I left off. So yes, I loved returning to work. I had been looking forward to it; I hated staying at home.

I was very lucky. I got a spot in the childcare centre of our choice. I had to take the spot two weeks earlier than I wanted as one became available, but that was OK as it worked out for us with a longer settling in period. In the first two weeks, I'd leave Alex there for an hour or two each day although I was paying for the full day. As he got used to the carers and the routine, the duration became longer. I could not be happier with our childcare arrangements. Being so close to my office means that I can see him at lunchtime. It also means that they can call me anytime, knowing that I can be there within ten minutes.

Balancing work and family life has worked out quite well for us. My husband drops Alex off at day care most of the time on his way to work and either he or I pick Alex up in the evenings. I now work from home, so I can easily have dinner ready by the time the boys get home. Even when I pick Alex up, we are able to have dinner by 6.45 pm, and Alex bathed and ready for bed by about 8 pm. We have a routine and it seldom changes. The housework is shared between us, and now that Alex is older, he can help too.

I never felt any guilt going back to work, as I like working and think I am a more balanced and sane mother because of it. If Alex were to be my full-time job, I think I would be much more impatient, angry and perhaps even resentful. It really helps that I am confident in the centre Alex attends and know that he is well cared for there. The carers love Alex and he has grown rather fond of them too.

The housework doesn't always get done but there is always food on the table and clean clothes to wear. We now have a cleaner who comes once a fortnight to do the floors and bathrooms. Everything else gets done when we have time and energy. Being able to work and be a mother at the same time depends on support from the children and your partner as well. You can't do it all on your own as there is no such thing as Superwoman.

Celia's Wisdom	I have learned that the best I can do is what is right for my family. I do not need to comply with someone else's standard of parenting and mothering to be a good mother and wife. It's OK for some families to have stay-at-home mums, and others to have working-at-home mums, and yet others to have mothers working outside the home, as long as that's right for that family and the wheels keep turning. Every family is unique.

Tips for returning to work

According to the Raising Children Network (2006), there are valuable things you can do to help you to balance your new family life. For instance, packing children's lunches and bags and ironing and laying out clothes can be done the night before so that the mornings aren't so rushed. Another great tip is to try batch cooking, which minimises effort during the working week and is something you can do with your kids on the weekend. Get them involved in cooking batches of meals and then freeze them for later use. If you find a rhythm, you should stick to it. Kids thrive on routines and tend to behave better when everything happens in generally the same way each day (which makes for a happier family).

If you are sending your child to care, you should have someone reliable whom you can contact at short notice for 'backup'. If your child becomes sick and needs to be collected but you're unable to leave the office, contact your backup and ask them to help you out. Having someone as backup can really help to relieve some pressure and give you peace of mind. You should also consider visiting your child at care (popping in for quick visits can be reassuring for some children), tackling any questions you have about your child's care as quickly as possible, developing a good relationship with your child's carer and letting them know in advance about any changes in your schedule.

It's also a good idea to try and leave work at work and concentrate on your children when you are at home. It can be difficult, but endeavour to switch off your Blackberry and shut your laptop down when you finish work. Wherever you are (work or home), be there, in the present. You cannot be everything to everyone all the time. If you try to live life at such a fast pace, you are more prone to burning out. Delegate wherever possible, both at home and at work, and when the kids are in bed (if you're not too exhausted) sink into a hot bath, read your favourite book or spend time relaxing with your partner or a friend.

Lastly, let go of the guilt: You are not harming your family by returning to work. A recent longitudinal study conducted by Cooksey et al. (2009) has found that 'Despite public opinion to the contrary [there is] little evidence of harm to school-age children from maternal employment during a child's infancy, especially if employment is part-time and in a context … where several months of maternity leave are the norm' (p. 115).

Mother guilt

Mother guilt is the all-pervasive occupational hazard of motherhood. Mothers want what's best for their children but 'best' is often unattainable and for this, mothers blame themselves. The range of issues and events mothers blame themselves for is endless; mothers can feel guilty about everything, from not having enough milk in the fridge, to giving their child a lollipop in the supermarket, to losing their temper and fearing they have scarred their child for life.

Hopefully, by reading these stories (and others throughout the book that refer to parents' feelings of guilt and self-doubt), you will realise that you are not alone. The trick is to figure out why you are feeling guilty. If you believe you have done something wrong (such as shouting at your child), then apologise and let go. You are only human. Of course, if you shout at your child often and you find that you are constantly feeling angry and frustrated, then you need support so that both you and your children remain safe and your quality of life improves.

If, however, you are feeling guilty for not living up to 'societal standards' of parenting (i.e. giving your child that lollipop in the supermarket), perhaps you should re-think your guilt. Societal standards are often unattainable and can put immense pressure on women to live up to the notion of the 'perfect' parent. But nobody is perfect. If you are still feeling as though you don't measure up, you are encouraged to read (or re-read) the introduction to this book, where the myth of the perfect parent is discussed in detail.

No such thing as a perfect mum: Accepting that 'good enough' is good enough

Keiko's story touches on so many issues mothers feel guilty about: 'losing it' when pushed just an inch too far, worrying about things you can't control, and worrying about things you think you can control.

Keiko's Story

I don't have to think too hard about the last time I felt guilty as a mum. In fact, it was yesterday morning. My husband had left for work, I was at home with my two sons who are three and four-and-a-half, and I was already in a pretty bad mood for some inexplicable reason. It was just a little trigger that set me off. Thomas, my eldest, demanded milk and biscuits—something I often give them—but yesterday I had a fight in me. I asked him to use his manners and he, testing the limits, said 'no'. Christopher joined in the request for biscuits, but he asked with a very whiney voice. This scenario went on repeatedly for about four minutes and eventually I cracked.

I stomped up to the kitchen, got them a biscuit and milk, anger rising with every jerky move I made. I threw the biscuits on the ground in front of them and yelled in a mean voice 'There, eat them, NOW—if you want to be rude then I'm going to be rude too'. Yes, it was a very immature parenting moment and unfortunately not a once-off. Thomas burst into tears and Christopher ate his biscuit. I knew I needed to leave the room and call someone.

Talking with my husband was calming and helped put things back into perspective. As I realised I was guilty of not looking after own my needs (will I ever learn this one?), my inexplicable bad mood became clearer to me. Together we worked out how I could get some 'me' time. I felt a big dose of guilt for not being the bigger, wiser and older person in the situation with the boys, but I did make amends with them.

I believe this sort of guilt, which rises quickly in me and falls away just as fast, is OK. Perhaps it is better described as remorse. Such remorse can give me the impetus to take responsibility and change what I'm doing. It is tolerable and probably even necessary, provided it is soon followed by self-forgiveness.

There have been times when guilt has applied pressure on the choices I have made. Not wanting to add to the environmental problems associated with landfill, I invested in some of the latest fitted cloth nappies for my first baby. Reading the websites when pregnant, it all sounded wonderful and my self-esteem was soaring as I thought about what a virtuous mother I would be. Unfortunately, Thomas proved to be frequent poo-er, with an average of six poo nappies a day; he was eventually diagnosed by my paediatrician as having toddler diarrhoea. Then Christopher was born. My soaking buckets overflowed and washing line was never empty. My life seemed to be all about poo. At this point, I gave up, went to the supermarket, and bought boxes of disposable nappies. I felt the guilt—not only because I was now (excuse the cliché) part of the problem rather than the solution, but also about the judgemental thoughts I had directed towards all those mothers with disposable nappies in their shopping trolleys. How humbling motherhood can be.

Perhaps the hardest blow inflicted by guilt was with breastfeeding. I diligently breastfed both by my sons months past their first birthdays, but to this day I question whether breast was best for Thomas and me. The first months were truly torturous. Not just as he fed, which would take an hour at a time, delayed by my fear of the latch-on and his little mouth not doing what a string of lactation consultants said it should. But between feeds my nipples would burn—I remember describing it as like having two cigarette lighters held under each nipple. And my breasts would ache—sounds weird, but it was similar to having a headache but in my breast tissue. I was told I had nipple vasospasm or Raynaud's phenomenon, a condition where the blood does not properly circulate around the nipples and they go white. It is exacerbated by the cold (Thomas was born at the start of winter). None of the suggested treatments made any difference. When Thomas was about six months old, the weather was warmer and breastfeeding him was finally on track.

I did not want to give up breastfeeding, as I so desperately wanted to give him 'the best'. I feared failure, being judged and the subsequent guilt. But ironically, this chapter in my life has still left me with some insidious guilt. Thomas feared separating from me from a very young age and today still struggles with saying goodbye. In my rational moods, I know this could be because of a multitude of reasons and I focus on working calmly with him to conquer his fear. But in darker moments, I worry that I caused his anxiety by struggling with him, literally, at the same time I was giving him his life-sustaining milk. A bitter thought fills me that no matter how hard I tried to give him the best, harm was still done. It's confirmed in my head: I'm a flawed mother.

But I know this punishing guilt is really unhelpful and keeps me stuck. How useless to torment myself with critical and shaming thoughts that solve nothing and only create misery in my life.

Keiko's Wisdom	Herein lies my antidote to guilt and my bit of wisdom. I believe the rhetoric that mothers need only be 'good enough'. I'm not perfect—nowhere near. I'm aiming to catch myself being a crappy mum (which I definitely can be) a little faster so I can quickly put things right, but I expect many slip-ups—forever really! And with that expectation, together with a bit of gentle compassion for myself, guilt visits, but doesn't stay too long.

Not guilty as charged: Learning the difference between good and bad guilt

Tanya talks about her feelings of mother guilt and how all-pervasive her negative self-talk can be. Her story illustrates the two types of guilt discussed in the introduction to this section: guilt for making a mistake and guilt for not living up to the expectations of society.

Tanya's Story

Mother guilt is definitely the most difficult aspect of parenting I have found so far and is also the one that is the hardest to talk about. I don't want to admit that I have lost it at my three-year-old for throwing a major tantrum because I turned the TV off. But I did. I picked him up, sat him on his bed and made him watch me as I picked up all of his toys and put them in a massive black garbage bag. He was hysterical and I was fed up.

The aftermath of that guilt was very intense. I felt guilty about what sort of a memory that might have created for him. Would he, ten or fifteen years from now, remember the day mum lost it and threw out all of his toys? Have I left deep scars on his impressionable young brain? And why did I react so furiously?

While this moment was one of the most intense I've had so far, bringing home his brother has brought with it a batch of guilt-inducing moments. When I first brought Ryan home, I didn't have much (if any) time to take Ben out for a play in the park or somewhere special because it was either too cold for the baby or he was sleeping or feeding.

Looking after two very young children, I became very sleep-deprived and was easily irritated. It wasn't necessarily about my three-year-old and his demands for my attention; it was more because I felt so inadequate as a mother and that I felt I had failed him somewhat. Why couldn't we go out? Other mums do. Why couldn't I seem to get out of my pyjamas before noon? Other mums do. Why couldn't I find time to draw or paint with my son? Other mums do.

Our relationship changed so quickly and so dramatically when Ryan was born that I was completely unprepared for it. I felt guilty that I wasn't coping and was taking a lot of my frustration out on Ben by yelling and (a few times) smacking the back of his hand. On those really bad days, I would cry at night because of the intense emotional pain I felt and the hatred I had for myself. Why had I become the type of parent I never wanted to be?

The guilt I have can be quite consuming. I see other parents with young babies and older kids and wonder if they ever have days where they feel the same as me or are they always as happy and calm as they appear to be?

I still have days where I feel out of control and try to remind myself that I am a good mum and that I am doing the best I can. My son is respectful and polite. He is fun to be with and most of all, he is happy, which tells me I can't be doing that bad a job.

Tanya's Wisdom	Admittedly, some days we fight about everything and by the end of the day, my patience has run out and I find myself starting to yell a bit. Yet other days feel near perfect.
	I am very hard on myself and I may be my own worst enemy but I am learning and I know I will always be thrown new challenges that ultimately can only make me a better parent. Perhaps if I didn't have any guilt, it would indicate that I didn't care and was unwilling to learn how to be the best mum for my sons.

When guilt has a purpose

As noted by Menesini and Camodeca (2008), there is a common agreement that guilt is an adaptive emotion; it is linked to empathy, responsibility and internalisation of rules. Put simply, 'normal' (or healthy) guilt can regulate your behaviour and enhance your social competence. In a way, it is like an in-built warning system that lets you know when you have acted against your own set of values and beliefs. For example, if you don't believe in corporal punishment for children, yet you lose your temper and smack your child, you will probably feel guilty. This is because the act of smacking your child does not fit with your own values. This type of guilt is quite handy (and healthy), as it can alert you when you're veering off course. It follows that if you feel a lot of guilt, you may well be veering off course quite a bit.

One useful example to illustrate the theory of healthy guilt is the issue of smacking your child, particularly if you have decided this is something you are not comfortable with. If you smack your child once because you have lost your temper, you will probably feel guilty. A good thing to do is 'note' your guilt, apologise to your child for smacking them and then let that guilt go. However, if you are smacking your child a lot, you will probably feel a more pervasive guilt. This is a 'red flag' and you should pay attention to it, especially if you are smacking in anger. Unchecked anger can cause serious emotional and physical damage to both you and your child. If you find yourself feeling angry a lot of the time, it is vital that you seek help so that your children remain safe. For further information and resources, please see page 256 of the Resources section.

Different shades of guilt: From the blackness of death to the colour of vegies

Kylie has moments of guilt where she feels she doesn't measure up to the standards of motherhood set by society, but she feels most guilty about her decision to bring a child into the world, knowing that her partner has cancer.

Kylie's Story

My biggest guilt is the fact that I brought a child into the world knowing her father won't see her grow up. I have suffered agonies over this and feel that I've been very selfish in this decision. I'm sure many would say 'At least she had a father' or 'At least she's making some memories' but what about the future pain I'm causing her by losing her daddy? And that day will come. Will I be strong enough to help her through this? Will I have answers to the questions she's bound to have?

But mother guilt also comes in more 'normal' guises for me as well. For example, I've caught myself losing my temper in a big way. After a frustrating day at work, I was too tired to pick up a cranky daughter who just wanted her mummy. I was under pressure to get dinner ready and do so many things that I just lost it. I ranted at her and stood her in the corner and when she came out and smacked me, I smacked her in return. It makes me blush even now when I think about it. We both ended on the kitchen floor in tears. It was pitiful. I apologised to Grace profusely for smacking her on the bottom and told her over and over again that I did love her, would go to the moon and back for her, but I had gotten too angry and had lost control. I told her it was no excuse, but I would work hard to rectify the situation, and try never to do that again. Bless her though, she appeared to shrug it off and forgive me; I don't think to this day that I've forgiven myself. I am more aware now, or at least try to be aware of what I'm saying and doing, and walking away from a situation with her so I don't blow a fuse. I count myself down to a calmer space to deal with the real issue in a better way.

On a smaller scale, I feel I don't feed her enough or encourage her enough to try vegetables and new meals. It's hard enough arguing with her father and half-siblings to eat anything considered healthy; I seem to have no energy to help her have better eating habits. I know I grew up on loads of fruit and vegetables and a huge variety of tastes. Am I letting her down by not doing this for her? I have mixed guilt about this. Some days I kid myself that she's getting enough fruit and veggies in her meals at childcare and that it's OK to have chicken nuggets or fish fingers for dinner and nothing else. Other days I cringe at myself for my parenting style and cringe more at the grandiose ideas I had before any child was in my care.

I think that mother guilt has a place in life. If it helps you learn from something you've done and you can change that part of you to be an improved version of yourself, then so much the better. Having said that, I have a tendency to chew over guilt for a long time and wallow in it before somehow suppressing it and moving forward. I don't often talk to other parents about feelings of guilt, or my guilt in particular, as it brings up so many more issues and can become quite a heated conversation.

I think I've reconciled myself to the fact that I'll always feel a level of guilt. It's up to me in how I deal and cope with it. I know I'm not capable of not feeling guilty, but I'm trying to put it into a better perspective so that I can continue moving forward.

Kylie's Wisdom   There are lots of parenting issues and parenting mistakes that cause guilt. People are unique, and as such, have different ideas and ideals when it comes to raising their children. You have to do what you think is best or right at the time. Sometimes, it is a lolly in the supermarket that gives you the peace you need to get the shopping done. Or a normally forbidden soft drink that helps you get through that long drive or difficult afternoon. One of my favourite expressions for difficult times is 'this too shall pass'. Let it go, let it pass. It will not make you love your child any less, or them you. And if you say 'no' to them, they'll get over that too. There are so many more important things going on in the world. Give small issues the perspective and time they require and not a moment more.

Think you're the only one who doesn't feel good enough? Think again …

I asked mothers to tell me if they had ever felt guilty about things they had done (or not done) as a parent. A staggering 99 per cent answered 'yes' (and I have my doubts about the one respondent who answered 'no'). My inbox was flooded with responses. Here is just a sample of what women feel guilty about …

Snapping and shouting when totally not necessary. I spend all day doing housework when I should be enjoying my son and playing with him. *The one thing that has made me feel guilty more than anything else is separating from my husband.* I feel guilt that sometimes I can't wait for my kids to go away. I completely regret and feel tremendously guilty about circumcising my first son. *Not doing enough for them and with them, making them do too much, 'spoiling' them (can you spoil a child? I'm still workshopping that one), being too uninvolved, being too involved* … Crying in front of my kids. Being too quick to anger and letting my frustrations get the better of me. *I feel guilty for feeling guilty.* I accidently hit my baby with a tin of formula I was getting out of his pram. I cried so much and I still feel guilty about it, even though it's been four years since it happened. I have felt guilty for employing the electronic babysitter (TV) when I'm just too tired to play. *I feel guilty about not being able to provide financially for my family and relying on my husband's income.* I feel guilty for not paying as much attention to my children as I think other people do. Sometimes I read a book or watch TV while my kids play. The following day, I'll make more of an effort, but I'm still not one of those fun moms. I feel guilty for not being able to breastfeed my baby and I feel guilty because she was starving (due to my milk not coming in properly). *I felt guilty due to baby number two arriving when my firstborn was only 16 months old.* I'm worried about my second baby suffering 'middle child syndrome'. I feel guilty because my youngest baby was always being dragged sleeping from her bassinette/cot so her older siblings could be taken to/picked up from kindy/family day care. *Mother guilt seems an endless game, one that I think I will probably suffer from until I die.* I feel guilty that when I come home from a stressful day at work that I can be short with my kids and not give them the time and energy that they expect from me. There is the guilt of not having the financial security that I would like for my children; of not having enough money to enrol my girls in the swimming lessons I would love them to have or the gymnastics/dancing that they would love to do. *I accidently hit my baby's head on the bedroom door when I turned around from the change table. She was fine but I felt like a bad mother for a while after that and was feeling unconfident about handling her.* Not being there for my daughter's first day of school, as I have to work. I still feel guilty for not following my parental instinct when TJ got chicken pox and listening to the doctor saying to give him paracetamol; then watching him a few days later having IVs and tubes placed and being told he was hours away from not making it. Every time I bathe him and see the scars I feel guilty. People asked me continuously why I didn't vaccinate him. I kept explaining that he wasn't due for it until the next week but I still felt so guilty, like I should have been able to read the future and get him done early. *I feel guilty that I wasn't able to give my children that 'perfect' family unit and that my marriage broke up.* I feel guilty that sometimes there just isn't enough time and energy for me to devote to them and keep a house and keep up with work. I feel guilty if I go out without my children and have to leave them with a sitter, so I tend not to go. *I feel guilty that I didn't pick up my daughter's visual difficulties until after she started failing at school.* One of the biggest things over the years that I felt guilty about was when the father of my two eldest children died. My little boy threw his head back and hit it on the corner of my cupboard door. He was screaming. I felt so bad that I wouldn't let him out of my sight for three days and I bought him new toys to try and make up for what happened. *I feel so overjoyed when day care days come around—how come I can't wait to 'get rid of' my child?* I have felt guilty for leaving my baby to cry, not leaving my baby to cry, feeding my baby to sleep, co sleeping … My latest is wanting to wean; it's my uncertainty of whether I really want to wean him, or am I just cracking from the pressure of society/family/and wanting a bit more space to myself? Serving up cold dinners of bread, ham, cucumber and tomato. Again. And again. And again. I need to nourish my children better! Luckily they don't seem to have rickets yet. *I sometimes push my child away in a cold, rejecting manner when I just feel selfish and unloving. Sometimes I can't stand the sense of neediness coming from my son and just shut down a little. I think those times are outweighed by the general warm loving and giving I do but still, I worry and feel guilty about it.* Putting on the TV for my four-year-old every day, often twice a day, and using it as an escape hatch when I can't be bothered to think of something more creative and really need to switch off from parenting. I have felt parent guilt for many things, the latest (and largest for me at the moment) is crying at bedtime. To pick up and soothe or controlled crying? I want a child who is capable of settling himself sometimes—I do not want to be his only comforter. But I feel guilty because I want to pick him up, and when I go in and cuddle him, only for him to fall asleep in my arms, I feel guilty that I let him cry that long. *I feel guilty that sometimes I long for the days when I didn't have a child.* Not changing a nappy in the middle of the night as I'm afraid I will wake my baby up and she won't go back to sleep. My girls will ask me something over and over again and because my tolerance levels are low, I snap and then feel instantly guilty for raising my voice. *I feel guilty for getting postnatal depression.*

As you can see, mothers feel guilty about anything and everything. Some expressions of guilt are normal and healthy. However, some can be quite damaging: feeling guilty for something that is not your fault or for not living up to societal standards (for example, not being able to breastfeed or needing to switch off from parenting) can play havoc with your mental health. Try to focus on all the good things you do as a mother. Write out a list if you need to and look at it when you're feeling guilty. It may help to reassure you that you're doing the best you can.

If your guilt is all-pervasive or overwhelming, it could be a sign of postnatal depression. In this instance, you should go to your local doctor and tell them how you are feeling as soon as possible, as you may need medical treatment. For a list of support services and resources, see page 258 of the Resources section.

Postnatal depression and anxiety

The postnatal period is awash with profound physical and emotional changes. It is also associated with mental disorders, ranging from the mild to the severe. The **baby blues** are on the mild end of the spectrum and are transient in nature, typically lasting for a few hours or a few days. When you have the baby blues, you may feel teary, cranky, restless or even a little 'dazed and confused'. Postnatal depression is more serious and won't just 'go away' like the baby blues. Postnatal depression has the same signs and symptoms of clinical depression but has the additional factor of time (meaning that it is depression directly associated with the birth of a baby and usually occurs between four to six weeks post-partum—although it can occur much later than this). On the most serious end of the scale (and fortunately the rarest, with a prevalence of one to two in every 1000 births) is **post-partum psychosis**. This condition exhibits the same symptoms as psychosis (such as delusions and hallucinations) but, like postnatal depression, is time constrained (in that it appears soon after delivery).

On paper, the description of postnatal depression appears quite cold and clinical. However, as the following stories illustrate, postnatal depression is more than the sum of its symptoms and classifications. It is real, it is scary, and it is potentially dangerous for both the women who suffer from it, as well as their children. Charlotte and Cait give heart-rending accounts of their illness in this section. Information on depression and what you can do about it is also presented.

No turning back: When postnatal depression takes over

Charlotte suffered from postnatal depression with her first baby, but was fortunate enough to realise she needed help and, with counselling and medication, she mended. She went on to have two more children and experienced postnatal depression on both occasions. Charlotte remains thankful for modern medicine and the help and support of professionals.

Charlotte's Story

*You wouldn't wish **postnatal depression** on your worst enemy. Really. You've been reading about all the stuff that happens to you when you fall pregnant, give birth and have a baby … and the changes and challenges you have to deal with. Well, postnatal depression makes the transition so much harder. It can make you decide that you really don't want to be a mother after all. But, as you find out, there is no going backwards, no returning your baby to the womb—you can only go forward, get help, be brave and soldier on in the knowledge that you will get better. Believe me, I know. I've been on that journey.*

I had my first baby in my mid-20s, a little boy born at the end of October. It wasn't an easy birth but then few actually are I now think. I survived, he was healthy, we thought 'Wow, we have a baby!' He was the first grandchild and the first baby in our groovy young inner-city gang. It was a big new adventure for us all. Was I prepared for parenthood? Probably not, but I was educated, well-read, and in love with my son's father.

I remember that first Christmas very well, because I was counting the days into the weeks until the magic six-week mark that everyone told me about. Six weeks held the promise that everything would be better and easier after that: the baby would start sleeping longer; feeding more regularly; I would have adjusted more to my new role; I would start enjoying being a mother. Unfortunately, no magic or quick or dramatic improvement took place for me. There was no timeline marked with a point that said 'Hooray, you have arrived at the happy motherhood station!' I looked the same as I did before. There was nothing to see on the outside. But inside, I felt terrible. I was exhausted. I was faking it. I was lost. Nothing made sense anymore.

Fortunately, I did realise I needed help. I picked up the phone and called an organisation that helps new mothers and babies. They had an office close by that I could go to where I was kindly and efficiently offered help. The nurse talked to me about my baby, what he was doing, what I was doing, how I felt about it, and showed me some things that would help with the practical care of a young baby. However, I needed more. I was referred to a psychiatrist and also offered the opportunity to be part of a group session for mothers feeling like I did, run by two psychologists who were expert in the field. That experience was invaluable. I am still in touch with two of the women I met in that group, over 18 years later.

The other thing I remember about those early months is the tears. Talk about 'cry me a river'; I got so tired of crying in strange people's offices, but that seemed to be the most honest expression of how I was feeling.

*Fast forward, three and a half years. I'd gone back to work, got comfortable in my role as a mum, stopped taking the antidepressants that I needed for about a year and was having lots of fun with my preschooler. In fact, things were so good it was time to have another baby. And so we did. Another son, long and skinny, with extra skin that he needed to grow into. A completely natural birth that was so quick, he was born less than an hour after we got to the **birth centre**. So many circumstances were different, and better. A planned pregnancy, more experienced parents, adorable three-year-old brother. So, did I fare any better? No. The depression this time, a devastating blow for me, was even worse than before. I couldn't sleep, I found my newborn impossible to settle, I felt like a total failure. After spending a month at my parents' house where I was almost immobilised by despair, the organisation that I had previously relied on for help and support again provided a lifeline and I spent a week living in at their mother–baby centre before, shakily, returning to my own home.*

*By the time I was pregnant again, it was seven years later. We weren't actually planning on any more children and now were living in the United States, far from the support that had helped me so much before. I was scared, but also older and thankfully wiser. I knew my situation had to be discussed and dealt with. My obstetrician referred me to a specialist in **postnatal** adjustment and her big thing was planning and preparation. Statistically I was likely to have postnatal depression again—it just seemed to be how the hormonal stew played out for me. And you know, I felt better seeing it as 'something that happened to me' rather than 'something that I did' (presumably wrong). I didn't want to start antidepressants while I was still pregnant (although that was recommended as a possible course of action) but did take them soon after. I was convinced by the argument that it is better (as in quicker and easier to recover) to not go so deep down into the hole of depression in the first place. And that was an enormous relief. I didn't necessarily feel great but I coped, and had a much more normal experience with my new baby.*

Charlotte's Wisdom	So what do I take away from this nearly 20-year parenting process, and all the happiness and sadness that went with it? Besides a ton of sympathy for sufferers of depression and other mental illness, I thank God for modern pharmaceuticals and the professional organisations

that helped me. Unfortunately, I still feel guilt and shame about what I went through. It is not something I choose to talk about frequently. I like to think my children have not been affected by my episodes of postnatal depression and that by getting help promptly the negative side effects to them were minimised.

If you can relate to this story, or more importantly, are in the thick of such an experience, please pick up the phone and talk to someone and get help. You really aren't alone, it is not your fault, and having a baby is not meant to be so hard that you want to run away from your life. My eldest son just started university and those awful (for me) early months of his life are just a small part of the kaleidoscope of experiences of motherhood.

Finding support for mental health issues

As mentioned in the introduction to this section, there are several mental disorders that are associated with pregnancy and birth: the baby blues, postnatal depression and post-partum psychosis. All of these conditions at the very least need support and understanding. Postnatal depression and psychosis require treatment by a health care professional, so it is important to recognise and understand these symptoms and seek help if you are experiencing anything that worries you. Talk to your local doctor, midwife or obstetrician and look up information on support services at the end of this book. Also read the information box on postnatal depression on page 154 so that you are aware of the signs and symptoms of depression.

When the wheels fall off: Recognising burnout

Cait's story illustrates just how difficult being a mother can be and how hard it can be to keep all balls in the air while keeping a smile plastered on your face. For Cait, her moment of recognition was when her dog died. Although it was most definitely not her fault, Cait blamed herself for it because of her use of diazepam; a prescription drug used (and misused) by some mothers who are not coping (otherwise known as 'self-medication'). Eventually, Cait was diagnosed with, and treated for, depression. Here is her story.

Cait's Story

*The wheels fell off when the dog died. I'd been wobbling along, convincing myself that I was doing OK whilst self-medicating on **diazepam**. But, when our spaniel picked up a paralysis tick and I didn't notice she was in trouble for 12 crucial hours, the seriousness of my situation finally began to penetrate the depressed fog I'd existed in.*

Ella died despite the vet's best efforts to save her. The Cavalier King Charles Spaniel is extremely vulnerable to tick poison, and honestly, even if I had picked it up earlier the outcome would probably have been the same. Probably. What really hit home was that I was so overwhelmed and so unable to see things clearly that I hadn't seen that she was in distress. I was devastated about losing her, but at the same time a voice in my head was screaming 'What if it'd been one of the children?' What if something had been wrong with them and I hadn't noticed?

I'd like to say that I hot-footed it to the doctor and got myself help. But while I was starting to acknowledge the problem in myself, the fact that I was totally overwhelmed and felt I needed antidepressants did not sit well with members of my family. When you are so depressed you can hardly see straight and you have people whose opinions you respect telling you that antidepressants are the Devil and you just need to pull yourself together, you listen to them.

However, during the Christmas/New Year break, I stepped back and took a long hard look at my family: one stressed out, overwhelmed husband, two deeply unhappy children desperate for the attention I had no capacity to give them, and one dead dog. I had two girls, then aged nearly three and four-and-a-half (18 months apart), a husband working full time in a demanding job, my own part-time demanding job as a published romance author with books due and being released with accompanying marketing demands, plus the cooking, cleaning, driving, gardening, worrying about the environment … you name it and I was pushing myself to do it, and under no circumstances was I going to let the world see what a mess I was in. I was always told that I could do it all and be it all, and that is precisely what I was doing/being. Only nobody mentioned that if you are going to do it all and be it all that you need A Lot Of Help. In fact I felt that if I admitted I needed someone to shoulder the workload with me then the world would figure out that not only was I not Superwoman, but I was also a big fat mothering failure.

So at Christmas I finally got myself to the doctor and told him exactly how I was feeling. It wasn't easy to own up to the fact I had been keeping it together by popping the diazepam that'd been originally prescribed when I slipped a disc in my lower back. He, like the rest of the world, saw me as a wisecracking, novel-writing mother of two, coping beautifully. His reaction, though, was 'Hey, it's OK. Let's fix this thing.' He prescribed me antidepressants, and cleared out all the samples in his office so I wouldn't have to start paying until we were sure they were the right ones for me, and he hooked me up with a wonderful counsellor.

Within a week I had had seven nights of real, actual sleep and had made the difficult decision that I had to leave work. A couple of weeks later I met my counsellor for the first time. She took one look at me, muttered 'Oh my God', sat me down and we workshopped a plan to get my life into a manageable context. I felt like I was getting better and better, but the counsellor was experienced in dealing with depression in women and saw only the black eyes and the lingering pole-axed expression. I wasn't going to be able to leave work for another four months (tip: never make yourself indispensible), and to try and alleviate some of my guilt over Ella's death we had a new puppy. So while the antidepressants were helping, I had actually managed to increase my workload, which was the source of the problems in the first place.

I met up with my counsellor again a week later and by that time I had organised a housekeeper (who tidied, cooked, cleaned, chatted and laughed a lot), sent the puppy to preschool where he was being trained for me, switched the kids from my work day care to one closer to home to stop putting them through hours in the car commuting, changed my work hours so they were spread across three days, got a man in to do the garden, organised a freezer load of healthy ready-made meals, and told my editor that she was just going to have to wait for the rewrites to be done on my next book.

Now, ten months later, I look back at how I was last Christmas and wonder what I was thinking, putting myself through it all. I don't regret trying to work and write and achieve the things I wanted to achieve, but what was I thinking when I decided I didn't need support? Working when you have young children does not have to be a gruelling, never-ending endurance event. But, if you try and go it alone then chances are you're going to put yourself under a boatload of pressure, which can be bad for you and bad for them.

Cait's Wisdom

Being a parent with young children and working is tough. Even with help it's still not easy, and without help … well, look at me, a sane(ish), rarely drinking, never-taken-a-drug-in-her-life type of girl—and I ended up guzzling half a bottle of wine a night, smoking up to a pack a day and taking diazepam, all to try and alleviate some of the stress I was under. I'm not even going to mention the comfort eating and the weight gain.

In approaching a return to work, or even if you are working already, it's a good idea to look at your salary and put aside as much of it as you can for supporting yourself; help at home, ready-made healthy meals (you can order them online), gardeners, cleaners, an ironing service, anything. Any little thing will help.

I know that making yourself and your own mental and physical health a priority is not easy. I know there are so many factors and constraints and that another dollar off the mortgage now means two dollars less in the future. But trust me when I tell you that floundering in a burnt-out depressed haze is so not worth those two dollars.

Postnatal depression

How common is it?

Rates vary, depending on how research is conducted and data collected (see Halbreich & Karkun 2006 for more on this) but the general rule of thumb is that the prevalence rate is between 10 and 15 per cent.

What are the risk factors?

Risk factors for developing postnatal depression include: a past history of depression and/or anxiety, a difficult pregnancy (and/or depression during the pregnancy), traumatic birth, family history of mental illness, problems with baby's health and difficulties with breastfeeding.

What are the symptoms?

Symptoms include: sleep disturbance (not related to the baby), weight gain or loss, crying, feeling irritable, feeling like you can't cope, having negative thoughts, feeling anxious about being alone or feeling overly anxious in general. Some women experience memory difficulties and difficulties in concentration and some women experience feelings of guilt, worthlessness, hopelessness and inadequacy. Some women feel they want to die. These are the most common symptoms.

Many women cry or feel sleep deprived and irritable when their baby is born, so how can you distinguish 'normal' feelings from those of depression? The rule of thumb is that a) the symptoms occur for longer than two weeks, and b) the symptoms greatly affect your quality of life. It is vital that you see your doctor as soon as possible if you think you may have postnatal depression, because if you have it, you need medical treatment.

Why is it so important to seek treatment?

Left untreated, the symptoms of postnatal depression can lead to: intimate relationship problems, family problems, difficulties finding employment (or staying employed), drug and alcohol overuse, anger issues and difficulty bonding with children. In the worst case scenario, it can lead to suicide or infanticide (when the baby is killed, intentionally or not).

What is the treatment?

As with most illnesses, postnatal depression should be treated holistically. Most women benefit from psychological (or 'talking') treatments, which can take the form of cognitive behavioural therapy or counselling (or both). Women diagnosed with postnatal depression may also need to take antidepressants.

Are there things I can do to help myself?

Yes. Although it's hard to take time out for yourself when you have a baby or child to care for, there are certain things you can do, no matter how small. Little things like making sure you have a shower every day, sitting down to eat your breakfast (and eating lunch and dinner as well) and walking all help. All of these can be done with a baby. For example, you can have your shower when your baby is napping, eat breakfast when your baby does, and go for walks with your baby safely in their pram. If you are able to, try to rest when your baby is sleeping; forget the housework—it can always wait. This is where support from others can also come in handy. If you have a partner, ask them to take over looking after your baby when they get home from work. This is not the time for you to do housework. Go and soak in the tub, watch television or get some sleep (whatever you feel like doing).

Ask trusted friends and/or family to look after your baby so that you can have some time to yourself, whether it's time spent with your partner or friends or time spent alone reading a magazine or sleeping. If you can afford it, hire a home-helper to come in a couple of days a week; ask them to do the dishes and the laundry and cook some nutritious meals that you can freeze in batches. Remember, when you have postnatal depression, you are in 'survival' mode: anything you can do to ease your workload and increase time for yourself is paramount. This, in conjunction with medical therapy (antidepressants and/or psychological intervention), can go a long way in helping you recover from postnatal depression.

Reflections on motherhood

Motherhood is an intense experience to say the least, and every mother experiences it differently. Here we meet three women, Miranda, Penny and Nette, all of whom love their children deeply and have learnt to adapt to the challenges and responsibilities of motherhood in different ways.

Behind slammed doors: Learning to parent

Miranda tells of her difficulty in learning to be a 'mother' to her son, rather than his friend—a life lesson for her in the importance of socialisation.

Miranda's Story

A few weeks ago, my eldest came to me in tears at an injustice he experienced at school. Apparently, his teacher didn't allow him to participate in an assembly because he had not turned in an assignment that was due. He had a list of people to blame, ranging from his teacher who didn't understand him, a handful of friends who distracted him, and ending with me as I didn't remind him. I listened to his account and my heart ached hearing of the pain he felt being singled out and excluded from the assembly. He had been embarrassed in front of his friends, he missed out on a fun experience, and he was angry the day had ended without resolution. He needed me to agree and champion his position.

When he ran out of breath and excuses, I reached out and took his small hand in mine. 'I guess you're going to have the assignment done next time.' I could see those words stung. He pulled his hand away and stormed off growling accusations that I didn't care about him, always took the teacher's side, and that I only cared about 'stupid school and stupid assignments.' With that, the door slammed and the room fell quiet. I felt a heavy blanket draped over my shoulders and it took every ounce of energy I had to return to the kitchen to finish the dishes. Minutes seemed like hours but my wounded child finally emerged from his room to apologize.

Before having children, I was completely certain of the role I wanted to play in my child's life. I knew the ingredients to being a good mom and I believed I possessed each of those ingredients in abundance. I saw myself as something of a superhero, ready to leap tall buildings for my children. In fact, not only would I clear the buildings but I would do so with grace and skill. When I learned I was pregnant, my confidence only increased. I was certain I would excel in my new life role.

On reflection, I realize that I lived in blissful ignorance of what it really means to be a parent … what it means to be a mom. I had no idea of the adventure I was walking into or the lessons that would sometimes be forced upon me as a result of a clumsily handled parenting situation. Before having children and during those first few years, I was the stereotypical new student that knew just enough to be convinced I was an expert.

I spent the toddler years measuring my own moral standards, analyzing the way I was raised by my parents and determining all the things I knew I would do better. To be clear, my childhood was as close to a Norman Rockwell existence one can imagine without a canvas to document the multiple idyllic childhood moments. But I had a list of things I would ban from my parenting that included statements such as 'Because I said so' and 'What will the neighbors think?' My sons and I would the perfect balance of friend and parent, confidant and mentor, champion and teacher.

However, that balance was impossible to maintain as flickers of their personalities emerged and I watched them actively engage in the world. Being their friend, their confidant and their champion wasn't really helping them navigate situations like my son not having his assignment done. It became painfully clear that in the real world, friends don't instinctively encourage responsibility, confidants are not obligated to hold you accountable, and champions may not care to be patient with you as you struggle to find your way through life's challenges. I had to face the facts: I am a human being raising human beings and it is my job to give them the tools to interact with other human beings. As my boy's champion, I was falling short of that duty. As their mom, it was my responsibility.

Along with this realization came another painful admission. My desire to be their friend, confidant, and champion only served me and my desire to be adored by my sons. I had defined myself as a mother only from what I wanted to be as a mother, without considering what my sons needed from their mother. Did they need another friend or did they need someone to give them the tools necessary for their future? If I continued on this path, I would be raising boys who adored their mother but would not necessarily possess the tools to navigate the world that awaited them.

When asking myself what I needed to provide my sons, the first answer was easy. I needed to give them a safe home, good nourishment, and adequate clothing. Beyond those basics, however, what did they really need from me? The answer was surprisingly simple: they needed a person who promoted fun and structure, supported individualism and responsibility, inspired creativity and accountability, and encouraged spontaneity and consistency. They needed me to teach them what it means to be a good co-worker, friend, neighbor, citizen, spouse, and father.

So, I can proudly say that my son is right; I do care about 'stupid school and stupid assignments.' It also broke my heart that he was embarrassed and missed the assembly. However, last week he finished his assignments and the morning he turned them in, there was a bounce in his step that brought a smile to my soul. Being a mom can result in angry kids and the occasional slammed door. But it has also resulted in my becoming a dependable human being, a compassionate person, and a responsible adult. Again … that is my job.

Miranda's Wisdom   Lessons learned from this experience continue as I watch my sons grow and develop their own opinions, friendships, and personalities and with each, I am blessed with spontaneous glimpses of who they will be as young men.

However, I am also provided with continual reminders that motherhood isn't romantic, glamorous or tidy. It can feel like a triage room; making decisions with little time to reflect and often too few resources to call upon. There is no rulebook to follow or tests to take at the end of each chapter to determine your progress.

The most precious gift I can offer my sons is the understanding of how to be adults, partners, and friends in a world where I won't always be there to wipe a runny nose or bandage a scraped knee. It is the future for which I am making parenting decisions, not the now. While that is so difficult to remember, it is ultimately what makes me their mom.

Exclusive membership: The 'club' of motherhood

Penny suddenly found that she had a ticket to the exclusive club of motherhood and her story explores how for her, being a mother meant learning how to grow and adapt.

Penny's Story

I remember just before the birth of my first child, I felt like I was looking into a great unknown. I gathered my girlfriends around me (most of whom were still single, and none of them mothers), and I had a slight sense of panic. Everything was about to change, and I didn't know what would happen or how. Would I be different? Would my life change? How much? I knew I was moving on, and I mourned leaving my old life as much as I waited with excited anticipation for my baby to arrive.

Now, five years on, as a mother of two, I am truly on the other side. Now I am the one who gives an encouraging, welcoming smile to the pregnant stranger on the street and empathises with the new mother struggling with her baby and stroller on the bus. I remember being overwhelmed by the outpouring of love and congratulations from all corners of the world, from people I barely knew, when my first baby was born. It was a celebration of a new life, and a welcoming into the club of motherhood. I feel that same thrill, that same joy, when I observe any new mother embarking on the journey.

So am I different? Has my life changed? Absolutely. Pregnancy and childbirth are profound experiences in themselves, and if you embrace motherhood, the love you feel for your child is like nothing you have felt before. Your priorities change. You are different, but of course you are still you, the you that was there before. You're a more tired you, a more distracted you, but you still like to chat to your friends, see movies and get to yoga when you can. The world does not end when the baby comes, though it does shrink for a little while.

Motherhood fast-tracks you into personal growth whether you like it or not. Raising children demands a selflessness that we achieve some days better than others. Your children are your best teachers and, if you are open to it, you will be challenged on every level—your thoughts, your behaviours, your feelings.

Recently I observed my first child on his own in the sandpit, as usual, when I picked him up from day care. After two years of part-time day care he was still without any close friends. I experienced such a pang of worry. I looked at the teachers, busy with the more demanding children (or so it seemed), and wondered 'Do they even see my boy? Do they make an effort to see his special qualities and draw them out? He's like an invisible boy ...' I was overwhelmed with a sadness that seemed disproportionate to the occasion. And of course it was, once I had time to reflect on it later that night. Something had triggered my own memory of being the shy little girl, who felt invisible and unrecognised. My boy was fine. He loved the sandpit and was quite happy there. This emotional reaction was all about me. Having children will push your buttons in ways you don't expect and may not especially welcome. One of the great challenges is not letting your issues get in the way of your child's experience of life. Which is especially tricky when you may not even know what some of those issues are.

Motherhood is about being willing to change and grow, or at least adapt. I can't seem to change into a morning person—I admire and envy larks, but relishing the morning is beyond me. However, I try very hard not to sit like a dark cloud on the couch clutching a cup of tea. I take turns with my husband to sleep in and I have established a routine when it's my turn to get up so I don't have to be creative before I'm ready. Sometimes TV is involved and I've decided that's OK. The 'whatever works' principle is a good one, within reason.

Motherhood makes you think about what is important in your life. This, perhaps, is the greatest gift of parenthood. When your life is all about you, it is easy to cruise along in pleasure-seeking mode without asking too many hard questions. When you have a baby who will grow into a child who will grow into an adult, suddenly everything becomes more significant. When you are raising a child with a partner, differences in values that once could be overlooked have to be addressed. Do you have a faith and how do you express it? What expectations do you have about gender? Is it more important to have money for nice things and holidays or more time to spend with the family? How much input should extended family have? What sort of schooling is best for your child? These are questions that will need answering and will demand some reflection.

Motherhood is not easy. As a stay-at-home mother, I have enjoyed some delightful years of 'being in the moment' with my gorgeous children, examining insects in the park, chatting in the playground with other mums and dads, getting crafty at home with empty boxes and pipe cleaners and telling lengthy stories about favourite toys. I have also endured days of frustration and tedium when I simply couldn't care less about boxes and pipe cleaners, insects and toys. I have wanted my children to go away and let me read the newspaper in peace. I have felt an increasing desire to 'do something worthwhile', as if raising children does not meet that criterion. As those days become more frequent, I realise it's time for a change, a new phase of motherhood. Fortunately my son is about to start school and my daughter will begin day care part time. My world is starting to open

up again, for study and work. But motherhood continues, with its challenges and its joys.
I wouldn't be anywhere else.

Penny's Wisdom	I believe in the notion that parents are caretakers, not owners of their children. Let your children be themselves. Try to be aware of your own issues about identity and achievement and not impose them on your children. Sometimes your child might 'be' in ways you might not recognise, understand or empathise with. That's OK, and as a parent your job is to raise them with love, compassion and space to develop into their own person.

Motherless mothering: How loss can shape you as a parent

Nette is a 'motherless mother', who lost her mother at the age of 16. Her story explores how this affected her own parenting and why she believes that a woman's past influences the way a she parents her children.

Nette's Story

It is impossible for me to untwine my relationships with my children from the one I had with my own mother. For when I pour my soul into them, when I give them all the love I have, am I not imbuing them with memories of my own mother?

For a long time, the process of my own mothering has been a desperate effort to either re-enact or rebuke the way I was mothered. She was loved, loving, gregarious, dedicated and funny. So, I try to embody those characteristics of hers that made her wonderful. She loved me, and the times we had together were for the main part fun. She would come home from work, dizzy, pour herself a vodka and put on the record player. Taking me by the hand, she would spin me round and round to Elvis. She was fun, and being in her presence felt sunshiny. Of course, she had her faults too, and initially, I did not realise that I was subconsciously rebuking them when I made decisions about my own children. She was dedicated to a fault—but to her work, not me.

Because of this, there were many times she was not there. So many times I would have to let myself in to an empty house, waiting for her to come home; an only child trying to amuse herself until mum arrived. And then, the ultimate absence—death. It was such a strange and isolating experience watching my mother mutate from strong and glowing to weak and sallowed. It took three years for her to die but no one (apart from dad and me) even knew she was unwell until her death. I was motherless at the age of 16—a crucial juncture in a girl's life and one I found I had to navigate on my own.

How can this be left unsaid when defining myself as a mother? It cannot. She devoted herself to her work; I devoted myself to my children, stopping a burgeoning career in its tracks. I wanted to be there for my children; no latch-keys for them. As much as I loathed pregnancy (for the most part), I bore three living children to ensure that they would not face life on their own. No matter what happened to me, no matter what will happen to me, they will always have each other. You may say that siblings might not get along and so that choice is moot. Yes, I accept there is that chance but it is highly unlikely, given the endless hours of social engineering, the lessons of friendship and trust I have imparted to my children, the import I have placed on love and family.

I'm sure that on some level, I'm still angry at my mother for abandoning me. I'm also quite sure that this is what drives my will to ensure my children will never be fully abandoned. I never want them to feel the trauma of being left alone.

My three children do not yet know that they have a sister, who died long before they were born. I was 28 when I sat aside the doctor, told I was due on the 26th of February. Auspicious, given that my mother died on the same day. 'Renewal', I thought. 'The universe is speaking to me. My mother is speaking to me'. For 20 weeks, I bonded with my baby; felt her kick, as if trying to connect with me, tell me something. I would smile and poke back, thinking about my mother, wanting to share this with her and feeling sad that she would never meet this child. Then at my 20-week scan, the news that she was 'incompatible with life', the offer of a lift home, being ushered out the back door so I wouldn't upset all the pregnant women awaiting their scans. She was born a few days later. I touched her face, she was wrapped like a cocoon. If I ever had any faith in a god or in the universe, it left that day. It wasn't a blinding flash of atheism, more a quiet slinking away of hope and trust.

How can this be left unsaid when defining myself as a mother? It cannot. You might see me in the playground hovering over my children, watching their every move and think to yourself 'She needs to lighten up—she's so overprotective'. I ask you, wouldn't you behave the same way if you thought for a heartbeat that something might go wrong—probably would go wrong? If your life had been shaped by loss, if against all the odds you had lost both your mother and your daughter, would you not be resigned to the fact that your other children were imperilled as well? If I so much as hear a thump and a wail, I feel my heart icing over—the cool of panic sets in as I race towards my children. For surely it was the thump of death or at least the sound of danger seeking them out.

Thankfully, they have never been in real peril but the thought always lurks in my mind. Just this Christmas past, my eldest daughter fell off a windowsill and knocked out two of her teeth. Shaking, screaming and bloodied, she was carried to the car by my husband—I was too terrified to touch her. Family had been over that night for dinner and all the kids were playing in the living room. I had sat with the 'grown-ups' in the kitchen, ignoring the urge to stand among the children, keeping danger at bay. I already had a reputation as an overprotective mum and I was desperately trying to prove that I was cool and calm. I fought my instinct so as to avoid judgement. I learned a hard-won lesson: follow your own instincts, not the parenting philosophy of others. I am the first to raise my hand and tell you that I am overprotective but I can't banish this flaw overnight. I am working on it. I realise my children need to have space to grow but equally I need space to get used to the fact that they might actually be OK without me.

I don't know what the key ingredient is to being a good mother. What I have learned is that mothering is a process. It is a pastiche of your past, both good and bad; a reaction *to your own experiences. I think a good mother knows herself and can point to her own flaws so that she might minimise the effect they have on her children. And a good mother forgives herself those flaws, recognising them as innately human.*

Looking at it differently, loss has shaped how I parent in a good way. I am so keenly aware of the brevity of life that I learned from an early age to 'stand and stare'. I can happily watch my children play for hours; I breathe in the giggles and the silliness of their capers, memorising the scent of their happiness and youth. I pretend to be asleep when they crawl into my bed, draw them close to me and wonder what they're dreaming about.

Like every mother on the planet, I have my bad days, when I am quick to temper and slow to cool. Yet I have lost enough to realise that life's blessings are right in front of me and even though I make so many mistakes, I know that my children feel loved and safe. I also know that the memories we are making as a family are happy ones. And that is good enough for me.

Nette's Wisdom	There are wonderful differences in our children, our families and our societies and I think the idea that there is only one 'correct' parenting style negates these differences. I have learned that I don't parent in any particular way or style (although some might label me a 'helicopter parent'). My style is just a mishmash of approaches and techniques that work for me and my family at any given time and for any given child.

We should celebrate our differences, and recognise that as mothers, we are trying the best we can. Most importantly, please, let's give each other the benefit of the doubt. Unless you know my full history and personality (and those of my children and partner), how can you pass judgement on the way I parent? The simple answer is that you cannot. So let's live and let live! |

Motherless daughters: Finding a connection

For many women, a natural response when they discover they are pregnant is to talk to their mother. Questions like 'How did it feel like to be pregnant with me?', 'What was it like to give birth to me?' and 'How long was your labour?' are usually on the top of the priority list. If your mother died when you were young, you no longer have the luxury of picking up the phone and asking her all of your burning questions. But there are several things you can try.

Firstly, did your mother have close friends or sisters who are still alive? If so, they might be able to fill you in on some of the details. If your father is still alive, you can try asking him too. Another thing you can try is to find out where you were born and who delivered you. Armed with this information, phone the hospital in which your mother delivered you and ask them how to obtain her medical records. As you are asking for your mother's records, you will probably have to prove her death (via a death certificate) and that you are closely related (via your own birth certificate).

Some hospitals charge a fee for this service and many hospitals take months to retrieve medical files, so it's best to start your inquiries as soon as you can. Medical records are usually quite comprehensive. If you're lucky, you will not only find out how long your mother laboured, you will also find out the type of delivery she had and how you and she were getting along in the first few days.

If you are unable to obtain your mother's records, have you still got documents of hers in a box somewhere, perhaps stored away in a cupboard or in the attic? Even if you're not sure, it's worth having a look. You never know what you might turn up. You may hit the jackpot: you may find her diary or even letters that she has received in which you are mentioned. If you look through all of your baby photos, you will soon find out whether she bottle-fed you or breastfed you; whether she carried you around a lot or whether you were often in a stroller. By studying old photos, you can sometimes get a sense of her parenting style.

If all else fails, try to take comfort in this: while the birth of your first child can renew your grief for your mother, it can also help to form a new connection with her. For the first time, you will be a mother like her and you may begin to see things through her eyes. The overwhelming feelings you have for your own baby will finally give you a profound insight into the feelings she had for you. What a beautiful gift.

For more information and support for motherless daughters and motherless mothers, you should read *Motherless Daughters* and *Motherless Mothers*, both by Hope Edelman. These, among other resources, are listed in the Resources section.

Why didn't anyone tell me that ...

- I would love my boys differently to my girls. Not more fiercely, just very differently.
- My fears for being the wrong 'personality type' were completely unfounded. Being a good mother and enjoying motherhood is about so much more than all the laundry being done, having a cutesy name for everything and making sure the dinner is on the table promptly at 5.30. My goofy and disorganised attitude works well and we're having fun!
- Motherhood is the biggest responsibility you can have.
- Motherhood is the easiest and the hardest thing. You can't just 'turn it off', even if you want to. For me, it also means being woken up five times a night, then at 5.30 am when asked in the most innocent and helpful voice 'Mummy awake?'
- Some days I would want to change my name to anything but 'mother'.
- Being a mother would push me to the extremes of emotion. I've never in my entire life felt so elated, nor so cross!

- Worry comes with the territory. Constant worry. Starting from when they're babies: 'They're not sleeping/eating/whatever', to 15 years later: 'Please God let her come home safely tonight'.

- Heartbreak is part of the job description. Seeing your child excluded by others, falling over and badly hurting themselves, crying when you have to leave them in someone else's care—all completely and utterly heartbreaking.

- I would feel so guilty! Never in my life have I managed to feel guilty about anything and everything but apparently that's entirely possible when you have children!

- Sometimes you don't fall in love with being a mother right off the bat. Sometimes it's a painful process of letting go of your old life and embracing your new one.

- Sometimes you wish for your old life back.

- There would be a Great Divide. Soon after I had my first baby, many of my closest friends (without children) dwindled away. They couldn't understand why I was no longer able to go out as often as I used to. It was quite crushing, losing some of my best friends. I wish someone had warned me.

CHAPTER SIX

Fatherhood

'It is not flesh and blood, it is the heart that makes us sons and fathers.'

Frederich Schiller (1781)

The concept of 'new fatherhood' has evolved over the past few decades. Increasingly, men are more supportive in their partner's pregnancy, labour and birth of their babies (Deave & Johnson 2008), are more emotionally connected to their children and more involved in the care of their children (Eggebeen & Knoester 2001). Palkovitz and Palm (2009) cite a growing body of literature that emphasises the transition to fatherhood as a 'critical juncture in men's development and in their contribution to the family wellbeing through father involvement and physical support' (p. 7). They go on to state that men's initial transitions to fatherhood predict different outcomes related to father involvement as the child grows.

It is clear from the literature that babies whose fathers are involved in their care are more likely to be securely attached to them and better able to handle unfamiliar situations. Furthermore, they display higher resilience, curiosity and an eagerness to explore their environment than those infants whose fathers are less involved. The parent-child relationship is a two-way street. It follows, then, that involved fathers also gain benefits: they feel more self-confident, find parenting more satisfying and feel more important to their children. Additionally, men who are emotionally supportive can significantly increase their partners' health and welfare. For example, women whose partners are supportive are more likely to 'enjoy a greater sense of wellbeing, good post-partum mental health [and] have a relatively problem free pregnancy, delivery process and nursing experience' (Allen & Daly 2007, p. 25).

As suggested by Palkovitz and Palm (2009), men vary considerably in the way they father and this depends on their personal characteristics (such as their age and income), relational factors (for example, how their partners view their abilities as a dad), whether or not their partner is employed and the age and sex of their children. It is also dependent on whether they are living with their children; fathers who don't live with their children are more likely to be less emotionally and practically involved with them (Henley & Pasley 2005). It is important to note, however, that many fathers who don't live with their children do not have less involvement by choice. In many instances, fathers want more access to their children but are unable to gain it. Following separation or divorce, children fare consistently better when they are able to maintain relationships with both their parents (Allen & Daly 2007).

As well as the increasing trend of 'new fatherhood', society is now recognising that fatherhood is not merely the domain of the 'typical' biological father. Fathers who are gay, for example, may be single biological parents or they may be living in a same sex relationship, where one man is the biological father or both are biological fathers. They may be fathers through other avenues as well, such as adoption and fostering. It is important, therefore, when thinking about or defining fatherhood that all fathers are considered. This is increasingly reflected in academic literature; it is crucial that social policy makers catch up.

In this chapter, you will read stories and snippets from men who talk about how they felt about becoming a father. Some felt a change in their sense of identity almost immediately (that is, when their partner became pregnant) and embraced that change. Some men found it more of a struggle becoming a father, particularly in how it related to their relationship with their partner. Recognising the amount of attention required by a baby from its mother, men still felt a bit 'left out' and some struggled with the lack of intimacy that ensued.

This chapter also addresses the challenge of balancing work and parenthood, which can sometimes be a different sort of test for fathers than mothers. You will also hear from fathers about how the relationships in their lives changed—not just with their partners, but with their friends, families and work colleagues. Lastly, several men reflect on fatherhood in general and offer their own advice and wisdom to other men.

Throughout all the stories, there remains an underlying theme: all of these fathers are emotionally engaged with their children and try to be supportive of their partners—giving their babies the best possible chance to grow into healthy, well-adjusted adults.

Identity

Like women, men experience a change in their sense of self upon becoming a parent. Some men feel a change in their identity immediately. Others take more time to start to come to terms with their new role in life. Whether the changes feel subtle or sudden, all the fathers in this section grapple with their change in identity and sense of self.

Father and provider: Grappling with the new role of 'father'

For Mike, the process of change was insidious; at first, he didn't even realise he was changing because it was such a slow and subtle process. It was only when his daughter reached 12 months of age that he realised that his sense of identity had changed.

Mike's Story

Honestly, I'd never considered that I might experience a change in my identity. I just thought that we'd have a baby, I'd still be me, and my wife Cathy would still be her. It never even crossed my mind that change was unavoidable, even though I should have known better.

When I met my baby, my first thought was 'Holy crap, I'm a father!' After that, I'm not sure. There was so much running through my mind that I felt a little overwhelmed by all of it. I do remember being instantly in love with both Clarissa and Brian when I saw them for the first time. I wish I could say that I had some deeply spiritual event when the kids were born, but the fact is, I just stood there with this goofy grin on my face. I didn't feel anything more complicated than happiness. That ought to be enough, I suppose. That feeling lasted for a long time, but after the first day or so, I began to adjust, and focus on more practical matters like getting everybody home, making sure the crib was ready, and so on.

I think I really began to feel a change when our daughter turned one. We had just moved closer to Cathy's family and were seeing them quite a bit more. What I noticed at first is that when they dropped by the house, they were usually there to focus on my daughter. In the past, since visiting us was more of an event, I was included more in the visit. Now, they could drop by on their way home from getting groceries, so nobody felt the need to chitchat with the grown-ups anymore. After our son was born, the trend continued. I began to feel like I was becoming 'Clarissa and Brian's dad', and not 'Cathy's husband' or 'Mike'. It just didn't seem that I was being valued as an individual any more. My worth came from the part I played.

At first, I didn't even realize that the change was happening. The changes were slow and subtle. Once I realized that who I was had changed, it was really too late to do anything about it. I didn't have any choice but to go with the flow. I wasn't all that pleased with the changes I saw, but I don't believe in crying over spilt milk. I think it's a waste of time and an admission of defeat.

The first thing I noticed was that I dropped a few places on my wife's priority list. Obviously, the kids are number one, which is as it should be. The spoiled brat part of me doesn't really like this, but the adult part of my brain is bigger and able to keep the brat under control. The biggest change that I've seen in our relationship has been, big surprise, in our romantic life. Before children, we had a far more active love-life. After both of the kids were born, things slowed down for a while, but I expected that, since having a new baby around the house is exhausting.

After our first child, things picked up, especially when we decided to try for a second baby. Once our son was born, though, it seemed like someone flipped our sex life switch to 'off' and glued it in place. I've found it frustrating because every time I say something about us not having time to just be husband and wife, Cathy agrees that we should do something about it, but never does. I think she sees me less as husband and lover, and more as father and provider. There's nothing wrong with those roles, but I still want and need to just be her husband more often than I am now. As the kids have gotten older, and as our daughter has gotten involved in activities in and out of school, there are even more demands on our time.

I don't know if there was a true shift in family dynamics or not. I feel like my opinions count for less now than they did before, but it's entirely possible that's just my fragile male ego talking.

I have at times wanted the 'old' me back but I don't think I'd want the old me back permanently. A few days would be OK. The old me didn't have somebody constantly wanting something from him all the time. But the me I am now is a much better person than the me I was several years ago. I miss some of the relative freedom I had before having children, but I don't think I want to go back.

Mike's Wisdom	So what advice do I have? First off, remember that the universe does NOT revolve around you! Has your role in the family changed? Absolutely. You are now a father, which is the most important job any man could ever have. Besides, your role in life ought to change every single day, as you adapt to events around you. If you don't change, you don't grow. If you don't grow, you stagnate and die.
	Don't expect yourself to be perfect. After all, our mistakes teach us a lot more than our successes, and it's really only the painful lessons that stick anyway.
	As far as a change in your sense of identity, remember that that's *all* that has changed; just your sense of identity, *not who you are*. The change is almost all internal. You ought to embrace it. I feel like I'm a better person with kids than I was without them. You should too. Be who you are now, not who you were yesterday. You're a better man today.

New roles: Different identity, same person

Theo gradually accepted (and embraced) his role as father, and felt that rather than defining him, being a father added another dimension to his sense of identity.

Theo's Story

I must admit that I really didn't consider how my sense of self or identity would change when I became a father. I do remember, many years beforehand, a friend talking to me about how after having his children, he came to think of his family not as his parents and siblings, but as his wife and children. I always remembered that statement and assumed that the same thing would happen to me (it did), but apart from that, I didn't really consider the more metaphysical issues such as 'sense of self'. I do remember, though, the somewhat daunting thought that came to us both post coitus—that this might just result in a baby! It was not a scary or unpleasant thought by any means but I do remember having the sense that something big may well have just happened.

The change was definitely gradual, and really began the first time my wife and I had sex without contraceptives. All of a sudden, we weren't a 'couple without children' anymore—physically, of course, we still were without children at that stage, but psychologically there had been a change. We were making love for a reason other than mere pleasure, and it felt different, more responsible, more adult in a sense, and it felt nice. We were entering a new phase and doing something new and significant.

In the months after that, various things dawned on me that cumulatively resulted in me identifying myself as a father. For one thing, I attended almost all of my wife's medical appointments, and people started to refer to me as 'the father'—which of course was a term that nobody had ever directed at me before. At first that felt very strange, but after a while I got used to it, which means, I suppose, that I started to see myself as 'father' and not just 'husband'.

On the other hand, I didn't think of myself as 'father' above all else, any more than I thought of myself as 'husband' or 'student' (I was studying at that stage) above all else. I was, and am, me; my identity is dependent on who I am and not on what I do or who I'm married to or what stage of life I am going through. Obviously all those things profoundly influence who I am and my sense of identity at any given time—but they do not determine my identity. So as my sense of identity changed, I didn't think of myself as a changed man or a different person. I was still me. My personality remained the same, my likes and dislikes and preferences remained the same, and in many ways, my priorities remained the same, albeit modified in some respects by the new responsibility I had. In other words, while becoming a father was life-changing in some ways, in other ways it was not. If, God forbid, I were ever to lose my family through death or other catastrophe, my sense of identity would change, but I would not (I don't think) become unrecognisable as me.

My sense of self-identity did change over the weeks and months after our baby was born, in two significant ways. First, I came to realise that I had a responsibility as provider for my family. But provision isn't just financial—it's relational. I had an obligation not just to be the 'breadwinner', but to provide for my wife and child emotionally and relationally. They didn't just need me to earn money—they also needed me to be there, and not just physically. The second thing that dawned on me was that being a parent was a blessing. It was fantastic. It was at times exhausting and frustrating (and even, dare I say it, boring), but the joy of being an integral part of family relationships and bonding with my children was just phenomenal.

So in that sense, my identity as a parent, and not just a man and a husband, grew, and I began to take relationships more seriously not just with my family, but with everyone.

More than ever now, I believe that relationships are what make the world go around. Relationships are not peripheral to what we do or who we are—rather, relationships are what we do and who we are, in a very significant and meaningful sense.

Of course, though, there were times when I looked back wistfully at simpler and more carefree times. It's too strong to say that I grieved for my old self. But having a baby is, in some ways, an inconvenience: you don't get to sleep when you want, go out when you want, see the friends you want (not as much, anyway), to spend your money in the way you want, or even to have the sort of relationship with your spouse you want. So at times I looked back on my relatively more carefree life in my 20s with a degree of nostalgia.

On a more practical note, my wife and I have always worked hard at helping each other to relax. For many years, each of us gave the other one sleep-in morning per week—a morning when one of us would get up with the children, while the other slept in. As our children have grown older, we've also each enjoyed cultivating friendships again. When one of us wants to go out with friends, the other will babysit the children. It is a love- and trust-based system, which works well for us.

Theo's Wisdom	Be yourself, and embrace being yourself. Don't feel guilty about needing a bit of time out. And try not to succumb to a 'grass is always greener' philosophy. Before you became a parent, there were genuine sources of joy and pleasure in your life which you may not be getting any of (or as much of) anymore. It's normal to miss some of those things, but try not to fall into the trap of thinking that there are no joys in your new life— because there are!

Dads on identity

- I was terrified when I found out Katie was pregnant. Life had been pretty easy up until then and I was in a nice, relatively stress-free, comfortable place. I felt terrible that I wasn't over the moon because I've seen the movies; I know how you're supposed to react. But it wasn't long before I got used to the idea that I was locked in. From that point on I started feeling good about it and excitement kicked in. I felt a real sense of purpose that I had never had before. Sure, I was still anxious but it was nervous excitement rather than the initial terror. By the time my daughter was born, I felt comfortable with this new stage in my life. Both Kate and I were in our 30s, so it wasn't like we were missing out much. We'd done all our partying and were ready and excited about the next chapter in our lives.

- I went with the flow; I was so busy that I didn't even think about what I used to do with friends, at work, down the pub, surfing and all that. I never grieved for my old self but sometimes I do miss being footloose and fancy-free.

- I was excited to step into the role of becoming a dad. All of a sudden, my life took on so much more meaning in the sense that I had serious responsibility ahead of me and if I screwed up it wasn't just me that would be affected. Becoming a dad made me dig deep within myself and address any feelings of inadequacy I previously had and to really think about how good a dad I could become. I did feel a strong identity as the 'father' of the family and was very eager to assume this role.

- I was happy to become a father, although there were times where I questioned myself as a father and as a person. Emotionally I was on a rollercoaster, having lows (arguments from lack of sleep) to highs (first smile) with everything in between! My old self was pretty cruisy, but having to look after a helpless baby became fairly stressful along with the changes in relationships and doubts about myself.

- I do fear that I will have forgotten how to be my old self by the time my kids are a bit older and self-maintaining. I don't wish to end up a fat slob defined only by my wife and kids and end up dreaming of retirement, a four-wheel drive and a caravan! I am happy to put the old self away for several years; I think it is selfish not to do this. I think it is unrealistic to try to be both at once. But I think I will need to dust off what I used to be occasionally and kick it over to be sure I can find it again one day. The travel, staying fit, sailing, seeing bands and shows; holding onto a shadow of the former glory will help ensure I am not completely transformed and can go back when the time comes.

- Something that stood out was driving Lizzy home. She was wrapped up and we were walking to the car when Susan said 'You can buckle her in'. We'd installed the car seat a few days prior, but I'd never really figured out how to use it as such. So I gently put Lizzy in the car seat and adjusted the straps. Strapping her in and taking her home was a big realisation for me—she was real, she was my daughter, and I was responsible for her becoming a good person and growing up.

Working dads and stay-at-home dads

While the concept of 'new fatherhood' emerges and continues to evolve, fathers are finding it increasingly difficult to balance their work and family lives. Gone are the days when fathers kissed their children and wife goodbye in the morning and came home (maybe) in time to tuck them into bed at night. Fathers are becoming more involved with the raising of their children and this often means that they have to rise earlier to take over some of the tasks of their partner (such as feeding their baby breakfast or packing school lunches). It also means, for many fathers, that a return from work does not necessarily signal the end of the working day. In fact, many fathers come home and take over their partner's household chores as well as the daily tasks of minding babies. While many men are eager to be more involved with their children, this has meant re-learning how to balance work and family life. Some men find this struggle very difficult, while others find it easier. Some men choose not to balance work and family life in the way men traditionally have, and instead stay at home with their children.

Challenging gender roles: When dad stays home to raise the kids

Simon made the decision to stay at home to raise his son, primarily due to financial reasons but also because he wanted to, viewing it as a golden opportunity to build a lifelong bond. Although Simon was happy with his choice, he found the unique isolation of being a stay-at-home dad difficult.

Simon's Story

Around the time of my first child's birth, I managed two restaurants and work seemed integral to my being. As well as an income, my job provided a form of self-identity and social validation, as it does for most participants in the modern economy. But then along came my first child, Liam, and within the space of a few months, all that I knew about myself underwent a radical transformation. Michelle's maternity leave was a golden period of sorts that allowed some initial leeway and breathing space to get our systems in place, and to know what we were doing as first-time parents. But as the leave drew to an end, a decision had to be made. Michelle out-earned me by a significant amount, so job stability and a higher wage were major factors in our decision.

In truth, I took on the stay-at-home dad challenge without much real hesitation. Choosing between the grind of restaurant life and the opportunity to spend more time with my boy was hardly worth deliberating, especially given our financial situation. Liam found it difficult to breastfeed, so we were already well down the path of formula and bottle-feeding by the time Michelle went back to work. There was also the hidden consideration, that of the two parents, I probably had a greater feeling for Liam's wants and needs. Michelle is his mother and I would never downplay her own special connection to her son, but I was very hands-on in the raising of my own brother and sister. When our baby was born, those instincts flooded back. Nursing, changing nappies and holding bottles felt like second nature; learned skills that I had acquired unknowingly when I was young, between football training and generally kicking around with my mates. For me it was just normal.

The role reversal allowed me to perform that most intrinsic human function of rearing a young child, a role only rarely and recently afforded to males, who for better or worse normally get lumped with the role of breadwinner within the family unit. That the main responsibility of nurturing and influencing our child would fall to me was a blessing. I still regard this decision as the best one I ever made as a father and this overwhelmingly positive experience was a factor in my decision to be the at-home parent for my next two children. I continue to be a significantly hands-on father today.

Attitudes to our parenting choice weren't really an issue among my friends, probably because no-one in our social network had children. For them, the novelty of a new child and the notion of a nuclear family was as different and fresh an idea as that of the father taking on the primary carer role.

The day-to-day grind of parenting (that bleary-eyed first year), however, was the main reality to be dealt with and it certainly didn't afford gendered speculations. You just did what you had to do to the best of your abilities, on a continual basis. Adding to our situation was the absence of family help, as both our families lived interstate. I found the first year a distinctly static existence which I wasn't completely prepared for; and although I loved every minute I spent with Liam, I was acutely aware of time and opportunities passing me by. For the first 18 months, it was basically Liam and me hanging out, waiting for Michelle to come home, at which time I would then go out to clear my head.

Stay-at-home parents, irrespective of gender, will likely experience negative views of their new found roles, and these feelings are not abnormal. But as an at-home dad, I felt distinctly alone in my experiences. The lack of mental stimulation was a big factor and often I felt frustrated at the lack of understanding people had for someone in my unique position. Nobody really got it, not even Michelle. By the end of the day, I was often an elastic band at snapping point, having had my patience well and truly stretched. As for connecting with other mothers going through the same stuff—I just didn't feel much in common with them. This was probably because in my mind they were doing something culturally acceptable and biologically 'normal'. I, on the other hand, was doing something that I had to do out of financial considerations.

Someone suggested that I join a playgroup. But being up to my eyeteeth in baby issues on a daily basis drove home feelings of emasculation, especially as I watched my male friends continue life as usual. Sharing these growing feelings with mothers didn't strike me as having the necessary cathartic attributes needed to remedy the situation, and there were no fathers' groups that I was aware of. Instead, I did a bit of part-time work which helped keep me sane, but nothing that involved responsibility and certainly nothing that could stand up to the 'What have you been up to?' questions that generally begin bloke conversations.

When Liam was about two, I had the feeling his social development had been hampered because I had eschewed the mothers' group. He'd spent some time in family day care and I'd taken him to parks and pools and other places where he'd mingled with his peers, but he had no real friends. His first birthday pictures were testament to this: a bunch of champagne-drinking adults and a child sitting around a chocolate mud cake. I felt guilty that this had occurred and although the nature of our experiences thus far had been overwhelmingly positive, they were also insular. I thought it only right to expand his experiences. The playgroup would be that place where we could go to rectify my issues and for a short time every week, I would put aside my inhibitions and relax, smile and think of England whilst he practised his social skills.

Along we both went, and while I introduced us I began to realise what I'd suspected all along: that there was little the mothers and I had in common. They were all very nice but there was definitely an awkwardness about the situation. Aside from our kids, there was little else to talk about. This is not a criticism of women or their conversations; it's simply that most women don't have an opinion on whether Murali is a chucker or whether it's just racism. For men, these innocuous subjects are vitally important entry points that allow a *sufficient amount of shit to be spoken before real matters of the heart can be attended to. The mothers' group wasn't a place where I could make more than polite small talk.*

My son saved me from the 'What does your wife do?' line of questioning by insisting I push him on the swing. While I pushed him, the thought occurred that our choice to reverse traditional roles wasn't something that these mothers agreed with. I got the feeling that it was regarded more with scepticism than positivity. Had we, in swapping traditional familial roles, crossed a line and challenged the primacy of mothers to raise children? Perhaps I was imagining it and being overly sensitive in an unusual situation. But I left feeling that the group was more for mothers to socialise than their children, who at that age don't really socialise anyway.

Of course, there were other outings in Liam's life where he mingled with little people and in those circumstances it was generally OK hanging with the mums. I actually found it pleasant talking about those things that mums talk about, but only on neutral ground and rarely beyond the level of small talk. The ease which mothers have with each other, as if they're part of a special club, is not something that men can access freely. Becoming part of that clique, where phone numbers can be exchanged and new friends made is difficult on so many levels.

Simon's Wisdom

Perhaps it seems as though I have a chip on my shoulder but in truth, I don't think I do. Having raised three children, I would strongly recommend more men do as I have, should the opportunity present itself. But be aware that there is a large gulf that exists between the experiences of men who choose to take on the primary carer role and that of women. With more understanding, perhaps we can do more to strengthen the position of men as primary carers and work towards undoing some of our social prejudices.

How many dads choose to stay at home?

According to the United States census data, the United States had approximately 5.5 million stay-at-home parents in 2003 (Randall 2008). Rochlen (Randall 2008) noted that '2006 census data indicate there are about 159 000 stay-at-home fathers [SAHFs]. The number of stay-at-home dads has grown over 60 percent since 2004, but getting an *accurate* number for just how many there are out there is very difficult. The census doesn't cover dads who are the primary childcare provider but who earned any income in the previous year, are part of a same-sex couple or are single fathers. It's a new phenomenon to even be counting stay-at-home parents.'

Academic research on SAHFs is limited but there is evidence to suggest that while they face social stigma from the general population, men who stay at home tend to experience positive reactions from family and friends (Rochlen et al. 2008a). Research has also investigated why some fathers stay at home. Rochlen et al.

(2008b) conducted a study on a relatively small sample of men and discovered that influencing factors ranged from the pragmatic and economical, to identity-related issues (for example, their wife was more invested in work), to childcare availability, to who was considered the most suitable caretaker.

If you are a SAHF (either by choice or necessity), there are certain things you can do to make your transition from work to home a smoother one. Firstly, like Simon, you may experience feelings of isolation—even if you do seek out playgroups and mothers' groups, you might feel very much on the periphery. However, if you live in a highly populated area, you may be lucky enough to go along to a fathers' group; if there isn't one available, you might even consider starting one of your own. You can also meet up with dads online—there are many forums and websites created solely for fathers (and some solely for SAHFs). This is especially helpful in you live in a remote area.

Everyone needs companionship and a sense that they are 'doing things right', so it is really important to seek out or develop your own networks of support. Another issue to think about is your return to work. If you plan to do so at some point in the future, it might be helpful to maintain contact with your colleagues and work networks. This may make it easier for you to re-enter the workforce. For a list of support organisations and websites for fathers and SAHFs, please see page 260 of the Resources section. For ideas on how to start your own fathers' group, see Appendix B: 'How to start up a support group' on page 225.

From worker to dad and back again: Balancing family and work

Michael lives and works in Australia and was not offered parental leave when his baby was born. He went back to full-time work four weeks after the birth of his son and found it very difficult leaving his family at home. Michael describes the difficult struggle of balancing work and family life, and how that struggle often leaves him feeling exhausted and 'running on empty'.

Michael's Story

I was employed full time during my wife's pregnancy and took four weeks of annual leave (parental leave is not offered by my employer) at the time of the birth. In many ways, those four weeks didn't feel like enough time, but I think this was compounded by the fact that our son spent almost two weeks in an intensive care unit in the beginning due to a lung problem. I felt a little cheated by that. Practical considerations had to be made, though, as I wanted to retain some leave to use in emergencies or just as a pressure valve during the first year, and I also wanted to start building my leave back up again in preparation for a second child in the not-too-distant future. It was very hard to return to work, and when I did go back, it was very difficult to concentrate on my duties. My mind and heart were very much still at home.

I don't think I've been on time to work more than half-a-dozen times during the six months since our son was born. Luckily, my employer is very considerate and flexible and this hasn't been a problem. While it's certainly a challenge to balance all of these commitments, I have coped pretty well so far.

I haven't noticed a significant change in my relationships with work colleagues. In some ways, those relationships have become more personal, as people are constantly asking about our son and how he is developing. An unexpected consequence of that, however, is that you find that you are always answering the same questions over and over again. Either it can get to the point where you want to avoid such conversations or simply long for someone to ask you about anything other than your baby — 'Well, I don't know much about animal husbandry … but I'm glad you asked.'

Walking through the front door after work is without a doubt the best part of the day. Seeing my wife and son after being at work gives me quite a boost. Sometimes, though, that boost can be short-lived. I try to do at least my fair share of domestic duties when I get home. I'm our usual cook and generally do any chores that are physical in nature, like carrying out the rubbish. These can be really draining, in contrast to helping to look after our son, which even when it's stuff like changing dirty nappies is still an opportunity for me to interact and bond with him. Thankfully, he is a very happy child, but on those rare occasions when he is cranky, it can be very trying too.

In addition to the domestic duties, I also help out with a contract job that we have taken on to help with finances. This work is physical in nature and can be frustrating because it can be a fair bit of work for not a lot of return. I sometimes resent this work, because I feel like it is cutting into the time that I have to spend with my son and even makes it difficult to find the time to do little things like mowing the lawn or giving myself a hair cut (one of the very few advantages of male pattern baldness).

Michael's Wisdom	In many ways, your work suddenly becomes your second job when you have a baby, as your primary job is now 'Dad'. While it's a great job to have, you have to be ready for the massive increase in time and energy demands. Balance can be elusive in a young father's life. I'm normally a very cheerful and calm person but when I start feeling overburdened, my behaviour can change quite alarmingly. If you don't take time to ease the pressure as it builds up, then you may find that you're not being the kind of father you want to be, and furthermore, you may not be the kind of employee or even person that those around you expect you to be.

Well-balanced: A supportive employer makes work and family life easier

Andre works in the United States, the only OECD country that does not have a comprehensive paid parental leave scheme (Institute for Women's Policy Research 2007). Fortunately for Andre, his workplace is very supportive, allowing him leave as he needs it. It is this supportive work environment that Andre attributes his ability to balance his work and family life more easily.

Andre's Story

I was in full-time employment when my wife was pregnant and took 12 weeks of unpaid leave when our daughter was born, which is the maximum allowed under The Family and Medical Leave Act. Looking back, that now seems to be far too long, but at the time, it wasn't. We were both nervous new parents and lived over an hour from the nearest family members, so Charlotte wanted me around as long as possible. When our son was born three years later, I only took a couple of weeks off, and by the end of that, Charlotte was inventing errands for me, just to get me out of the house.

Fortunately, I've never had issues with balancing work and family. If I've needed the time to take care of family matters, I've gotten it. I am a paramedic, and our Director is of the opinion that you need to know your family is OK, so you can have your head completely in the game while on duty.

How I feel when I get home from work really depends on the day I have had. I work a 24-hour shift, so I may get home after being awake and running for the preceding 26 hours, or I might have been able to go to bed early the night before and sleep through the night without interruption. As for household chores, we've always split them up, so having kids didn't really change much. I have done most of the cooking since we got married, and we both do cleaning and laundry as we notice it needs doing. Bathing and feeding were always traded off, but if one of us had to work the next morning, the one staying home had the duty that night. I've always felt that this was a good way to split things up. I suppose I did feel a bit more tired during the baby days, but I learned pretty quickly to nap when the kids did.

When the kids were really little, I did feel like a bit of a pay check extension. The first year or so is really mom's time. It seemed like all I did was come home from work just in time to see the beginning of nap time. This passed once the children weren't sleeping quite so much.

My relationships with my colleagues stayed more or less the same. Nearly all of my co-workers have kids, so we had a bit more common ground. The emergency services community is a pretty tightly knit one, so we tend to treat each other like an extended dysfunctional family anyway. It's like working with a whole group of weird uncles that nobody ever talks about.

Andre's Wisdom   The main thing I've learned is that every parent is willing to offer advice. I had an enormous number of offers to help from all of my co-workers. Taking some of them up on those offers was one of the smartest moves I've ever made. The best advice I can offer is this: try to remember that a job can be replaced far more easily than a family. Think about your priorities (if you have that luxury).

Relationships

Many people think that having a baby will improve their relationship with their partner, but the opposite can often be the case. The truth is that having a baby can test your relationship with your partner to the absolute limits. Functioning on little (or no) sleep, learning how to care for a newborn, and trying to be supportive of your partner while balancing paid work can leave men (and women) extremely exhausted and irritable. Women's bodies go through enormous changes during pregnancy and after birth. Many women feel uncomfortable during pregnancy for a variety of reasons. After birth, women may feel sore, have stitches and be breastfeeding. They have a lot of physical recovery to go through, and if they are breastfeeding, some women still feel as though they are sharing their body. All of these issues can lead women to feel a drop in sexual desire. Men, on the other hand, while tired, have not undergone such enormous bodily changes and may feel more desire than women. This can be problematic for both parties.

While the desire for intimacy rates highly on men's wishes for their relationships, they also talk about their relationships with friends, colleagues and family. Some felt a more intense relationship with their family of origin, while others felt distanced. Some men lost many friends, while others managed to maintain some sort of relationship with their existing friends. All the men contributing to this section felt a discernable change in all of their relationships, but these changes were not always negative.

Oh baby: When a newborn leads to a sexual dry spell

David found that while his relationships with his family and friends changed when his wife became pregnant, it was his relationship with his wife that changed the most. David had always felt that their sexual relationship was an important part of who they were as a couple and so was greatly affected when sex was withdrawn.

David's Story

Our relationship was still quite new when we fell pregnant, and the news changed my relationships with my family, as they felt we were rushing into it. My parents were concerned and felt that they were too young to be grandparents, despite being well into their 40s.

My relationship with my friends had already cooled when I started seeing my partner; they still wanted to party and go out, while I was seeing and feeling something real and important in my new relationship. They could not see that my main focus was my partner and my soon-to-be family. My friends felt that was too serious, which was hard for me at first but not really a major issue in the total scheme of things.

My relationship with my partner, once we knew that she was pregnant, was something that was overwhelming and scary. We were going from two young people enjoying ourselves, to a family unit, with responsibilities and ties that were not there before.

Throughout the pregnancy, the change that was the most prominent was the sexual side of things. She had morning sickness and issues with her self-esteem as she was putting on weight. I wasn't the most understanding about it all; I found it hard realising that the sexual side (which had been a strong foundation of our relationship) was all but gone. I guess I hoped that after the nine months were over, things could go back to the way that they were. It was a frustrating, difficult thing to live with on top of all the other changes that were happening at breakneck speed.

After our baby was born, my first reaction was an overwhelming sense of tiredness but there was also a sense of disbelief that this child was actually mine. My life as I knew it was changed forever. The past was gone and things could never be the same, my responsibilities were now glaringly obvious, and things would now be forever different; these were the intimidating thoughts that were running through my head.

The first six weeks after the baby was born were a massive change for me—I felt lost, depressed in a way. I felt like it was hard to get any attention because everything was all so busy. The feeding, the deprived sleep, being separated from my partner and baby for work, the lack of the sexual side of things, indeed the lack of intimacy altogether, was really hard to adjust to.

Weirdly, the person that I loved was now not just a partner but a mother, the mother of my child, the person that had gone through all that pain for me. I did get angry about not being able to get my own way with things as much but knew that there were changes that she was going through too. I wanted to contribute and let her know that I was there, but it was hard. My friends were now non-existent too. They didn't want to be a part of the whole family thing; they were still partying and enjoying themselves—they didn't want to be weighed down by a man with a baby.

I found the sexual side was something that I really missed and wanted. In the last months before the birth, we didn't have sex. Then I had to wait until the six-week check up. I know it sounds selfish but it just really got to me. It was like something was missing, something that was really vitally important to me—to us. After the six-week mark, we did attempt sex but it felt awkward. My wife was so nervous; she was worried about how she looked and how it would feel for her and how it would feel for me. She hated the first attempt at sex and I felt awful. I know that she was adjusting but to be rejected at the first attempt in so long was depressing. I felt like it might always be that way; I was worried that the pain that she was feeling would stay there for a long time and that we may never get that side of things back on track. It was something that we talked through a lot, but to actually tell your partner how hard it is, and to be wanting them and the intimacy so badly and not getting it, was just one more thing to have to get used to.

I know that for a while our sex life suffered; we didn't have sex much for about eight weeks. Then it slowly got back to the way it was. It did feel different; I know it did for both of us. It was good that we could talk and that she was so understanding. She always made me feel wanted, it was just that the actual physical side took time to get back on track.

David's Wisdom	Through all of this, I guess it is important that we always try to remember the positives and let go of the negatives. Sometimes it's a hard road, and you can feel overwhelmed, but it does get there in the end. You have to learn to be strong, have belief in yourself, and try to deal with obstacles as they come along. Try not to take it personally if your partner doesn't want sex; she may have many reasons for abstaining and none of them might be to do with you. Talk to her and find out what her issues are and try not to take the lack of intimacy personally. Things do tend to work out OK—different but OK.

Separation at birth: When a new baby places strain on your relationship

When his partner became pregnant, Dean felt immense changes in all of his relationships: with his friends, his colleagues and his family. He also felt a shift in his new family's dynamics; he found it increasingly difficult to relate to his partner. The sheer exhaustion from working ten-hour days and then being 'handed the baby' created a tense atmosphere. Eventually, the lack of intimacy and the endless arguments forced Dean and his partner to separate.

Dean's Story

We didn't plan to have a baby, so our daughter coming into this world was a surprise. Consequently, there was little time for consideration of how our relationships might change. One of the biggest changes that I felt was with workmates and people my own age—they seemed happy as single people or as a couple; once children were mentioned, looks of horror came across their faces. An event that stuck out in my mind was when I was undergoing training on a new computer package at work. My blank looks were annoying this particular person, and when questioned about my attention to the training, I smiled and said 'Work doesn't really compare to having kids ... there's bigger things in the world than work'.

Regarding family relationships, Olanthe was the first grandchild for both of our parents and as such, the relationship between our parents and us felt like it changed—from a parent/child relationship to more of an adult/adult relationship—my wife and I were no longer seen as children.

Mandy and I were excited about Olanthe, and our relationship changed from spoiling each other and spending lots of time with each other as a couple, to one of preparing for Olanthe. It was a bit strange to start with—getting the house ready for someone that was only tiny—but once we saw the scans it was more real and believable.

Meeting Olanthe, I felt amazed. I couldn't believe how much hair she had (I was expecting a bald baby) and once she had spent some time on Mandy's chest bonding and getting her cord cut, she was given to me to weigh on the scales. I remember holding a wet, crying thing that I just wanted to squeeze to bits. I had no idea what to do except cuddle her. I remember thinking how small she was, how she was alive, and how I was now a dad to her. I just remember thinking to myself how much of a huge learning curve this next part of my life would be. I think the first three to six months of your first child's life would have to be the most stressful times due to the huge learning curve. We were much more confident with Olanthe after six or so months, and I can only guess that the second (and third) are a little bit easier, due to experience with the first child.

After four weeks' leave, I went back to work in a male-dominated world which greatly contrasted to my home life with Mandy and Olanthe. Usually, I would do a ten-hour shift and go home, expecting five minutes to just sit down and chill out, but this got varying reactions. The most common were 'Olanthe's crying, sort her out, I'm having a rest' and 'Olanthe's asleep, I'm going to sleep, do the dishes and clean up the mess'. I tried to understand where Mandy was coming from, having ten hours on her own looking after a baby that didn't come with a manual, and tried to reason with Mandy about where I was coming from too. On my days off, I tried hard to spend a lot of time with Olanthe so Mandy would get a break but regardless of that, our relationship was getting rocky, due to our misunderstanding of what the other person did (or didn't do).

Before pregnancy we had a healthy sex life; during pregnancy it was irregular (perhaps once a month in the first three to four months then none after six months) and there was no sex life for six weeks after the birth. When we did have sex that first time, it was disappointing, as our relationship had changed. Sex had gone from something fun that both of us enjoyed, to a chore for one of us. Overall, we had sex perhaps a dozen times in the 18 months after Olanthe's birth. This lack of emotion, positive attention and love was one of the reasons for our separation.

I did look at my partner differently after Olanthe was born. There were times where I saw her as a mother (which was predominant) and the odd occasions where she was my lover. I think a lack of sleep was a major factor with our behaviour moving from a happy couple to two irritable, tired parents who fought a lot. Because of this, she changed (in my eyes) from a fun, outgoing person to one that was forever grumpy, hated our house and location and was short-tempered. As a result, my behaviour changed from a generally happy, outgoing person to someone who didn't enjoy being at home, and I became a quiet person who didn't speak out of turn lest I get in trouble.

My relationship also changed with my mates. As both of us were relatively young to become parents (both of us were 22), we found ourselves stuck between our friends who didn't have kids and 30-something people who had kids of a similar age. As such, we found it difficult in a smaller town to find people our age with kids around our child's age.

*Regardless, our relationship with friends certainly changed from news of the pregnancy onwards. My partner ceased drinking and smoking immediately, and our social life went from regular parties and going out to pubs to essentially nothing. So our regular 'drinking buddies' soon lost interest as our interests changed. We tried to make friends at the **antenatal** classes at the hospital, but moving again within three months of the birth made it hard to keep and maintain existing relationships.*

Dean's Wisdom	Be understanding of what your partner is going through—no matter how tired or grumpy you are, there's a good chance they are too. For the working parent, find the time to give love and attention to the carer parent as they've just had all day of baby/child interaction with no adult conversation. The Wiggles, Shrek and In the Night Garden all get to you in the end! So spend some time at the end of the day with your original loved one.
	From a dad who went through separation 18 months after our child was born, if you break up with your partner, realise that although your relationship with the other parent may have ended, your relationship with your child will never end. Another thought is to keep things nice when the kids are around, particularly as they grow older. Kids pick up emotions and vibes—and no child needs to grow up dreading 'handover days'.

From husband to dad: Swapping quantity with quality

Dhruv experienced a positive change in his relationships when his baby arrived, particularly with his wife. Although he recognises that his sex life is not what it was, he sees this as a normal part of life and believes that it will return when things settle down. He has maintained relationships with his friends, particularly those who are dads, but doesn't have much time to put into socialising while looking after his wife and baby.

Dhruv's Story

Prior to and during my wife's pregnancy, I felt an odd mix of excitement and trepidation regarding how our baby was going to change my life and specifically my relationships. On one hand, I was very optimistic and thought a baby would only make our lives better and more fulfilling. On the other hand, I was scared that nothing would ever be the same again, especially in terms of my friends who weren't parents themselves, and that a baby could create a divide between my wife and me.

I knew that I would love and care for our child and in some way that might take away from the amount of time I could spend demonstrating my love for my wife and looking after her—and obviously the reverse would be true too. I felt confident that we could manage that, but I have to admit that I didn't realise how hard it would be to be a good husband while striving to be a good dad. It's simply an issue of time and energy—both are in shorter supply once you have a baby and you have to be willing to accept that the focus of your relationship with your partner has to shift from quantity to quality, and you actually have to work hard to achieve that quality time. In terms of friends, I made peace with the possibility that I might drift away from some friends.

After our baby was born, sex was pretty much out of the question for an extended period because my wife had to have an emergency caesarean. She needed time to heal and that was fine. Since then, we have found very limited opportunities to make love. Because we do not have a lot of support in terms of family living locally, we haven't been able to spend a lot of time together without our son. That makes it hard. As such, sex seems a bit rushed and erratic. There have been times when we've had to abandon our fooling around because our son has woken up. On a personal level, I haven't been too upset about these obstacles. This might also be because I'm so tired that I haven't felt too amorous anyway. I understand why these things are happening and I am confident that our sex life will not only return to normal, but may even be better for this experience. I certainly won't be taking sex for granted anytime soon.

I think I look at my wife slightly differently now that she is the mother of my child. I have always loved and cherished her, but now I see her as a much more central figure in our family life. Instead of just two people who negotiate things as a couple, our family life has become a three-ringed circus that requires, among other things, a ring master—and that's my wife. She's not just my partner, she's the central cog in our family. I used to just be thankful that she loved me, but now I'm also indebted to her for giving me this brand new, little person who now means more to me than all the other things that I used to think were important combined. I have always felt fiercely protective of my wife, so that hasn't really changed, but I guess that is another aspect of how I feel about her—I'd do anything to make sure she and my son remained safe and happy.

I was fortunate that a number of my friends had babies around the same time as us. That said, however, there are certain sacrifices that you make because of a baby. You have less disposable income to spend doing things with mates and there are time pressures too. That has put a strain on some friendships. I firmly believe, however, that if some friends can't understand these pressures and tolerate them, you have to accept that you'll probably drift away from those mates. I only have room in my life for one baby at this point in time, so I won't be spending too much time worrying about mates who behave immaturely. Besides, I have been enjoying my new family so much that I haven't even really noticed it, and I am also much more likely now to make new friends with other fathers (especially new dads). There's even a chance that those friends who drifted away might drift back into my life when they start families themselves.

Dhruv's Wisdom	Naturally, there are many things about a baby's arrival that change a relationship. At this point in time, with our first child being six months old, I'd say a baby has done much more to improve my relationship with my wife than harm it. Together we are guiding a new life. I see our child as a physical representation of our love and commitment to each other,

and a vessel that we can fill up with love. While we had shared interests before, now we share the greatest interest of all—our son.

Not all changes are so obviously positive. Both my wife and I now have to share the attention and affections of the other person with a very attention-hungry baby. Amidst nappy changes, feedings and bath times, there are fewer opportunities for those little pampering things you used to enjoy giving and receiving. There is also an obvious and significant impact on your sex life.

I think husbands really need to be on the lookout for ways that they can be supportive. You can't succumb to jealousy and, conversely, you have to make sure that you don't neglect your wife as you're heaping love onto the new baby.

Most of all, I think mothers and fathers need to view each other as teammates and try to work together and support each other. Along the way, that's going to require empathy, tolerance and patience.

Made in Manhattan: Life as a single dad in New York

Tom was a high-powered executive who was financially successful but had almost no relationship with his two small children once he and his wife divorced. He had to make a conscious decision to be a father to his kids.

Tom's Story

When my wife and I divorced, I had to look for another place to live. I eventually found a killer bachelor pad penthouse on the corner of Commonwealth and Massachusetts Avenues, but it took quite a while for me to settle in.

My ex-wife and I agreed that the kids would come to my apartment every Friday night. I put bunk beds and a matching wooden toy chest in what would become their room. Each week I'd pick up Seamus and Kerry, and all their gear, and drive around my city neighborhood looking for a parking spot. The kids were usually grumpy and hungry by the time I finally parked the car and loaded them into their double stroller. I'd put their bags on top and start pushing. I was driven by adrenaline, trying to make this all OK for them. By the time I had reached my building, unloaded the kids, and got them through the door and into the lobby, I would feel as though I had climbed Mount Everest. I'd tell Kerry to hold Seamus's hand, and then I would go back outside, collapse the stroller, and lug it up the stairs and into the lobby before corralling the kids into the elevator. From the elevator, the kids would run ahead down the hall. I'd catch them just in time to open the door to my apartment and lead them up a final flight of stairs inside. Then it was time for me to make dinner.

The first night I had the kids on my own I gave them baths, slipped them into matching footie pyjamas, tucked Kerry into her bunk, and then warmed a bottle for Seamus. In my bedroom, I turned off the lights and rocked him gently while he drank. I inhaled deeply. It was the scent of my son that changed everything—his scent and the sound of him suckling his bottle, the softness of his skin and the sensation of holding him as his body gradually went limp with sleep. I looked down and realized that this—being a father— was my deepest satisfaction. Chasing Kerry around the house at five the next morning, catching her, and tickling her as she screamed with joy confirmed it.

In the days that followed my kids' first overnight visit, I realized just how much work I had to do as a dad. I feared I would never be a decent parent no matter how hard I tried. When they were at my apartment, my childhood fear of heights returned. I often had nightmares of the kids falling out the bay window. Kerry didn't help matters. Even at age three, she loved to taunt me by standing on the ledge inside that window with her nose pressed against the glass, looking out at the city and giggling at my discomfort. To set my mind at ease, I nailed two-by-fours across the bottom of the window.

I didn't want to see my kids just on weekends. During the week I took them to a playgroup in one of the buildings on Newbury Street. I sat in a circle with the moms and their kids, singing, wrestling, and generally acting goofy. As I rolled around on the floor, the moms didn't know what to make of me. But they gradually accepted me, and I got to be with my kids. On Saturdays I took them to the top of the Prudential building, only a few blocks from my apartment. The carpeted floors and large, soft furniture were ideal for some safe roughhousing, and the observation deck was a large square track, where the kids could wear themselves out by running around and around. There were rainy days when we couldn't see a damn thing, but we still went up there, just to have something to do together.

Care objects were very important to the kids as their little minds tried to manage all the moving around. Kerry had a blanket she slept with every night. Seamus became attached to a stuffed Pal dog from the PBS show 'Arthur'. Pal took on identifying textures and wear marks as he was beaten, barfed on, and laundered. He was one of a kind and not replaceable. I became obsessed with knowing where Pal and 'Blankie' were at all times. As the end of each visit approached, I turned the apartment upside down with drill-sergeant precision to ensure all the kids' stuff was accounted for.

Then one day Pal disappeared. I scoured under beds and behind furniture. The apartment wasn't that big, so coming up dry convinced me that the crisis was indeed serious. After several nights of listening to my tearful son on the phone bemoaning the loss of Pal, I slunk over to FAO Schwarz and purchased another.

I brought the replacement Pal to my office. I tried to duplicate, in a single day, years' worth of wear marks. I took a baseball bat to the pristine doggie, and then I threw the six-inch-thick Handbook of Fixed Income Securities *at him. My partners in our venture firm couldn't figure out what was going on. My door was shut and I didn't respond to any calls or emails all day. On the walk home, I took the now-limp dog and rolled him in sidewalk sand. When I got to my condo, I threw him in the washing machine for an extra-heavy spin cycle.*

That night I stood apprehensively at my ex-wife's front door with the new, but suitably worn, Pal. But before I could present him, I learned that the original Pal had been recovered: Kerry confessed to smuggling him home and hiding him inside the folds of her mother's curtains. When I returned to my apartment, I stored the spare dog in the back of my closet, just in case.

Tom's Wisdom	It's never too late to start loving your kids. As men, we are hardwired to be good fathers. All kinds of things can get in the way, but you need to move past them. Even if you only have limited time with your kids, like I did at the beginning, make the most of it. That doesn't mean doing anything special. It just means being with them. Holding them. Reading them books. Tickling them. And loving them.

Tips for single or divorced dads

Tom is the founder of the 'Good Men Project', which is a book, film, series of events and an online magazine about what it means to be a good father, son, husband and worker in modern society (for more information on The Good Men Project, please see page 261 of the Resources section). Tom outlines some general tips for newly divorced dads:

- Show up for your kids on time, every time.
- Keep heated discussions with their mother/co-parent private.
- Be hands on; play with your kids.
- Spend time with extended family to keep your kids connected to their relatives.
- Make your space a home for your kids with special toys.
- Develop a routine with the kids at your house.
- Even if your time with the children is reduced because of the divorce/separation, make the most of it.
- Never give up on your love for the children.

Another great tip comes from RJ Jaramillo, founder of Single Dad (www.singledad. com), who says that the first 90 days of being a single dad are a time of crisis. This is the time when men are most likely to feel completely overwhelmed and liable to make bad decisions. He has found that having newly single men focus on specific, learnable skills—such as learning how to cook or really understanding their finances—can make all the difference as to how they cope during this time of crisis.

Dads on relationships ...

- With my partner, having a baby stretched our relationship to the limits. We were both not in our home countries and with no family around, we felt isolated. The transition into parenthood was a huge obstacle for us (especially with the arrival of our firstborn, who arrived six weeks early) and combined with the change in routine, set the scene for a lot of arguing. Because of our desire to make it work, in the end it has made us both stronger people and better parents. With my mates, it pretty much stayed the same, probably because in the beginning (when I was fighting with my partner so much) I didn't really cut out any Friday night sessions with the guys and continued to come home drunk. I eventually realised the error of my ways and am lucky enough to have friends that have stuck by me through thick and thin.

- My new life is definitely more fulfilling than my old life. I've become tremendously involved with my family—both immediate and extended, perhaps to the detriment of some of my friendships. I'm annoyed at myself for being slack in this department and I want to fix it but I find I get pretty much all I need from contact with close family and very close friends.

- Becoming a dad has changed my relationships a bit. My mates without kids just don't get it. With my partner, there is less time together—we spend far less time on the relationship. I think that having a child certainly tests beliefs, standards, morals and rules across relationships that would never be tested otherwise. I should add that our son is the first grandchild for both our families, which has meant increased (and intense) interaction with our families, something that we had to get used to.

- The most obvious change in relationships was with my workmates—many of whom were around my age (early 20s) and were still in the dating/pubbing/clubbing scene. When I explained my absence from 'the scene' (for example, I was preparing for a baby and providing support for my partner), they seemed incredulous and generally made jokes about how my life was over.

- I left Melbourne (where I had been settled for some time and have family) at about the time I became a dad. I felt more connected with my family (especially my father's family) and not so interested in Shanghai (where we ended up) when we got there.

Reflections on fatherhood

Like women, all men experience fatherhood differently. In the following stories, men reflect on how they feel about fatherhood, and on what it's like to be a dad.

What is the secret? Humour, common sense and compassion

William takes a light-hearted look at what it is like to be a father. He believes that if you possess common sense, compassion and a good sense of humour, you are off to a great start.

William's Story

Nobody can really prepare you for being a dad. You pretty much have to make it up as you go along. There are lots of magazines, books and websites for moms out there, but not for dads. There's a reason for that. It goes back to the whole 'I'm a man and I don't NEED instructions!' thing. It's a good thing we don't, because kids don't come with any. So, what have I learned from being a dad? I've learned that I've got a lot to learn, and none of it is particularly easy.

First off, nobody ever told me that most days, the hardest part of parenthood is keeping a straight face. Let's face it, when you investigate noises like THUMP 'Ow!' THUMP 'Ow!' THUMP 'Ow!' coming from the other room, and find your son is trying to get out from under the dining room table by standing up and walking out, it's tough to be the figure of authority when all you really want to do is laugh. If you and the kids aren't laughing a lot, one of you (probably you!) is doing something wrong. Lighten up.

Patience is also a really good idea. I sometimes forget that things I see as relatively simple tasks, like pulling your pants up after using the bathroom, are still new concepts to the kids. It can take some time for them to master complex fasteners like snaps and Velcro that require exceptional manual dexterity to operate and demand intense concentration to avoid injury. Take a deep breath, let them try to do it themselves for a while, and relax. Nobody learns a new skill overnight. You also need to be patient with the kids' questions. And believe me, there will be questions. Lots of them. You know the old saying 'There are no stupid questions?' Not true. There are a whole bunch of stupid questions, and my kids have asked virtually all of them. Repeatedly. My secret is to give equally stupid answers. That seems to satisfy them, but I think my daughter is beginning to catch on. She keeps checking my answers with my wife, then says 'Quit joking me!' Her brother is still gullible enough to think I know what I'm talking about, so I'll mess with his head for a couple more years. I'll stop when we start getting calls from the school, or when the kids figure out they're the ones that get to pick my nursing home some time in the future.

Something that runs hand in hand with the patience thing is time. It took me a long while to realize that kids perceive time the same way dogs do. That is to say, not at all. Assigning a relatively simple task like picking up a pair of dirty socks and carrying them to the laundry basket can take in excess of an hour. Learn to add 'Right now!' to the end of every order. It doesn't help, but you'll feel like you're doing something to speed the sock-picking-up process along. You also need to know that when you promise something to a kid, they assume you're going to deliver on that promise immediately. Keep your mouth shut until you're in a position to deliver, or you'll regret it. That is, unless you like being harassed about a trip for ice cream for six solid hours.

Speaking of food, my wife and I have been asked how we got our kids to eat so many different things. That one is actually easy. Neither of us is a fussy eater, and we enjoy trying new things. When we had our daughter, we decided to not dumb down our diet. We did season a little more lightly, but otherwise we ate the same stuff we always had, and so did she. That must have been the secret, because now both kids will at least try whatever we put in front of them. Simple but effective, which is how I like it. If not making a big deal about what's on the plate doesn't work, lie. Make something up, the more disgusting sounding the better. The kids may not eat meatloaf, but 'pate du snouts de aardvark' will disappear quickly.

William's Wisdom	So, what's the real secret of being a dad? The real secret is that there isn't a secret. To be a good dad, all you need is the same things it takes to be a good person. You need common sense, a sense of humor, and compassion in more or less equal amounts. You might get away with a little fudging on the proportions, but if you're lacking any one of these qualities, you're going to have a rough go of it. Parenthood is the single greatest responsibility placed on a man. When you have kids, the future of the world is in your hands. Don't screw it up.

What I want my partner to know is ...

- That I still need you to myself once in a while. I love the kids to death, obviously, but sometimes I want to spend time with you and without them.

- That I really am trying as hard as I can, despite my many mistakes and despite the fact that sometimes my instinct is to do things the opposite way that you would. Despite anything you might think to the contrary, I honestly worship you. The feeling of your skin against mine as we sleep at night is the greatest comfort in my life.

- That often I try to act like I know what's best for my family but inside I can be scared that I might mess up.

- By having you in my life, you make me stronger every day. Stronger to be a better husband, stronger to be a better father and stronger to be a better man.

- I love you and I choose to spend my life with you; it doesn't change because we have children. My priorities have shifted and as a dad, I understand the impact I will have on their lives. I want to ensure that I spend as much time that I can with them so they develop into amazing people. It doesn't mean you're not as important, but I only have a certain amount of time to pour into them before they leave; and the time I have is precious—I won't ever get it back.

- I hate that I can't fix your depression. Sometimes, I fall apart, usually when the pressure piles up. The kids are melting down in the back of the car, my boss has just sent me a curt email about the shortcomings of my work; a little devil starts to whisper in my ear. I start to think that you're not trying and I feel sorry for myself. When you're very sick, it's a daunting feeling bringing up three small children by myself. I can't braid my daughters' hair. I want you back. I want you better. Not just because of the kids but because you are my other half, my love and I miss you.

- When you're up to your eyes in nappies and tantrums and suffering from lack of sleep and you think you can't take one more full cup of milk spilt over you—hang in there! Someday soon, you and I are going to get the hell out of here for a whole week and escape by ourselves to somewhere beautiful, like Venice! We'll stay in a romantic hotel and laze around drinking coffee in little side street cafes and go for romantic walks in the evening and get to feel like normal adults again … for a little while.

- I need you to know that I can't do everything your way because I am not you. Yes, I understand that you spend all day with our baby while I'm out at work but I need to learn how to bond with him myself and I can only do that if you let me be. Does it really matter that I put him in an outfit that doesn't match? Is it so essential that I change his nappy exactly the same way as you? I just want to learn how to be a father to my son, and while I really do appreciate your advice, I would like the opportunity to figure some stuff out for myself, just like you got to do.

- The truth? I miss you! I love our new family—it's made me a better person and our relationship stronger. And I know you have a lot of physical healing and emotional adjustment to get through, but I can't wait to have you back in my arms; to be intimate with you again.

- I love the family we have created more than anything. The 'accident' we made three years ago was the best thing I ever made. I would go back and live it again if I could. I wouldn't change it for the world.

- I would love for you to learn how to switch off when our baby is in my care.

Soccer-mad dad: Being a dad to three boys

Gavin loves being the father of three boys, but still feels like he's learning how to be a dad as he goes along.

Gavin's Story

The first thing to say (and it's been said many times—if you are a 'dad to be' you are probably sick of hearing it) is that you have absolutely no idea what it's like being a dad until you actually are one. People might tell you and you might think you have an idea of what to expect, but nothing can prepare you for the feelings you get when you become a dad. I'll never forget the feeling I got when our first son Adam was still in the womb. He was not even born but the ultrasound showed he had a dilated kidney. I had no real clue what this meant and we needed a follow-up test so it must have been serious. In hindsight now (as a dad of three boys) it was nothing, but I felt something that night that I had never felt before: unconditional love (and worry—sick to the stomach worry) for my unborn child.

Are you a dad before your child even takes a breath? I don't know, but looking back I remember experiencing different feelings for the first time, and there was no turning back from that. These were also very different feelings to those that you have for your soul mate; a different kind of love. Then they are born and the journey begins anew. I'm six years into fatherhood and still feel like I have no clue what I'm doing. I still feel like a kid myself but feel like I must be doing something right (even though my six-year-old currently has a cast on a broken arm).

I have been speaking to a mate of mine in England and they recently adopted a six-year-old child. It is weird to suddenly find your friends having an older son than you, when two months ago they were a childless couple. He's been saying how hard it is being a dad. I absolutely agree, but he's trying to be a dad to a six-year-old 'immediately'. My respect goes out for taking this on. I was able to give him advice on how to be a dad to a six-year-old as I had six years of practice and 'grew' into (and with) my child. I have another mate who has a 12-year-old. I look at his kid and wonder how on earth he does it, but then my wife reminds me I have six more years to 'learn' how to be a dad to a 12-year-old.

Recently, my wife and I were talking to our next-door neighbour, Jack. He is about 45, on holiday and 'completely bored'. He'd detailed the car (twice), maintained his flat, cleaned out the fridge and had no idea what to do next (except voluntarily go back to work a week early). My wife told me that he didn't have kids. They have their moments when you want to strangle them, believe me, moments when you are the most embarrassed (or in the eyes of everyone around you—the worst) parent in the world … but at that moment I felt sad for Jack.

What is it like to be a father? On the surface, and as a sports mad person, having three boys is pretty cool—I have ready-made left and right wingers, and a centre forward for the Socceroos when Australia hosts the World Cup in 2022. I can relive my childhood by exposing them to (far too much) Star Wars stuff. My life at the moment is Obi-Wan Kenobi and Anakin Skywalker and I love it. We can do 'boy' things that really get on my wife's nerves (making farting noises and laughing hysterically is an example). Being a dad to boys is special but I am also sad that I will never have the opportunity to walk my daughter down the aisle, or watch my wife plait her hair or go girly shopping with her.

Being a dad is fun. It is constantly changing, challenging and evolving and no day is ever the same. It is anything but boring. Looking into your child's eyes when they are recounting (or making up) a story about Batman is truly amazing, and when they laugh hysterically together at something that was never funny until they thought it was is one of life's best feelings.

Having said that, from a selfish perspective, there are plenty of experiences that you have to miss out on by being a dad. This can be hard, especially when you see smug childless couples heading off to a Pacific island on a whim or going to ski for the weekend in Austria. There are times as a dad that you want to press the 'pause' button on life so you can catch your breath and find just one hour to do something you like doing. I have seriously considered 'pretending' to go to work but then calling in sick and checking into a hotel for the day just to sleep, maybe watch a movie uninterrupted or read a book. But the ironic thing is that I'd be bored in ten minutes. The idea seems great but I'd be wondering all the time what my family was doing.

Gavin's Wisdom	It's incredible as a dad to look at your kids and reflect: Wow … we made them all by ourselves. Bigger wow … we are totally responsible for these little people. As they get older, they will begin to have memories of their lives that will hang around even when they are old. This means that whatever I am doing and the experiences I am making for them, they will thank (or not thank) me for. That is a powerful thought. My greatest hope is that when they are grown, they will be grateful for their childhood experiences.

What I felt when I first met our baby …

- I was out of my mind with relief and excitement. I felt a little apprehension when Tom came through birth without so much as a squeak and was all floppy. No screaming like in the movies; it was like we caught him napping. It was an incredible learning curve and every move he made was riveting.

- The birthing experience was an amazing and fascinating thing, yet it was one of the most disgusting things I have ever seen. It is always portrayed as a beautiful thing, but it really made my stomach turn. I'm still trying to comprehend how our darling boy fitted in there!

- Oh wow, I felt much pride, hope and excitement. I knew from the moment I first met Lila, and again with Mia, that our lives were going to become so much richer. The birth of each child immediately put where I was, at that moment in time, into perspective.

- Awe, wonder, amazement … lots of positive emotions! My first glimpse of my daughter was during the labour; her little head was visible and I was amazed that she had hair. A few minutes later, she was given to me so I could put her on the scales to weigh her. I held her close and treated her so gently as I laid her down—even though she was a healthy size, she still felt like a feather. Over the next few days, I learned how to change nappies and bathe my daughter, but the main thing that I kept telling myself was 'This is my daughter … I made her'.

- I felt proud and content in the first few days. I tend to get asked this question a lot and I think the expected answer is 'It was the best day of my life', or 'I dropped to my knees and wept'. I felt these emotions to a degree but I think it's sad if that was the best day of your life. What about all the following days … first words, first hug, first kiss, first 'daddy', seeing them play with other kids? I have plenty of 'best days of my life'; I wouldn't dream of singling one out.

- I'm not sure what I was expecting but the reality was not at all what I imagined. I think I watched too many stupid Hollywood movies where the husband is all overwhelmed and ends up fainting on the delivery room floor. Initially, I felt relieved that it was over and everyone had made it through safely. Maybe it's the way the male brain works: a) wife OK, b) baby OK, c) doctor smiling—right, turn alarm bells off now. Later on, when it was quiet and I was sitting down with her in my arms, all wrapped up in her little blanket, I remember feeling overwhelmed with love and the need to protect her.

Charting a new course: When children bring new perspective to your life

Troy's whole outlook changed when he became a father. At first he was worried that his struggles with the big questions in life would hinder his ability to be a good dad, but he soon found this was not the case.

Troy's Story

The day I first held her in my arms was the most surreal experience of my life. Here, nestled in the crook of my arm, was a little creation that only months before had been a faint blip on a monitor screen. How had this come to be? Where had this little life come from? Although biology could explain some of it, I felt a strong sense of the miraculous at play ... my daughter had arrived. And she was the most beautiful thing I had ever laid my eyes on! I must admit, those first few early hours early on a late autumn morning were some of my proudest. Even though I had tried to imagine the moment, had gone through it many times in my mind, the reality was so much more intense. Here was a life I had helped to create. My second daughter's arrival only three years later still held me in awe. Holding my hands to my mouth as I first saw her little face, then her little arms and then the rest of her following. Amazing.

It was always in the back of my mind, somewhere, that one day I would have children. I knew it but it always felt like that would be later, sometime. I'm sure I was imagining when 'later' arrived, my life would have such sense and meaning, that I would have cast off my nagging sense of doubt and would be living life with abounding energy and wisdom.

So, it was a surprise to me that I felt so ordinary, so human, when my wife and I started talking seriously about having children. My first thoughts were 'How can I be father of any true worth when I still don't have all these answers to my own questions?' This was something that resonated within me for quite some time during my wife's pregnancy. Don't get me wrong, I was excited that this child was coming. I was just coming to terms with what it meant to be a father and role model for this young life. Wasn't I supposed to be the one with all the answers?

Then a very wise friend suggested to me 'You are the perfect parent for this child. You are enough just as you are.' This was a turning point for me and still is a great reassurance as I grow as a father. If my child is the hand, then I am the glove, moulded perfectly to their form and temperament. I don't have to have all the answers because as my children grow, so do I. It's an incredible partnership. And anyway, it's the love I show towards them that they really cherish.

Those first few months with my new daughter were quite an interesting time. While I had this intense desire to connect with my child, all she really needed from me was to pass her to mum. And while I really wanted to connect with my wife, all she really wanted to do was sleep between three-hourly feeds. I think after the euphoria of holding your child in your arms for the first time, the following months can seem a little less 'magazine glossy' and more 'newspaper typeface'. The advice that I now give other fathers-to-be is 'Fill up your endurance tank prior to a new child. Be prepared for the family to draw from you physically, spiritually and emotionally for the next six months.' It is a tough job, but thankfully one we were made for.

When my second daughter was born, it was a different experience again. Now I had a three-year-old daughter who was used to having her daddy all to herself having to 'share' with her newborn sister. While the feelings of awe and wonder at this new life were the same, I now had to devote equal time to both. My endurance tank needed to expand to meet the new challenge. While I wasn't ready to begin with, I have found that as time has passed, I have been equipped appropriately. It does take time for the family to adjust to the new groove and sometimes we still skip, but life is in the learning.

As I have seen my children grow, it never ceases to surprise me how one little thing they say or do can impact me in such a deep and profound way. The first smile is deeply beautiful, the first laugh is pure joy, and the first words left me speechless. To see them grow in their understanding of the world and people around them, to be there as they walk for the very first time … the simple things that I have taken for granted in my day-to-day life suddenly become wondrous milestones—Kodak moments I have on my phone, close with me always.

I have noticed how both my daughters are like little sponges and will soak up everything and anything that we say or do in our daily lives. And I mean everything. It is both endearing and confronting when you hear your child speak in a manner that you have. (Just make sure all those things you say about people in private are words you are happy to have spoken in public by your children!) Becoming aware that these children absorb everything they see me do and hear me say has burdened me in a good way. All those things that I have always wanted to do and be have taken on a new perspective now. My choices now have a family ramification. I liken being a father to being the captain of a ship. I want to chart a good course, and that challenges me to explore deeper things. I want to live a life that speaks volumes to my children rather than having to speak at volume.

As a father, I have found the things I thought were important pale into insignificance when I consider how important my daughters are to me. Material possessions are now only as important as the value they provide in supporting our family. Holidays are now just as important for building family memories as they are for a little rest and relaxation. Family and friends are like gold, displaying the colourful fabric of the world up close and personal. I could never really understand my parents' love or sacrifice for me until I became a dad. For now, I have just seen a glimpse but I can say sincerely say that my parents did a great job. And as my daughters grow older, I hope that one day I can hear them say the same to me.

Troy's Wisdom

My experiences as a dad have taught me that I have a relatively short time to influence my daughters in how to live life well by honestly and openly living it myself first.

I would say that the thing that stands out the most is that being a dad is a journey. Every step is a new experience—sometimes of joy, sometimes of doubt—but I am constantly learning new things about my children and also about myself. Learn to ask questions and be open with your journey—other parents are a great resource and sometimes even a great comfort.

What I would tell other dads ...

- One of the main things I've learned is that you get what you paid for; with children, you get what you put into them. Also, there are few things more precious than, or as worthwhile as, a child's forgiveness. My daughters have taught me that it takes a big man to admit mistakes and that when I admit I'm wrong, I will be forgiven.

- Being a parent is very hard work but you get untold satisfaction, love and contentment back every day that makes it all worthwhile. Don't take anything for granted and try to modify your behaviour and actions constantly as you learn new things. Remember things that you did and didn't like about your own childhood and use that information with your kids. Involve yourself with your kids as much as you can and try new and interesting things all the time. Work hard at your relationship with your partner—support each other.

- I am eternally grateful for the unconditional, powerful love that I have for my kids. Early on during the pregnancy of our first child, I was petrified that I wouldn't love him as much as I should. Mum always told me that I needn't worry because you just do. She was right.

- Babyhood is the most tiring and most rewarding time of your life as a parent—kids grow up so quickly. Try to spend lots of quality time with your kids and always tell them that you love them. Perhaps the biggest realisation I had was that there are different types of love. You can fall in and out of love with your partner, but the love you have for your child is never ending and knows no bounds.

- Treat your child with respect; talk to them as if they understand and don't get angry with them if they do the wrong thing. It is very important to talk to your partner about how you want to bring up a child. Write it down and stick to it. Then continue to give each other feedback as you go. We are all learning and we need to be told (constructively) if we are doing the right or wrong thing in any given parenting situation.

- Patience and calm are priceless. The whole process of fatherhood is emotionally charged. It brings out the best and worst in friends, relatives, husbands and wives. Bite your tongue and let people show their colours; you learn more when you are not speaking. Never, ever pass up the opportunity to watch your baby grow; your relationship with your child will be the better for it.

- Fatherhood isn't an easy job and even though the military coined the phrase 'the toughest job you'll ever love', I believe that applies wholeheartedly to my approach to parenting. I can be there and not really be engaged in their lives, or I can pour myself into these kids and allow them to see a glimpse of what a great husband and father a man can be. That's what I desire for my kids and that's what has changed more than anything else for me in regards to becoming a father.

- Whatever you're feeling, whatever you're going through … it might not be universal, but it's normal. Some parents—both fathers and mothers—get depressed. It's normal. Others have a bit of trouble bonding with their babies for a while. It's normal. Still others totally immerse themselves in their new baby and thrive on their new role. That's normal too. Just because you're not going through what others are going through does not mean that those other parents are normal and you're not! You're normal too. As long as you're looking after your family to the very best of your ability (whatever that ability level is), you're doing fine.

- If you want sex, you should know that for many women, having a man who is helpful, brave, engaged and supportive (including in practical ways such as cooking, changing nappies, giving baths, washing up, cleaning the toilet, washing the clothes and so on) is the biggest turn-on!

- Being a father is the best feeling in the world. To have someone who looks up to you no matter what is such a wonderful responsibility.

- Being a father is wonderful. Relax, enjoy and absolutely make time for your child. If you don't, you might not realise just how wonderful it is.

CHAPTER SEVEN

Families come in all shapes and sizes

'Call it a clan, call it a network, call it a tribe, call it a family. Whatever you call it, whoever you are, you need one.'

Jane Howard (1999)

What image comes to mind when you think of 'family'? Is the image of two parents, two children and perhaps a pet? If so, you are conjuring the image of the 'nuclear family', a phrase made popular by anthropologist George Murdock in 1949. Murdock conducted a worldwide study, comparing 250 cultures and the types of families that existed within them. While he found that half of the family types were centred on extended family forms (also known as 'joint family systems') and one quarter were polygamous (where the husband has more than one wife), he theorised that the 'nuclear family' was universal. This controversial theory is still contested by academics today.

So what exactly is family? The nature of family has been studied across disciplines and cultures (mainly from sociological, economical and ecological perspectives) and has been proven flexible, culturally diverse and adaptive. That is, there is no rigid definition of family; while the family is an enduring social *construction* across cultures, the key organising structure throughout history has been the household, rather than any fixed notions of who might actually be a part of that household (Koons 2005).

The concept of family in the 21st century naturally differs depending on which society you study. Looking at Australian demographics, the average household size is projected to decline from 2.6 people per household in 2006 to between 2.4 and 2.5 people per household in 2031. In 2016, Australia's average household size (2.5 people) is predicted to be the same as New Zealand and Japan (both 2.5), and larger than England (2.2) and Scotland (2.1) (Australian Bureau of Statistics 2010). In 2006 in Australia, approximately 81 per cent of children and teenagers under 15 years old lived with two parents. Australian statistics predict that of all family types, the number of couple-families without children will overtake the number of couple-families with children by 2031.

This decline in the traditional concept of family (married couples with children) is also reflected in United States statistics, as Americans are living longer, marrying later and many are choosing to remain childless. According to the United States Census Bureau, in 2008, less than one third of the population were living in a 'traditional' household. A similar trend has emerged in the United Kingdom. British statistics found 17 million families living in the UK in 2004. However, of these families, just over 12 million of them were headed by married couples—a number that fell by half a million between 1996 and 2004. Lone-mother and cohabiting couples increased significantly over the same period (Office for National Statistics UK 2005).

While it is possible to identify trends in familial structure with the help of census data, these statistics cannot convey the richness, complexity and diversity of families in the 21st century. In this chapter, we meet many families, all of whom have different household structures. You will hear from single mothers and fathers, married couples with children, same sex couples with children and from parents raising children with extra needs. While on the surface, they may seem diverse (and they are), they all have a common focus: their children. As exemplified in the following stories (and reflected in academic research), the structure of these families does not dictate how well a child is loved or nurtured. In fact, structure (i.e. two-parent, one-parent, same sex parents) seems to have very little to do with how well a child is raised. What is important is the environment, and every family that follows has gone to great lengths to ensure theirs is a happy and loving one.

A wise option: The story of a single mother

Ciara was in a relationship with her partner who verbally abused her. That abuse escalated to physical violence and Ciara decided to end the relationship. She tells us how she copes as a single mother and what her relationship is now like with her ex-partner.

Ciara's Story

Growing up, I never wanted to have children. And I certainly never thought that I would be a single mum of two at 37 years of age. But life sometimes has a way of throwing you a curveball.

I got pregnant with my daughter at 32 and it was totally unexpected. We were living in Brisbane at the time, and my first decision was to move us back to where my family were in Perth so that I would have some support. I had been in a relationship for about three years, and it wasn't a great one. My partner was verbally abusive, but that was as far as it went. He wasn't very supportive throughout the pregnancy, and the only appointments he went to were the scans—the fun appointments. I had my daughter by elective caesarean at 39 weeks. I went into labour the day I was due to have her, and once again, my partner was totally unsupportive. I was in pain and he said 'It can't hurt that much'. I was furious, but in too much pain to say a lot about it. Once my daughter was born and was placed into my arms, I fell totally in love.

As soon as we were home, Mark went back to work—he took just one day off, for the caesarean section, so I was left to care for a newborn baby and do the housework. Thank God for my mum! She came over often and would just hold my daughter to give me a break, hang a load of washing out or clean up the kitchen and lounge. Mark was completely unsupportive about breastfeeding so I decided to bottle-feed my daughter. I still feel some resentment over that.

Things between Mark and me deteriorated to the point of physical abuse, and when my daughter was eight months old, I made the decision to leave. I rented a house for the two of us and moved all of our furniture out, without telling my partner. He wasn't happy, but it didn't change my mind and I told him why we had left. I was fine coping alone—I had been doing it since Daisy was born anyway!

Mark later contacted me and told me that he had been to the doctor and was prescribed antidepressants for bipolar disorder. He wanted to see Daisy. I agreed, and over time, we became friends again, and decided to give our relationship another shot. I conceived my son.

At 14 weeks, we had an argument and he tried to kick me in my stomach. I managed to turn and protect my baby, but his foot caught me in the back. I locked myself and my daughter in the bedroom and decided that was the end, and called the police to remove him from my house. I went back to raising my daughter alone, pregnant with my son, and my ex moved back to Brisbane.

I also had an elective caesarean section for my son and my mum came with me. Various friends and family members came to the scans with me, and my best friend was with me at 16 weeks when I found I was carrying a boy. I was over the moon and figured I'd cope with two—I had coped with one, after all. Mark was insistent that he was coming to the birth—his words were 'You can't stop me; I have a right to be there'. I told him he most certainly did not have any rights, and I would instruct the hospital he was not to be allowed in, and did not give him or his family the date of his arrival. I also named him myself. He had no input.

After my son's birth, an interstate friend visited for two weeks and she took over all the housework so I could work on establishing breastfeeding and spending time with Daisy.

She was an invaluable support person during those tough first weeks. I also had support from my mum and my grandmother. I am a very proud person and rarely ask for help, so during this time, I had to swallow my pride and ask for the help I needed. I wouldn't have survived without those people in my life.

Splitting my time between a newborn and a toddler was harder than I had thought, but I was fortunate in that my son was an easy baby. Daisy was a lot more work, and soon after my son was born, she was diagnosed with autism, which was a great blow. However, I managed to squeeze as much time as I could into every day, and when my son was sleeping, Daisy got extra attention. I didn't get a lot of sleep, but I plodded along.

I did not receive any child support until Daisy was five. Consequently, Mark has a rather large debt that he is slowly whittling down. He doesn't see the kids, and that's his choice. I gave him the opportunity and met up with him once a week, but that only lasted six weeks before he faded out of their lives once again. I do feel angry for my children that they don't have two parents involved in their lives, but they barely know him. I also feel angry that I can't look forward to time out, with my kids going to their dad's for the day or weekend. I feel angry that I can't organise going out somewhere easily, and I envy those that have ex-partners who are only too happy to have the kids so they can go out. However, my mum and my ex in-laws are very involved in the kids' lives and I can ask them to babysit without too much trouble.

It's hard being 'it' for your kids — you are the one always there when they hurt themselves, when they have a bad dream, when they're ratty and tired, when they need to be bathed and fed. But I still know that what I did was right. And while it's hard being 'it', I am also 'it' when they learn to walk, talk, draw a picture, or have a great day at preschool, and I was 'it' to get all the hugs and kisses.

You can be a single parent. It's not ideal, but sometimes it's the only wise option.

Ciara's Wisdom	You are far better off raising your children in a house with one happy, safe parent than in a house with two parents who are fighting, either physically or emotionally. You are stronger than you think you are and you can do it alone. When it comes to your kids, you will do anything possible to keep them safe. And remember that you deserve far better than violence; you are worth more than that.
	Use every bit of support you possibly can and swallow your pride, as I did, and ask for that help. Yes, it can be hard financially, physically and emotionally being 'it' for your kids, but it means you are safe and you don't have to walk on eggshells. Don't be too afraid or too proud to seek help from the government and child support agencies. Charities are there if you need them too. Seek counselling to help you through it. No one deserves to live in a violent relationship, and how can you love someone you are frightened of? Remember that children learn from what they see, and the lessons you want to give them do not include bad treatment of a partner, by their partner. You want their memories of childhood to be of a safe, happy home, with a mum who loves them.

Domestic abuse: What it is and what you can do about it

Your partner apologizes and says the hurtful behavior won't happen again— but you fear it. At times you wonder whether you're imagining the abuse, yet the emotional or physical pain you feel is real. If this sounds familiar, you may be experiencing domestic violence. (Mayo Clinic 2009)

Domestic abuse is carried out by both men and women, however men are by far the most common offenders. It crosses all socio-economic and cultural boundaries. Abuse is generally grouped into three categories: physical, sexual and/or emotional. Examples of *physical abuse* include: being slapped, having something thrown at you, being hit with something, being kicked, dragged or beaten up, being choked or burnt on purpose, and/or the use of threats or weapons. Examples of *sexual abuse* include: being forced to have sex when you don't want to, having sex with your partner due to fear they might harm you if you don't, and/or being forced to do something sexual that you find degrading or humiliating. Examples of *emotional abuse* include your partner: trying to stop you from seeing your friends and family, insisting on knowing where you are at all times, ignoring you and treating you indifferently, getting angry if you speak with another man, being suspicious that you are unfaithful, and/or expecting you to ask permission before seeking health care (Garcia-Moreno et al. 2006). This list is not finite—there are other examples of abuse (for example, financial abuse and using your children against you); trust your instincts. If it feels wrong, it probably is.

If you are in a *same sex relationship*, you may be experiencing domestic violence if your partner threatens to 'out' you, tells you that if you leave the relationship you're admitting that same sex relationships are 'deviant', or if they portray violence as normal, or mutual and consensual.

Ellsberg et al. (2008) emphasise the diverse and detrimental effects abuse can have on women who are abused. While many women sustain injuries, abuse is consistently linked to a broad array of negative outcomes, including gynaecological disorders, adverse pregnancy outcomes, irritable bowel syndrome, gastro-intestinal disorders and various chronic pain disorders. In addition to physical problems, women also experience negative emotional outcomes, such as depression, anxiety, post-traumatic stress, phobias, alcohol and drug abuse and suicide; there is also an obvious negative impact on children's emotional and physical wellbeing. It is therefore crucial that you seek help if you think you are being emotionally, physically or sexually abused by your partner.

Especially salient to women is the fact that domestic abuse can begin (or increase) during pregnancy, and may continue or worsen after the baby is born. This puts both the woman and her children at risk, as children who grow up in an environment of abuse are more likely to be abused and display behavioural problems. As adults, they may think that abuse is normal and may even perpetuate the cycle of abuse. Many women believe that seeking help will place them in further danger but the opposite is true: seeking help is the best way to protect yourself and your children.

You can begin with baby steps, by talking to a trusted friend or health care professional, and the sooner you do this, the better. The longer you stay in an abusive relationship, the more your self-esteem is eroded and the less likely it is that you will seek help.

Although it is best to leave an abusive relationship, doing so can be dangerous. Below is a safety plan, which you might like to follow if you are thinking about leaving:

- **Create an emergency plan**: Phone a women's shelter or a domestic abuse help line when your partner is away or at a friend's house (organisations and help lines are listed in the Resources section on page 261). Pack an emergency bag and hide it or leave it with someone you trust. Make sure you include important documents like passports and birth certificates, as well as health care cards, cash and any prescription medications. Know exactly where you will go and how you will get there, especially if it means you need to leave in the middle of the night (for example, if you have a car, make sure the tank is always filled). Know what your partner's 'red flags' are: learn to watch for the signs that trouble is brewing and have in mind a ready-made list of excuses for you to leave the house before he or she resorts to violence. You should also consider using a code word that you can use to alert neighbours, the police or your friends that you're in trouble.

- **Be careful with communication**: Technology is so advanced now and abusers may use this technology to their own advantage, as it helps them gain greater control over you. When you make phone calls, be cautious, as your abuser may listen in to your conversation or may check through your phone log for texts and calls (they can also go through phone bills). Also, be cautious on your home computer, as spyware might be checking what sites you are visiting and emails you are receiving. It's better to play it safe and use a computer at work or at an internet café. Always change your password and make it a strong one; use numbers, symbols and capital as well as lower case letters to make it harder to break. If you must use your home computer, clear your browsing history. You should clear all of the sites you have visited, as well as any cookies that have been installed on your computer and temporary internet files. To learn how to do this within your web browser, go to <www.google.com> and type, for example, 'clear history in Internet Explorer'.

- **Try to remain calm**: Leaving your partner may be a scary thought, especially if he or she has threatened you with violence or threatened to harm your children. You can feel trapped and helpless. But remember that you are in much more danger if you stay. There are many shelters, legal services and help lines that can help you to live free of fear. Remember, you are not the cause of your partner's behaviour, you and your children deserve a happy and safe life and you are not alone: there are people and organisations waiting to help you.

Domestic abuse is dangerous. It can lead to serious physical and emotional harm, and even death. Ciara and her baby were lucky to escape harm. But what if you suspect that a friend is being abused? People who are being abused may exhibit a number of telltale signs, and while it's difficult to know what's going on behind closed doors, you may pick up clues from the following types of behaviour. According to Smith et al. (2009), when people are subject to domestic abuse, they seem overly keen to please their partner (such as going along with everything they say or by constantly letting their partner know where they are), they may get frequent calls from their partner or they might talk about their partner's jealousy or quick temper. If they are being physically abused, you might see visible evidence of injuries, which they may describe as the result of accidents, or you might notice that they frequently call in sick to work or miss important occasions, and they may dress so that their injuries are covered (for example, they might wear sunglasses indoors). People who are abused usually have very low self-esteem and may show major personality changes (for example, a friend or colleague who was once outgoing may now be withdrawn and quiet). They may even be depressed or suicidal.

If you suspect a friend, colleague or family member is being abused, try to talk to them in a private place. Tell them that you are concerned for their safety and tell them the things you have noticed that worry you. It's also important to convey that you're there to listen and that you will help in any way you can. It's definitely not a good idea to put pressure on them or place conditions on your support. Don't wait for them to come to you—you should go to them. And remember, domestic abuse can take place in both heterosexual and same sex relationships. For more information and support about domestic abuse, see the support services listed on page 261.

Leaving home: When being single is better for baby

Daine and his partner had a baby when they were young, and stress, increased financial burdens and lack of family support led him and his partner to separate. Here, Daine talks about his tough decision to leave, what it is like to be a single father and how co-parenting has worked for him.

Daine's Story

I separated from my wife approximately 18 months after our son was born. There were many factors in the separation, which included the stress involved with learning how to be parents for the first time. Other issues at the time included financial (increased financial burden and job changes); family (dealing with grandparents and their ways of parenting, getting conflicting advice from other family members and different families); moving from the country back to the city, and personal issues between us. We drifted apart over time with the realisation that we only had our son in common, making my decision to leave hard, but justified. We both agreed over the years that it was better for a child to have two happy, separated parents than two parents constantly arguing and fighting in front of them. Unfortunately, we had become the latter.

We mutually agreed for my partner to look after our child for ten nights in a fortnight, and for me to care for him the other four nights. We have an equal say in our parenting roles, responsibilities and decisions, and have a mutual respect for each other due to our love for our son. My ex-partner has since entered a new relationship and I have a new girlfriend, so we are now negotiating the minefield involved with having our new partners in our son's life. I believe that my ex is fantastic with our son's care and development, and I try my best to be a good role model.

I can't afford a place of my own at the moment, so I live with my parents, which means they help me out when I'm looking after my son. My wonderful girlfriend is caring and understanding, as she is in a similar situation, and other family members help out too. Their support means respite at the end of the day when my son has been 'full on' and I'm physically tired from running around, or lifting him onto slides and play equipment. This is when gran and granddad can have an hour or so entertaining while I have a chance to recharge my batteries and continue with the evening's activities. When there is no support around (for example, during the middle of the day), I find that I need a few minutes alone to get away from the situation and think about other things—best done during nap time!

I give financial help to my ex-partner in the form of child support, which is about twice as much as the minimum. Other single dads at work don't understand this (they think I'm getting 'screwed over') but I can see that my son is cared for, loved and given the best support for him to grow up. So, in my mind, that extra money is going directly to him for a good place to grow and develop, and I'm happy with that.

I don't feel angry about my situation; the feeling I get most is sadness. We all grow up expecting to have mum and dad with us in the same house, then find a partner and settle down. Instead, my son will grow up having a mum here and a dad there, probably with other partners and possibly with step-siblings. That's what makes me sad—as a kid growing up that's what you expect, and I feel like I've failed my son in not being able to provide him with that. Having said that, I console myself with the fact that our arrangement is better for our son than having his parents constantly fighting with each other.

There isn't as much a stigma associated with being a single dad as there is being a single mum—some mates reckon it'd be easy to 'pick up chicks by walking around the shops with your kid'. Having said that, questions do get asked ('Giving mummy a break?') and there is an uncomfortable silence when I explain that mummy is somewhere else and it's a daddy–son day. I cope by trying to be the best dad I can be, being attentive to my son and his needs, and ignoring the looks I get at places like the shops. Even in this day and age, people look at you in a certain way when you are paying your child a lot of attention. What they don't understand is that I don't get much time with my child so I want to have quality time with him.

I know that my parents will always be there for me, for support, guidance and time out when I need it. I know that my family will help when they see it's needed or when I ask, and I know that my ex's side are just as willing to give my son the love and attention he needs.

Daine's Wisdom	Just believe in yourself—there are days when you think there is no light at the end of the tunnel, and something as small as a laugh, giggle, smile or a hug can melt your heart and make you believe again. No matter what happens, your children love you unconditionally and it's things

like that which make you realise that the world isn't going to end if you don't have time to make your bed in the morning. Enjoy the time when they are babies and toddlers; they grow up fast and it's over in a flash! Remember the 'firsts' for they will bring you endless joy and happiness.

Lastly, being a single dad can be hard—it's definitely hard to leave your child, knowing you will only see them on designated days. However, I truly believe that it is more important to ensure the wellbeing and safety of your child (both physical and emotional) and if that means you need to leave a relationship that is full of conflict, then that is what you must do. In the end, it worked out best for our family—we've learned how to co-parent and lead separate lives; it has been best for us and best for our child.

One child family: When only doesn't equal lonely

Kathy had a difficult pregnancy with her daughter and, nearly three years after her delivery, still feels as though she needs time to recover. While she doesn't rule out another pregnancy, it is not a choice that she is currently considering.

Kathy's Story

Growing up, I came from your typical family at first … then it started to fall into the 'broken' family category. My parents divorced when I was young and my brother, four years my senior, really rebelled against everything and everybody. He and I never got along well and he left home at quite an early age. From that point on it was mom and I and she did a wonderful job on her own. I always thought I would have a big family and remember once saying I wanted four children. It's amazing how things can change once you have the first one, especially after a dreadful pregnancy.

I would be lying if I said that my pregnancy with my daughter didn't scar me emotionally somewhat and affect my choice of how many children I would have. But I think I would also be lying if I said that I didn't think I could do it again.

My pregnancy was not planned, but was welcomed. My husband and I got married and within two weeks, we were pregnant. The pregnancy was very difficult, and seemed like it would never end. I don't think a day went by that I didn't complain. I had severe morning sickness until week 18, so much so that I could barely function and had to quit my job that I had loved. The feeling of the all-day nausea and vomiting really threw me for a loop.

My daughter is going to be three soon and by now, it seems that most people I know have already had another child or are pregnant. I definitely feel like I am in the minority. I have felt the pressure to have another child since my daughter turned a year old. I can honestly say the pressure to have a second surpasses the pressure to have a first. I was pretty angry about it for a while, not quite understanding what the rush was, why I was not allowed to enjoy my one and only daughter and think about the rest later. Why rush it? I started to do some research on only children, looking into all the myths that surround one-child families. I also spent a lot of time talking with my friends who had more than one child. I am not oblivious to the fact that children with siblings have a live-in playmate but I am also not oblivious to the fact that no matter what the age difference between siblings, sometimes they do not get along and may never get along.

Call me crazy but three years is not enough 'recovery' time for us. I am still learning daily how to be a mom and all the wonderful facets of my daughter's personality. I love this time—our time—and don't think that we are any less of a family because we only have one child. I am not a working mom who doesn't want the burden of another child, I am not an older mom who needs to worry about her biological clock ticking, I am just a very realistic mom who faces the challenges and joys of parenthood with my daughter every day and knows her own shortcomings. I don't see anything negative about wanting to give our child 100 per cent. I feel she is completely deserving of us and it should be this way for however long we want. Our sole focus is our daughter; I don't have anyone else to worry about and there are no other children to soothe or bodies to clothe or feelings to mend … we just have her.

We like it this way and want it this way until we feel more ready (although never fully ready I am sure) to open ourselves further and invite another child into this closely knitted pack. Maybe that time will never come.

Kathy's Wisdom	Despite what anyone says, a family is a family no matter how many children. Many world leaders are only children and any research you do, you will see that 'onlies' are at no disadvantage. As long as the child is loved, socialized and never made to feel like they aren't enough, then it's a wonderful thing.

Same sex parents: When two mothers raise a baby

In many ways, Ingrid and Jane's family life mimics that of any 'traditional' family: they face the same worries, pressures and juggling of roles. Where they differ is how people react to their family unit.

Ingrid's Story

My partner Jane and I take it in turns to get up at night when Brendan cries, although I am breastfeeding, so regardless of who is on night duty I end up with him at 5 am when he wakes up hungry. Usually these days I just bring him into bed with me so we can both go back to sleep.

We happen to live in a part of town where the maternal and child health service has a high staff turnover. As a result, we have never met the same nurse twice. For all of our appointments there has been a different nurse to meet. I don't mind this so much, as they keep good records so there is always continuity in the care Brendan receives. But it can be a bit confronting for us, as a same sex couple, to have to 'out' ourselves again every time we meet a new service provider. It would be nice to be able to just see the one person who knows us and who we know is supportive. That being said, the nurses have all been fantastic. One nurse in particular was really excited to meet a same sex couple. She gushed to me how she thinks gay people make wonderful parents. Her brother is a gay man and by all accounts has the most delightful 18-year-old.

I started back at work full time six weeks ago, and Jane quit her job so she can stay home and care for Brendan. So far, Jane is enjoying being a full-time mum. Most days she and Brendan walk the dog in the morning then head out in the afternoon to visit people or wander around the shops. On Mondays they go to playgroup. On Friday afternoons they take care of my four-year-old niece who loves Brendan more than anything else in the world.

Jane says she sometimes feels like a phony when she is out and about and strangers stop to talk to her, assuming Brendan is 'her' child. It's not that she doesn't feel like his mother. It's just that people assume she has been through the whole 'birth' experience and this assumption will, on occasions, edge its way into conversation. Also, because Brendan is mixed race, people will often ask about his father. For me this is easy to answer because Brendan's father is Asian and I am white. However, Jane is also Asian. So she has more explaining to do if people want to know why Brendan looks mostly white. I once asked Jane if she would feel like a 'phony mum' if she had an adopted child. She answered that it would be different in that situation because she could just explain to people that the child was adopted. However, as it is, to fully explain Brendan she has to make it clear that he has two mothers.

It is amazing how often strangers comment or ask questions about babies. When babies are involved, people are forward in a way they never are with adults. I quite like this most of the time. I love how babies somehow help people let their guards down. People smile at you more when you have a baby. Jane and I sometimes answer the questions that strangers ask with the 'full story'—the two-mothers explanation. But mostly, if a stranger in the supermarket wants to know about Brendan, I just give brief explanations and often let people assume that his father is my partner. I never lie. I just don't elaborate and they fill in the blanks. It's tiring to have to explain your sexuality to strangers. You risk being judged harshly every time and some days I am just not up for that. But when Brendan is old enough to understand the conversation, I will be more upfront. I want him to be proud that his family is different.

Going back to work has been a bit of a challenge for me. I love the work. I have the sort of job where I spend my days writing and thinking—using my brain a lot. I really missed this type of thinking work while I was on maternity leave. So it is great to have an opportunity to think again (although this often occurs through a sleep-deprived fog). But I am in tears some mornings leaving Brendan. By Friday evening, I miss him so much I can't bear to put him to bed. I just want to hold him all night.

I think as a same sex couple Jane and I have had to learn to be brave. Most people we know or have contact with are really accepting of us and, of course, everyone loves Brendan. But there is still a lot of discrimination out there, which obviously Brendan is *going to pick up on as he gets older. Challenging this on a day-to-day level, just by being open about who we are, is hard sometimes (especially when you are operating on not much sleep). But it is important to stand up for your family and to demonstrate to the world that you are happy to be who you are. As far as I am concerned, this is what will ensure Brendan becomes a confident and resilient adult. So I remind myself of this every day: be brave and proud and happy (sounds a bit cheesy, I know, but it is important).*

Ingrid's Wisdom

What advice would I have for others in my situation? Definitely get out there and meet other parents, especially same sex parents. It makes a world of difference to your day to have like-minded others to talk to. Thanks to the wonder that is the internet, making connections with local lesbian and gay parents can be quite easy (depending on where you live).

Also, take it easy. Just as soon as you think you are on top of your baby's sleeping, eating and crying, something changes and it all goes out the window. It is not the end of the world if you do all the things the books and the nurses tell you not to do. At four in the morning, when you have had only five hours sleep over the past two nights, what the books say is meaningless. Do what you need to do to look after yourself. Babies don't need perfect parents. They just don't. They need happy parents who love spending time with them. And happy parents come in all shapes, sizes, colours and genders.

Same sex parents

We live in a time of change and of increasing acceptance, but while the world has gradually accepted that individuals have differing religious beliefs, ethnic origins and abilities, most countries still do not accept that people have different sexual orientations. Nine countries punish homosexuality with the death penalty, a number of countries deny LGBT human rights by blocking free expression and assembly and 75 countries (that's one third of the world's countries) still have legislation that criminalises consensual, same-sex sexual acts.

Unfortunately, the same discrimination and stigma are often applied to LGBT parents. The *Declaration of Montréal* (International Conference on LGBT Human Rights 2006) states:

We fall in love, and establish relationships and families – however configured. For many of us, these relationships and families are the most important parts of our lives. Unless they are legally recognized, our rights to equality and dignity cannot be fully secured. Indeed, many countries are willing to grant us equity in every area of our lives except in relation to our relationships and families, to ensure that our relationships and families are stigmatized as inferior. As a matter of simple equality ... LGBT individuals and same-sex couples who are parents, or wish to become parents, [should be] entitled to equal rights. (p. 6)

The Declaration goes on to assert that equal rights can be achieved only when there is legal marriage for same sex couples, similar partnership rights for LGBTs in de-facto relationships and equal access for all to every option for parenthood (including adoption, fostering and medically assisted reproduction).

As evidenced in a recent literature review (Short et al. 2007), family studies research specifies that it is family processes (such as relationships within the family and the quality of parenting), rather than family structures (e.g. number, sex and cohabitation status of parents) that contribute to determining children's health and wellbeing.

However, same sex parents continue to face prejudice, mainly through the 'presumption in much legal and social policy that lesbian and gay parenting is suspect, second-rate or harmful to children' (Millbank 2003, p. 541). Some of the more commonly expressed 'concerns' documented by the American Society for Reproductive Medicine (ASRM 2006) include the notion that children need fathers, that children of LGBT parents will be socially isolated (teased), will have gender identity and/or sexual orientation problems (that is, gay parents produce gay children), and that children of LGBT parents are at increased risk of abuse or other mistreatment. ASRM (2006) found that 'the evidence to date … cannot reasonably be interpreted to support such fears' (p. 1334). Likewise, the American Academy of Pediatrics reported in 2002 that 'no data have pointed to any risk to children as a result of growing up in a family with one or more gay parents' (p. 339).

As the stories in this chapter reflect, families are increasingly diverse. As well as the 'traditional' family structure of two heterosexual parents, families can be intentionally childless, have single parents, separated or divorced parents, same sex parents, step-parents or be blended families and may also have been created with the assistance of reproductive technology.

The desire for children is a human one, not one limited to heterosexuals. Societies that continue to reject LGBT parents ignore the growing body of evidence that children's wellbeing is shaped by the parenting process, rather than parental structure. Children thrive in an environment where they feel loved, safe and happy. There can be no doubt that children benefit from the love of people who care deeply for them, whether their carers are straight, gay, single or married.

Large family, large hearts: Learning the art of family management

Helen has seven children with her husband Romeo. They are happy with their large family but tire of the assumptions made about them.

Helen's Story

We have seven children ranging in age from age 2 to 26 years. I experienced a teen pregnancy at age 17 and became a single mother; this baby was not planned but was very much loved and wanted, even though everyone around me encouraged me to have an abortion, telling me my whole life was ahead of me and that I would ruin my life. How far from the truth they were; having my children have been my greatest life-changing moments.

I met my Romeo (yes, his real name) when I was 24 and we wanted a baby together straight away. Romeo's dad was very old when he was born; it was like he had a great grandfather for a father so he wanted to have children young—and we managed to have three by the time he was 22. Our son Zak was born six weeks early on my 25th birthday and Romeo only informed his strict European parents of my pregnancy when I was 32 weeks along, so they only had two weeks' notice.

Child number three was a bit of a surprise (although very welcome) and this was when some of the comments started about large families. It seems as though in Australia you are expected to only have 2.1 children as that's the national average. Later, I was able to please our former Treasurer when he said 'One for the mother and one for the father and one for the country'; well, I doubled that and then some!

I always wanted at least five children; I actually visualised it and put it in the back of my mind and thought I'd be the last of my crowd to get hitched and get pregnant as I was a keen traveller. I was the eldest of five (one half-sister, one brother and two step-brothers) and I belonged to a large Irish Catholic family and loved the big family Christmas and New Year gatherings with the multitude of cousins.

I think the best thing about having a big family is that there is so much love to go around and things are always interesting. The different personalities are amazing to watch and interact with; each child has their individuality, their own quirks and attributes. I love that we share a lot and have good times with lots of laughter. I am looking forward to those big family Christmases in years to come—I'll bet we get loads of grandchildren out of seven children.

I don't really see any negatives about having a large family, although I will say it can be difficult at times to manage things logistically. For example, when we have to be in two or three or even five different places at the exact same time—it's difficult. However, we have become masters at juggling and multi-tasking, and we just accept that sometimes there will be clashes. While we are very energetic and lead extremely full lives, we sometimes simply cannot do everything that is available to us.

People can be so nosy and aren't shy about offering opinions or assumptions about our large family, from our carbon footprint to our food and utility bills. We dislike this and find it quite odd but people really do think it costs a lot more. We beg to differ. From our experience, we notice that we spend less on shopping than most two-kid families we know and our bills are very cheap. We shop cleverly and we know how to cook up a storm and eat like kings and queens on a budget. I have become a whiz at buying bargain designer clothes for my kids and preserving clothing to pass down. You don't have to dress your kids in rags and op-shop clothing when you have a large family. I am always finding spectacular stuff in the sales.

We still get to travel a lot; we don't always fly as a whole family but we drive from Adelaide to Brisbane a couple of times each year to visit family and friends and do house swaps with my brother. I travel all the time to conferences and workshops. It's quite an exciting life; not one trapped at home with kids under my feet like some people have assumed.

Helen's Wisdom

We have had to learn how to juggle, practise good time management and patience, multi-task, budget—pretty much all the skills you need to run a business; I guess that's how we manage to run such a large family. We also try and impart these skills to the children so that they have real skills for the real lives they will lead out in the big world when they leave home.

When you have a large family, there is never a dull moment and there is always enough love to go around, always something to do and experience. I love having a big family and I wouldn't swap the love and the laughter we share for the world.

'Average family': When traditional roles cause strain on the marriage

Although Sadie is besotted with her children, she feels let down by her husband, who, she believes, is not involved enough in their daily lives.

Sadie's Story

We are one of the 'average' families of mum, dad and two children living in the one house, with the same biological parents for both children, aged six and four years. I am fortunate enough in that I don't have to work. When child number two came along it was a joint decision that both parents working and juggling childcare would be too difficult, so I would stay home. But even though it looks like I'm living my dream, at times it feels more like a nightmare.

For me, the biggest challenge with parenting has been the divide between my husband and me over expectations and levels of commitment to our new roles. The support I longed for in a parenting partner I find more often in my parents and friends. It would be easier for me to accept my husband's lack of interest and involvement but unfortunately, the dream I had never ceases to crave fulfilment, so I always feel some disappointment. I know my husband loves his children but his interest stops at a having a cuddle while watching television or the occasional wrestle or pony ride on the floor when he is in a very good mood. I continue to ask for the practical assistance I need with day-to-day care but this is often the source of conflict, no matter how minor the request. I wonder if I lived in a time like my parents if we would be happier with our roles. Did husbands just go to work and wives did everything at home? And were they happier because they expected no more than this arrangement?

If we did not have children together then I believe neither of us would wish to continue the relationship, or perhaps if we did not have children we would not have the conflicting attitudes. Who knows? It remains uncertain as to what would be the better outcome for the children—to have their parents together but living in conflict or to have a separated family? This decision is one that I battle with daily. There is never a right answer. The effect of separating the family unit on our children and me would be life-changing. The obvious emotional turmoil suffered by everyone involved, not to mention the financial losses and changes in lifestyle are all considerations that have kept me in a relationship that is less than I would have settled for before having children. The biggest fear that binds me to stay is the threat of dividing child custody. The thought of not seeing my children for a number of days each week is not one I could contemplate at this stage in their lives and mine.

When we first decided to get married, we were both keen to have children straight away. I was 32 and the prospect of not having children possibly clouded my thinking about spending more time establishing the marriage. I would highly recommend to my daughters that they get to know their partners more before they commit to parenting with someone. I don't regret having my girls as they are absolutely amazing and the best thing in my life, but I would love to share more of that amazement with their father.

I realise now the importance of examining how your partner was raised by their parents. For us, the expectation of what it meant to parent is quite different. We did discuss our values and beliefs, but not the actual practical day-to-day raising of children. Maybe this can only be worked out in practice. My husband believes kids should amuse themselves and their routine should fit your own. I interpret this as him wanting to do his own thing and the children work around that. He had a domineering father who believed that kids should work, not play. My husband balanced this by spending his spare time playing with his friends and as little time as possible at home. I think now he associates spending time with his own children as work and therefore something unpleasant.

I love spending time with our children and get most of my pleasure from their excitement and enjoyment. I do get tired of the practical chores of raising children mostly alone though and find I have to balance this by planning fun times that remind me how lucky I am to be doing this. Time shouldn't be an issue but it is. I usually find the most difficult days are those when I have become preoccupied with all the jobs that need doing instead of enjoying what I have.

I really do believe we are meant to share the experience of raising children. But maybe this can come in any form, a husband, or a grandparent, or a friend—whoever appreciates how much joy you get from a child. I have some wonderful friends who continue to motivate me to appreciate each moment, just by enjoying the children with me. My attitude completely changes when I am focusing on the positive moments and so does my reaction to the other challenging times.

I cherish the moments my husband and I can appreciate together. I am sure that it is different for every couple and possibly different depending on the age of the children. Maybe the more important thing is to make sure you keep focused on the positive parenting moments to ride you through the tougher ones. Maybe that's the same in our relationships as well.

Sadie's Wisdom

When my own daughters grow up, I will stress that picking your partner to marry and have a family with is one of the biggest choices you'll ever make and can completely affect how you will be able to parent. The only way to know someone is to spend a few years, if possible, developing your relationship as a couple before you extend that relationship to children. The more you discuss your expectations of a father and mother, including how each of you were raised, the more able you will be to decide if that person has a compatible parenting style. Parenting is such a special experience and the best way to enjoy it is to make sure you keep focused on the joys it brings and even more so by sharing these with another.

Pure love: Parenting a child with different abilities

Parenting Liam has been a difficult and joyful learning process for Pat and her husband. Pat talks about what it is like raising a son with extra needs and how it influences their family life both positively and negatively.

Pat's Story

We were planning a homebirth for our first child and had chosen to have minimal testing, so we didn't know that Liam had Down syndrome until he was born. The labor didn't go well, and I ended up being rushed to the hospital and having an emergency caesarean section. He was really struggling so they rushed him to the NICU (Neonatal Intensive Care Unit). I had been under general anaesthesia so I wasn't aware there were any issues with my baby. When I came out of anaesthesia, and my husband came back from the NICU, I could see that there was something wrong. He told me it was a boy, and that they thought he had Down syndrome.

The next day they did a blood test which took a few days to come back. It confirmed their suspicions and we got the diagnosis. However, he has always been a little bit different from other kids with Down syndrome. I would go to Down syndrome parent groups and come home crying because I felt like he wasn't doing as well as the other kids, and I knew he couldn't handle what the other parents said we should be doing with him. For example, there was a child who could write his name at four years old—at four, Liam was only just able to make marks on a paper. On the other hand, his language was always a relative strength and he was pretty interactive. So, we wandered along, providing him with the services he needed, but without much support for ourselves.

Finally, when he was around eight years old, I became aware that children with Down syndrome could also have autism. We made an appointment with a doctor who specializes in dual diagnosis. It took a while to get the appointment, but he did diagnose Liam as being on the autism spectrum. We later went to the Down syndrome clinic of the Children's Hospital and underwent a more rigorous screening and got a diagnosis of autism. In addition, he has multiple developmental delays and scoliosis (the hits just keep on coming!) for which he underwent corrective surgery this summer. He also has a fabulous sense of humor, a smile that would warm anyone's heart, and is very good at math. He loves music, videos and his little brother. Our family is very supportive and they are Liam's biggest fans (except his younger brother, who struggles with having a big brother that can't do many of the things that he already can).

Liam was in school when his brother Jack was born, so we balanced their care pretty much the way everyone does—you do the best you can and you get very tired. After my maternity leave of five months, Liam would go to school in the mornings and Jack would go to the babysitter while my husband and I went to work. Balancing therapies and early intervention is more of a struggle since we both work. But somehow you just make it work with the resources you have (time, money, willpower, whatever).

We have been fortunate in that the people around us have been very understanding. One of the benefits, so to speak, of having Down syndrome is that people know you are disabled (many people in the Down syndrome community would not agree with me on this). However, comparing our experience to the experiences of kids who just have autism—with no obvious external signals—it has been much easier. Many people think kids with autism are just throwing tantrums, when really they can't help themselves. People often stare and make comments. We don't usually have that problem. Now that he's a bit older (13), people tend to be a little bit less comfortable if they can't understand what he's saying to them. When he was little, they were more patient because it isn't uncommon not to understand a little child.

Because our first child had special needs, we have had to learn a lot about parenting since having our second child, who is typically developing. There are so many differences between what you need to do for a disabled child, and what you need to do for a typically developing child. I actually think the typical kids are harder!

I love Liam more than life itself. Every time he does something new or learns a new skill, he is so proud of himself and we are so proud of him. He has no guile, he doesn't manipulate. When he's happy, he's happy—and when he isn't, you know that too.

As I mentioned, he has a fabulous sense of humor. One day, I was in the supermarket and a woman was yelling at me from down the aisle 'Mrs Smith! Mrs Smith!' I thought 'Who is this woman?' It turns out she was Liam's aide that day and had such a fun time with him, she had to tell me about it. Apparently they were working on telling time. Every time she would point to the clock on the page and say 'What time is it?', he would look at her out of the corner of his eye and say 'Time to go home?' She was telling everyone about it, because he was totally aware that he was making a joke, and it really was funny. That was a great experience—and it isn't the only time people have had to tell me about something Liam did.

Due to the autism, Liam has high levels of anxiety and can't handle new situations very quickly. We can't go to a lot of places since he gets overwhelmed by loud sounds, birds, and large dark spaces (like a theatre). While that is getting better, it still limits our freedom. It's very challenging because we'd like to take our other son to see a lot of things—so we either have to split up (one parent/one child) which isn't satisfying, or we don't go. Sometimes my mother will come places with us, so that she can take Liam if he gets overwhelmed. I think this is going to continue to be a big issue for us, even as Liam is better able to handle certain circumstances; our desire to do things will outpace his ability. This is very sad to me.

Also, he perseverates (he says the same things over and over). It's very difficult to talk to him when he's doing that, and it hurts to have to finish the conversation before he's ready because he is just saying the same thing again and again and again. And again. 'Mommy, and again. Again? Again? Mommy, again?' You can imagine how frustrating that can become, and how upsetting to have to say to your child 'You've told me that already, now I have to move on.' Otherwise, you might stand there for 15 minutes.

It's very easy to be overwhelmed and frightened by the idea of having a child with a disability. And there can be a lot of work involved. But you do connect with your child very deeply — even a child who doesn't have typical social or communication skills. Somehow you know them. Liam has brought us a lot of joy and a lot of laughs, in addition to the challenges.

A lot of parents are looking for perfection in their families. They have an idyllic picture in their heads of what life should be like. They want to have perfect careers, be perfect parents whose children are outstanding students with good hair and good manners, have a perfect home, be dressed perfectly, be perfect hosts and gourmet chefs, with an enviable knowledge and collection of wine. Much of this is hard to accomplish at all with children, but having a child with a disability immediately changes the picture. Marketing is perfect — life is imperfect. Cut yourself a break and do what's important and what you enjoy. Forget about perfection; forget about the image of what your life is supposed to look like. It's too stressful, for no good reason. Do the best you can do and have a sense of humor about what you can't.

Pat's Wisdom	Every family has problems. Some of them are more visible, like having a child with a disability. But if your child didn't have a disability, you would still have issues to deal with. Sometimes I get jealous of friends whose lives seem easier than mine, but I remind myself that their fate isn't mine. And I'll look at what's making me jealous about their lives, and try to improve that area of my life, which is obviously lacking something when that happens. It might be travel, it might be doing social things locally, or going out to eat easily, or keeping the house neater.
	Another lesson I've learned is that no-one understands you like another parent of a child with a disability. You can say anything to them, and they get it, without trying to make you feel better with platitudes. I hate when people say 'God doesn't give you anything you can't handle' — really? Then maybe I should have been weaker in my life so my child wouldn't have been born with a chromosomal anomaly. 'You must be very special for God to give you this child'. Great — had I known that, I would have robbed a bank before he was born to make me less good. So, get thee to a support group. Or connect with other parents at your school.

Why didn't anyone tell me that ...

- Parenting will never work unless you and your partner invest 100 per cent each.

- I should have talked more with my husband about division of roles before the baby was born. Now that we have two kids, I am left to do everything while he plays on the computer.

- Having babies does not fix relationships on the rocks. It just makes them that much worse.

- People would often stare and make comments at my child with autism. They just don't understand that he is not simply throwing a tantrum, he can't help himself.

- We would often have to explain ourselves as same sex parents. Constantly talking about my sexuality gets a bit draining.

- I knew many people's reactions to our family would be adverse but some people have really gone to town. What do they think we do? Run gay nightclubs from home? We are just two men raising babies. One of us goes to work and thinks about what to cook for dinner, while the other stays at home and looks after our boy, taking him to playgroups and doing the same thing that most parents do. Trust me, if you got a peek into our lives, you would probably yawn!

- When I made the decision to have three children, I would get disparaging remarks from so many people, even my own family. 'Why on earth would you want three children?' 'Isn't two enough for you?' 'You're very brave, aren't you?' And from my own father: 'Well, you've made your bed, you lie in it'. What bizarre reactions!

Epilogue

Having reached the end of this book I hope you have become convinced of the key message that there is no one way to bring a child into the world or to raise it. What counts is how much you love that child; everything else will follow. These stories will ideally pave the way for parents to begin actively supporting each other's choices.

Parenting in the 21st century has become polarised and contentious but it clearly doesn't have to be that way. I think it's important to recognise that men and women are raising individuals and therefore their parenting styles will necessarily differ from one another, according to their own needs and the needs of their children.

I hope these stories will provide a sense of support, connection and optimism. So many mothers and fathers out there wonder, on a daily basis 'Is this normal?' The short answer is 'yes'. Everyone feels anchorless at times, bored, unappreciated, guilty. It's also normal to feel angry, depressed and even slightly out of control. These are the kinds of subjects unlikely to arise at your local parents' meeting or playgroup, yet to know that this is a universal experience can be a lifeline for many and one I hope you will hold on to should you need it.

In addition, I am continually amazed at the lack of full representation in parenting books. Why aren't fathers, single parents and gay parents included in mainstream parenting books? Surely we live in a society where everyone is equal and absolutely everyone has the right to create a family. I sincerely hope that *Why Didn't Anyone Tell Me?* contributes to rectifying this situation.

It has been an amazing privilege to work with so many parents in the creation of this book. Reading their stories has caused me to laugh and to weep, to feel angry, shocked and inspired. Having read these stories you will now know for sure that there is no parenting expert. Only you are the expert on your own children so please don't let anyone make you feel bad about your parenting choices.

I hope you have enjoyed *Why Didn't Anyone Tell Me?* I am currently working on my next books, all based on narrative. If you have any comments or suggestions, or you would like to contribute, please contact me through my website <www.becgriffin.com>.

Research

Interpreting research: A 'how to' guide for parents

'That's the nature of research—you don't know what in the world you're doing.'

Dr Harold E. Edgerton (Bruce 1994)

Written by Dr Rachel Glasson BMBS (Hons)

In centuries gone by, parenting was a skill passed from generation to generation by example and practical experience. Larger, extended families meant that most young adults had already been extensively involved in looking after younger siblings before they contemplated becoming parents themselves. In the late 19th and early 20th centuries, along with the rise of science and medicine, the first 'parenting experts' appeared, as the average family was becoming smaller and first-time parents began looking beyond their own parents for advice on how to raise their children.

At the turn of the century, a fairly rigid and authoritarian method of parenting was advocated by experts such as Dr Luther Emmett Holt (1894), who discouraged parents from kissing or cuddling their infants and emphasised the importance of imposing regular routines and habits. As society changed after World War II, a more relaxed approach came into favour as one of the most recognisable names in child psychology, Dr Benjamin Spock (1946), published a child-rearing manual which encouraged parents to pick up their babies and enjoy them. Thus, the confusion began.

Since then, there has been an explosion of both scientific knowledge and technology, which can leave the average parent bewildered and confused. The widespread availability of the internet in the Western world means that there is a vast amount of information about all aspects of parenting— from breastfeeding, sleeping, settling and discipline to feeding, clothing and education—available right at our fingertips. Increasing numbers of research studies have been conducted on many aspects of child rearing, often with conflicting results. A simple search may turn up a number of impressively scientific studies which completely contradict each other, leaving parents struggling to make decisions based on conflicting advice.

This appendix does not aim to explain away any of the controversies that exist in the world of evidence-based parenting. Rather, it is an attempt to equip parents with tools that will assist them in navigating the ocean of research and recommendations that exists out there, and through which we all must somehow sail.

When advice becomes judgement

Parenting is a highly emotive subject, one that is fraught with guilt and anxiety. There are so many questions that new parents continually ask themselves, so many things to consider—sleeping, feeding, comforting, childcare, vaccinations—and in each area, there are many schools of thought, often with conflicting points of view.

When a particular method has worked for you, it is natural to want to tell everyone about your success and to recommend it to every parent—if it worked for you, it has to work for them, right? Although sharing experiences and stories is one of the best ways parents can support one another, attempting to convert others to your parenting beliefs is dangerous. Even though you mean well, it is so easy to tap unwittingly into the deep well of guilt within most mothers, who fear they are doing everything wrong. It is a short journey from 'Why don't you try ...' to 'Oh, you shouldn't do that ...' where advice turns to judgement and hostility. Many of the stories in this book contain tales of judgement heaped upon parents who dared to use a parenting method that others found controversial. It should make us all wary when we are tempted to tell others how we think they should raise their children.

Also, beware of anecdotal evidence being quoted as proof for why a certain method is better than all others. Just because it worked for one family, or even one child within a family, does not mean it will work for others—even in the same family. Anecdotal evidence is typically given more weight when it concerns a negative outcome: horror stories of what happened to so-and-so's baby when they tried this or that may easily put parents off trying what is a perfectly safe and humane solution to their problem. Try to bear in mind that each child is different; their parent knows them best and does not need to hear nightmarish tales of woe when they are in need of support and encouragement!

Research studies and their relevance to everyday life

As parents, we all want to do the best we can for our children. We want to give them the best possible start in life, sometimes in reaction to things we feel were missing from our own upbringing. Research studies aim to answer important questions—such as whether or not to vaccinate, what is the best method of soothing a crying baby, is breast milk really better than formula—with scientific evidence that parents can trust.

The first problem most parents encounter is the sheer volume of information available online. For example, if you type 'baby feeding' into a search engine, you get over 12 million results; 'baby sleeping' produces a staggering 34 million. Even if you limit your search to research studies, you will encounter a second problem: not all studies produce valid results. There is so-called scientific evidence out there that is false, and it can be used to validate a practice or belief that is potentially harmful.

The third (and largest) problem is that the average parent is not equipped to identify which studies are scientifically sound and which are not. The result is that parents may find themselves convinced to trust research that is biased or invalid, and when the health or wellbeing of their children is involved, this is a serious problem indeed.

When good research turns bad

There are various groups who will use faulty research—knowingly or not—to push their ideas and methods on others through the internet. The first of these groups is generally people for whom a certain method of parenting has worked, and who zealously seek to convince others to try it. They may even cite scientific studies to support their methods or beliefs, but there is no guarantee that these studies are valid. Many research studies may seem to prove their point, but in reality, they are deceptive. They may fool all but the experts—and therein lies the danger for unwary parents.

The second is a group who have a vested interest in promoting a certain treatment, drug or belief. This group includes, but is not limited to, drug companies and legal firms. They may prey upon parents' anxieties—the link between autism and the MMR vaccine (see below) is a particular case in point—in order to convince them of associations that are neither proven nor real. The consequences of this kind of behaviour can be grave.

Evaluating research

In order to produce scientifically reliable results, a research study needs to have a number of specific qualities. Checking for these is a simple and effective way of being able to gauge whether or not to trust the conclusions being drawn. In order to produce a valid recommendation about a certain treatment or method, a study should ideally be:

- Sufficiently powerful to demonstrate that an outcome is not due purely to chance. This generally means having a large number of subjects in the study. Beware of any piece of research where the number of subjects (n) is low.

- Reliable—the outcome that is being measured, or the results, should be able to be reliably recorded. Measurements, or the presence or absence of something, are reliably recordable; patient or subject recall about events, or subjective responses (such as feelings) are very difficult to standardise. Memory is particularly unreliable and any study which relies on people remembering when a symptom started or how something felt should not be trusted without careful scrutiny.

- Prospective, rather than retrospective—subjects should be enrolled in the study and *then* undergo the treatment or have an intervention; looking back at historical data and trying to make associations is not as reliable.

- Randomised and controlled—there should be a similar group of subjects who do *not* have the intervention/treatment who are evaluated as well as the test group. Subjects should be randomly assigned to the control or intervention group, in order to minimise bias (i.e. the chance of putting a certain type of person in either group, thus skewing the results).

- Reproducible—it should be possible to repeat the study and have the same finding. If the results are not reproducible, it raises the possibility (unfortunately not unheard of) that they may have been somehow falsified.

- Impartial—all financial interests and funding must be declared, as well as any potential conflicts of interest. Beware any study that is funded by a drug company, particularly if its conclusion relates to a drug they produce. Similarly, any advice or recommendations by a doctor who has been paid by a drug company or legal firm should be treated with suspicion and regarded more as an advertisement than a true medical opinion, unless it is backed up by solid research findings.

Any research study that does not have the above qualities may not be able to prove its hypothesis with any reliability. It may be able to make associations or identify trends, but it should NOT be taken as evidence or proof of anything.

Fatally flawed research

To illustrate, let's consider a hypothetical research study proposing a link between eye colour and tooth decay. A group of investigators examines a large number of school-age children and records three outcomes: the presence or absence of dental caries, the number of affected teeth in those with caries and the colour of each child's eyes. The result: they find that brown-eyed children are more likely to have dental caries than blue-eyed children, with an average of three teeth affected. The conclusion: they propose new guidelines for childhood dental hygiene and advise that parents with brown-eyed children should be educated that their children require more frequent check-ups in addition to regular brushing and flossing. The study is partially funded by the Dental Association of England.

What's wrong with the above findings?

Most obviously, a relationship between eye colour and predisposition to dental caries is difficult to postulate. There is no obvious connection—one could postulate a genetic link, but it would be hard to believe and costly to discover.

That aside, these results are questionable for several good reasons. Firstly, there are any number of outside influences which have not been accounted and adjusted for. Diet, dental hygiene habits, socio-economic status, the presence or absence of fluoride in local tap water—all of these could have affected the results, absolutely independently of a child's eye colour. Perhaps more brown-eyed children were from low socio-economic backgrounds, or they lived in an area without fluoridated drinking water. This kind of bias must be eliminated in order for the findings of the study to be meaningful, but as far as we know, it has not been accounted for.

Secondly, the conclusion reached is suspicious when one considers the financial interests of the Dental Association, which has in part sponsored this study. It is clearly in their best interests to give anxious parents cause to seek more frequent check-ups for their brown-eyed children, and what better way to do so than to publish research studies such as this one?

Of course, this hypothetical study is a frivolous one and most parents would not think twice about dismissing its conclusions. The danger arises when bad research is published on topics which are serious business.

A prime example of this is the study published in respected medical journal *The Lancet* in February 1998, which caused a global health crisis despite being scientifically unsound in many obvious respects.

Autism and the MMR vaccine: A controversial association

In 1998, a study was published in *The Lancet* which caused an almost immediate furore amongst parents (Wakefield et al. 1998). It linked symptoms of autism (behavioural regression) with the administration of the MMR (measles, mumps and rubella) vaccine, leading parents all over the developed world to panic and vaccination rates to plummet, despite the study being full of flaws. Its impact was enormous, but no-one could replicate the findings and indeed six years later, the editor of *The Lancet* published a statement of its intention to fully investigate the actions of the authors (led by Dr Andrew Wakefield) who undertook the 1998 study, largely as a result of investigations by a *Sunday Times* journalist named Brian Deer (Deer 2010).

The outcome was an unprecedented, complete retraction of the 'utterly false' study by *The Lancet* from its published records (the first ever retraction in its nearly 200-year history), in February 2010. The British General Medical Council's board of review found that Wakefield had acted unethically in the conduct of his research, had falsified results, had introduced bias by seeking out patients, and had shown 'callous disregard' for the 'distress and pain' the subject children had undergone as a result of invasive investigations for his study.

Yet the damage done by this single, appallingly flawed study remains: the investigation also found that 'the Wakefield study has been a key piece of evidence cited by many parents who do not vaccinate their children because of autism fears' (see Park 2010). How long it will take to undo the damage done to parents' confidence in vaccines is unknown; meanwhile measles outbreaks are once again on the rise and in 2006, the first UK measles death in over 14 years was recorded (BBC News 2006).

More recently, worldwide outbreaks (in Australia, the United States, New Zealand, Switzerland, the United Kingdom and Ireland) have caused widespread concern, specifically because of the lower rate of vaccinations (Public Health Agency of Canada 2010). Dr Steven Donohue of Queensland Health said that only 90 per cent of people in Queensland (Australia) had been immunised against measles. 'That is a pretty big opening. We are on the edge of a situation where, if vaccination rates drop even just a little bit, it could lead to a very serious outbreak.' He goes on to explain that 'Measles is not a trivial disease by any means. People can develop pneumonia. About one in 1000 will get encephalitis (brain swelling) that can lead to permanent brain damage. It can kill you. It is a very serious disease' (Kellett 2010).

The flaws exposed

We can use the checklist given above to quickly evaluate how much importance to assign to the Wakefield study.

- The study only examined 12 children—a very low number—who presented to a specialist unit for investigation of gastrointestinal symptoms including diarrhoea and abdominal pain. This is by far too few patients to even begin to prove an association, given the incidence of vaccinations, bowel disease and autism in the general population.

- The outcome, being the close temporal association of behavioural regression and vaccination, was parent-reported; most claimed that signs of autism had appeared within days of the MMR vaccination being given. This method of result collection—asking parents to remember when something started—is notoriously unreliable, and it was later found (from their previous medical records) that many of the children had shown behavioural problems and abnormalities weeks to months before the vaccination was given.

- Financial interests were not declared. It emerged that not only had Dr Wakefield been given a large sum of money to conduct his research, he had also been paid by a law firm representing parents with autistic children who were hoping to bring a class action against drug companies who made MMR vaccines. Further, he had patented his own single measles vaccine and had used his own study as 'proof' that single vaccines (rather than the combination MMR) were safer for children.

- The children were not randomly selected, but were mostly contacts of the law firm for which Dr Wakefield worked and were sent to him with the specific purpose of being enrolled in a study aiming to link the measles virus (part of the MMR vaccine) to their gastrointestinal problems and blame it for their behavioural problems. This kind of selection bias renders any results or conclusions completely invalid.

The bottom line

Although scientific research into parenting issues is a valuable tool to help us all raise our children in the best possible way, the final checkpoint should always be your family doctor or paediatrician. They have a responsibility to keep abreast of current literature and to be able to critically evaluate research studies in order to know whether they are sound or not. If it concerns your child's health and wellbeing or if it affects the wider community (think vaccinations) then the safest way to be sure that you are putting your trust in valid conclusions is to ask an expert.

If you want to find reliable scientific evidence on certain parenting subjects, then the best place to look is not Google but rather the Cochrane Collaboration (www.cochrane.org). It contains a database of systemic reviews of the medical literature, aiming to assess critically the evidence for and against various interventions. Cochrane reviews are the best source of reliable information about health care topics, but may only identify that there are no top-quality studies (randomised, controlled trials) on a certain topic. There is unfortunately very little information about general parenting methods, because these are almost impossible to study in scientifically rigorous ways.

Putting it all together

No one would disagree with the statement that parenting is a difficult process. Children do not come with instructions and there is a huge amount of advice and information out there on every aspect of their care. In the end, there is no such thing as pure evidence-based parenting, and there probably never will be. Often, we still have to rely on the wisdom of those who have gone before, and a useful recipe for caring for your baby might be: common sense, love, and a little research … and trust your instincts.

How to start a support group

'It is one of the most beautiful compensations of this life that no man can sincerely try to help another without helping himself.'

Ralph Waldo Emerson (Kelly 2003)

Re-printed in part with kind permission from the Schizophrenia Fellowship of NSW Inc (2007), *Group Leader's Manual*, Sydney.

What is a support group?

A support group is an association of people with similar problems and interests, working together to provide each other with information and support. Support groups are an important part of our society and evidence has shown that they play an integral role in helping people to connect, share problems and even lobby for systemic change (Reay-Young 2001).

If you decide to start a support group because there are none in your area concerning your cause (for example, you may wish to start a fathers' group or a group for parents whose children have autism; the list is endless), it is important to bear in mind that the success of your group relies heavily on recognising and meeting the needs of its members. Aside from being committed to doing something about your cause or issue, people will be joining your group for all kinds of reasons. For some, it may be an effective avenue of forming friendships and gaining mutual support, while for others, working to achieve something through the group (for example, better LGBT legislation) may be their main priority. It is important to recognise these personal needs of the members and make sure that, to some extent, they're met within the group. A group that is concerned solely with one task may find it has a problem of dwindling members.

Why do we need support groups?

There are many benefits in belonging to a support group. Any list of such benefits could never be all-inclusive. At the very least, each support group has its own particular strengths due to its membership. However, some of the benefits that can be gained by belonging to a support group are:

- unique support, understanding and strength given by people who find themselves in similar situations. To know that you are not alone in the difficulties you are facing and that there are others with similar circumstances who can offer help and support is comforting knowledge. The feeling of 'belonging' has great value in itself.
- the chance to learn from the combined wisdom of others who are experienced in coping with day-to-day problems.
- the opportunity to make new friends and to create your own social networks.
- the satisfaction gained through helping others.
- the promotion of greater factual understanding as opposed to your own subjective (personal) understanding. A major obstacle for many people is a lack of information; belonging to a support group has the potential to provide you with a wealth of useful information.

The collective voice of a support group can also be a powerful tool for advocacy. Perhaps you need a playground in your suburb. Maybe you want to lobby for your right to birth at home or advocate for LGBT individuals and couples who want greater equity in the eyes of the law. Starting or joining a support group can help you to influence policy and lobby your government.

The support group should offer an environment that is non-judgemental, open, constructive and focused on every member gaining benefit from the group. Its philosophy—indeed its very reason for being—is one of empowering its members.

Creating a start-up committee

The start-up committee is your core group of two or three individuals who share your interest in creating a support group. The members of the start-up committee should be willing to invest their time and energy to help organise and develop the group. Committee members should make a commitment to the group and contribute whatever talents, skills, resources and information they have that will lead to your group's success and growth. Members should agree to share the work ahead and take responsibility for their participation. Some issues your start-up committee might like to consider are:

- overall picture and goals of the group
- how the group will operate
- organisational plan of the group
- focus of the group.

Since the start-up committee will be the strength of the group and will guide its future course, its members should be chosen carefully.

Preparing for your first meeting

For a successful first meeting, you could plan an interesting, basic educational program, perhaps with a guest speaker. You might like to consider the following points:

Publicity	How are you going to get your message out to the community?
Venue	Does your proposed venue need to be booked well in advance?
Speakers	What topics are you aiming to cover? How will you find your speakers?
Agenda	What issues do you think will need to be addressed?
Duration	How much time will you need for everything to be covered?
Refreshments	Will you be providing tea/coffee and light snacks?
Information	What kind of literature will you have available for guests to read?

Publicity

It is a good idea to have as many people as possible attend your first meeting. It makes a good impression on your potential members and can promote more interest in your group as the word spreads. It's a good idea to think about how you will publicise your group. Common methods include: press release distribution, poster/leaflet distribution, interviews and announcements on community radio, invitation mail-outs and local newspaper advertisements.

Venue

Obtain a central location (local community centre, service club premises or church hall, for example) that is easily accessible. Some aspects of the venue that you will need to consider are: the room (size, ventilation, lighting), the cost and equipment (tea and coffee making facilities, chairs and tables, etc.).

Speakers

It is important to choose your guest speaker carefully, as they are a potential drawcard for your group. You need to work out what issues you would like to be addressed and then obtain a relevant speaker. Places to try are local community health centres, hospitals, or anywhere that you might find a speaker for the topic on which you wish to present.

Agenda

Most public meetings follow a pattern and you may wish to model your agenda on the following:

1. Welcoming statement
2. Explanation of what the meeting is about and why it was called
3. A brief outline of the form you want the meeting to take
4. Presentations by the invited speakers and/or video about the issue and how it can be pursued
5. Meeting open for questions and contributions from anyone else present
6. Discussion of resolutions for action
7. Planning of future meetings
8. Appeal for financial support
9. Closure of meeting.

The agenda reflects how the meeting will be run and what issues will be raised. Take your time when writing this, as a poorly planned agenda will result in a disorganised and therefore unsuccessful meeting.

Duration

In general, it is best to try to keep the meeting to two hours. Any longer than this and guests are liable to become bored, disinterested or tired. Break the meeting up into sessions (as per your agenda) and be sure to have breaks for tea and coffee. Concentration usually lapses when presentations are longer than about 50 minutes. A good idea to keep up a high level of interest is to have your speaker present his/her topic and then allow for question time (as reflected in the agenda above).

Refreshments and information

The provision of refreshments and literature is useful in that it gives guests a chance to settle in, pick up some basic information and meet others attending the meeting. Other members of your start-up committee can circulate among guests and make them feel welcome, explaining something about the group or the program to be presented. To ensure the smooth running of your first meeting, you should ensure that a few people arrive early to set up the room and greet people as they arrive. Someone should also be appointed to note down comments and ideas as they arise. You may wish to consider taping your first meeting so that it can be played at your follow-up committee meeting to help you with your evaluation. If you decide to do this, make sure to check as soon as the meeting opens that everyone present agrees to the taping.

Plan, plan, plan!

It cannot be emphasised enough that running groups and public meetings needs thorough planning and attention to detail. The process may seem a little daunting at first but you will soon find that running your meetings becomes like second nature to you.

A final word

A word to the wise: there is no need to re-invent the wheel. Make sure there are no similar support groups in your area before going to great lengths to start your own. The information listed in this appendix can be used to start any support group but it is not prescriptive; you may wish to have a very simple, informal gathering at your house every couple of weeks. If this is the case, all you need is common sense and kindness. If you are interested in starting up a lobby group or a group for people who are in need of information and support, then the ideas above may be helpful to you.

There are many large organisations that support the development of local groups. It is always a good idea to try this avenue first, as many such organisations have a plethora of resources that you can use. This is especially the case for health conditions. For a list of large, national organisations please see the Resources section.

Glossary

acid reflux	A condition in which, after eating, there is a regurgitation of stomach contents up the oesophagus (the tube that connects the mouth to the stomach). Acid reflux disease is also known as gastro-oesophageal reflux disease (GORD).
active labour	Active labour is when labour really gets going. It is generally described as having longer, stronger contractions that are less than five minutes apart.
amniotic fluid	The fluid that surrounds the unborn baby in the womb.
anovulation	Failure of ovulation during a menstrual cycle.
antenatal	The period between conception and birth. Also known as 'prenatal'.
APGAR	The APGAR score is a system used by health professionals to assess the general physical condition of newborns and is based on five criteria: heart rate, respiration, muscle tone, skin colour and response to stimuli. Infants are given a score between 0 and 2 for each of the criteria; a perfect APGAR score is 10. The observations are conducted one minute and five minutes after birth.
artificial insemination	Also known as AI, artificial insemination is the process of inserting male sperm into a female via a variety of techniques.
assisted reproductive technology (ART)	ART is the umbrella term that refers to the use of eggs, sperm or embryos that have been donated by a third party ('the donor') in order for an individual or a couple ('the recipients') to become parents.
augmentation	The process of speeding up labour.
baby blues	The baby blues is a common but temporary state soon after childbirth when a new mother may have sudden mood swings or feel weepy and lonely.

Baby-Friendly Hospital Initiative (BFHI)	A worldwide program of the World Health Organization and UNICEF to improve the role of maternity services and increase breastfeeding rates globally.
birth centre	Birth centres are staffed by midwives and are usually attached to major hospitals. Birth centres offer a more homely environment. The strongest form of pain relief available is usually pethidine.
birthing stool	Used for many centuries, a birthing stool is a stool that is made low to the ground, allowing women to squat (or sit) during the labour process. Most importantly, it is designed with a hole in the middle for a baby to fit through.
blastocyst	A ball of cells produced one week after fertilisation.
blighted ovum	Also known as anembryonic gestation, a blighted ovum is where conception has occurred but the embryo does not develop.
breech position	The baby is facing bottom down (instead of the head down position).
camping out method	Parents sit with their babies until they fall asleep and gradually remove their presence over a period of time.
cascade of intervention	A term used by some to describe the way obstetric inductions (or augmentations) can sometimes lead to further, and escalating, obstetric intervention, such as surgical delivery or caesarean sections. This is still an area of controversy and studies continue.
cervix	The lower part of the uterus that joins with the top of the vagina. The cervix dilates to as much as 10 centimetres to allow a baby to be born.
Chlamydia	A human, sexually transmitted infection caused by the bacterium *Chlamydia trachomatis* that can detrimentally affect fertility.
clomid	A fertility drug that stimulates ovulation.
colic	A term attributed to unexplained crying fits and general distress in young infants and caused by acute abdominal pain and intense spasmodic cramping.

colostrum	Breast milk that is accumulated during the last stages of pregnancy and secreted within approximately one day of giving birth. It is nutrient rich and supplies the baby with 'food' until breast milk 'comes in' around day three to day five.
comfort settling	A technique used to teach babies to sleep (not to be confused with the 'cry it out' method).
controlled crying	*See* 'comfort settling'.
co-sleeping	An umbrella term that includes baby sleeping in the same room as the parents and/or in the parental bed.
delivery suite	A labour ward room in a large hospital where women can choose to deliver their babies. Delivery suites are staffed by midwives, obstetricians and paediatricians.
diazepam	Diazepam is a benzodiazepine that used to be called 'Mother's little helper' in the 1960s.
dilation and curettage	An operation performed on women (in which the cervix is dilated and the lining of the womb is scraped away). Often carried out when miscarriage has been missed or is incomplete.
doula	An experienced health assistant who provides physical and emotional support both during birth and post-partum but does not have midwifery or medical training.
ectopic pregnancy	The fertilised egg implants outside of the uterus, usually in the fallopian tubes. An ectopic pregnancy is not viable and can be extremely dangerous.
endometriosis	A disorder in which tissue that is supposed to form only in the inner lining of the uterus grows in other parts of a woman's body. Can cause pain and infertility.
epidural	A spinal procedure whereby anaesthetic drugs are delivered via a small catheter inserted into the epidural space in the back. Other drugs can also be introduced through the catheter, such as pethidine.
episiotomy	A surgical incision made in the perineum to enlarge the vaginal opening during birth.
fibroids	Benign (non-cancerous) growths in the wall of the uterus.

forceps delivery	Forceps (like big salad tongs) are inserted in the vagina and used to grasp the baby's head so that it can be manually eased through the birth canal.
frenulum	The membrane which attaches the under-surface of the tongue to the floor of the mouth. *See also* 'tongue tie'.
genetic counselling	Genetic counsellors consult with parents about the possibilities and probabilities of passing on certain genes to their children. In some cases where there is a family history of disease, such as cystic fibrosis, parents will be tested for genes via blood tests to determine the likelihood that their children will develop the disease or condition.
gestational carrier	A type of surrogate who carries the baby for the recipient and who has no genetic ties to the baby.
gestational diabetes	A condition in which women develop diabetes during pregnancy.
hands-on settling	A teaching-to-sleep technique whereby the caregiver offers the baby comfort in the form of patting or rocking, while the baby stays in the cot. This is often used for very young babies (usually up to six months).
homeopathy	A method of alternative treatment that involves treating a disease using heavily diluted forms of remedies that when used in large doses reproduce the symptoms of the disease.
humidicrib	Also known as an incubator. A type of plastic box that controls temperature, commonly used for premature infants.
hypnobirth	Type of hypnotherapy used in childbirth.
hysteroscopy	An examination of the inside of the uterus via an endoscope (slim tube) inserted through the vagina and cervix.
Implanon	A type of birth control for women in which a small rod is inserted under the skin of the arm to prevent conception for up to three years. It does this by suppressing ovulation and increasing the viscosity of the cervical mucus, reducing sperm motility and penetration.
induction	*See* 'augmentation'.

Intrauterine Growth Restriction (IUGR)	Refers to inadequate growth in utero. Specifically, babies who are estimated to weigh below the 10th percentile are considered for a diagnosis of Intrauterine Growth Restriction.
in-vitro fertilisation (IVF)	A process by which egg cells are fertilised by sperm outside of the womb.
laparoscopic surgery	Keyhole surgery that is used to examine the interior of the abdominal or pelvic cavities.
let-down reflex	An involuntary reflex during breastfeeding which causes milk to flow. A let-down reflex, or milk-ejection reflex, is the process of milk being made available to a baby by propelling the milk into the ducts and nipple of a woman's breast.
LGBT	Term used for lesbian, gay, bisexual and transgendered people.
linea nigra	A dark, vertical line that can appear on the belly during pregnancy.
live-in service	In Australia, a 'live-in' service refers to organisations that allow parents and their babies to live-in for a short period of time (usually one week), while they are helped by trained early childhood nurses.
low-lying placenta	The placenta is situated quite low in the uterus and in some instances, covers (partially or wholly) the cervix, otherwise known as placenta praevia.
luteal phase	The second half of the menstrual cycle when fertilisation and implantation occurs.
maternal pyrexia	Fever during, or shortly after, labour.
meconium	Viscous, dark green material that is the first faeces of the baby. Meconium-stained waters can indicate foetal distress.
mucous plug	Also known as 'the show' and an indication that labour may soon begin; the mucous plug is a thick layer of mucus that covers the cervix during pregnancy.
nuchal scan	This is an ultrasound conducted at around 12 weeks of pregnancy to detect if there is a high probability for Down syndrome. This test is often conducted in conjunction with a maternal blood test.

oocyte	Immature egg (or ovum).
ovulation	Part of the reproductive cycle in which an egg is released by a mature ovarian follicle.
oxytocin	A hormone mainly involved in the reproductive system.
palpation	A method of physical examination in which a part of the body is felt (usually by the hands of the health care practitioner) to determine its size, shape, firmness and location. Palpation is conducted routinely during pregnancy.
pap smear	A sample of cervical and uterine cells are gathered and examined under a microscope to detect precancerous changes.
perinatal	Generally refers to the period from 20 weeks gestation through to the first month after birth.
perineal massage	Practice of massaging the perineum in preparation for childbirth. It is thought to help soften and stretch the perineum and thus avoid tearing during delivery.
perineum	Region between the genitals and the anus.
peritonitis	The inflammation of the peritoneum, which is the tissue layer of cells lining the inner walls of the abdomen and pelvis.
pethidine	An opioid painkiller offered during childbirth.
pica	An eating disorder that can present in pregnancy that causes women to eat non-food items.
placenta accreta	A condition where the placenta attaches too deeply into the wall of the uterus.
placenta praevia	A condition where the placenta implants on or near to the internal opening of the cervix.
Polycystic Ovarian Syndrome (PCOS)	An endocrine disorder that affects approximately 10–15 per cent of women, leading to menstrual abnormality. It is one of the leading causes of infertility.
postnatal	*See* 'post-partum'.
postnatal depression (PND)	The same as clinical depression, the main difference being that the depression is time-related to birth (with onset occurring anywhere up to one year post birth).

post-partum	After (post) birth.
post-partum haemorrhage (PPH)	Excessive bleeding after birth.
post-partum psychosis	A condition experienced after birth that exhibits the same symptoms as psychosis, such as delusions and hallucinations.
pre-eclampsia	A disorder of pregnancy that is characterised by high blood pressure and protein in the urine.
prenatal	*See* 'antenatal'.
progesterone	A hormone involved in the menstrual cycle.
reflux apnoea	A type of 'mixed' apnoea. Apnoea is defined by the cessation of respiratory airflow. Babies with gastro-oesophageal reflux may have regurgitated contents that obstruct their airway, thus causing apnoea.
sacroiliac pain	The sacroiliac joint is in the pelvis between the sacrum (the triangular bone at the base of the spine—the posterior part of the pelvis) and the ilium (the uppermost and largest pelvic bone). In pregnancy, hormonal changes relax the connective tissues in the body and can cause sacroiliac pain.
SIDS	Sudden Infant Death Syndrome is the sudden death of an infant under one year of age.
sperm ducts	Also known as the 'vas deferens', the sperm duct carries sperm from the testes to the urethra.
sperm washing	A process for men living with HIV/AIDS who wish to have children, that concentrates and separates the fertilising sperm from infectious seminal fluid.
subchorionic bleed	A mass of blood between the pregnancy membrane and the wall of the uterus.
syntocinon	A synthetic hormone used to induce labour in women.
TENS machine	A non-pharmacological form of pain relief. Gentle electrical pulses are sent through electrodes that are taped to the skin.
tokophobia	Fear of childbirth.

tongue tie	Tongue tie is a congenital malformation where the frenulum membrane is too tight and therefore restricts the movement of the baby's tongue, making it difficult for the baby to latch correctly.
transition	The phase of labour where a woman moves from the first stage of labour to the second, pushing stage (the third stage is when the placenta is delivered). Women often describe this as the most intense period of labour.
transverse	The unborn baby is lying in a sideways position.
uterine atony	Failure of the uterus to contract after delivery.
VBAC	Vaginal birth after caesarean.
ventouse	A device that helps to 'pull' the baby out during delivery. It consists of a plastic cup that is placed on the baby's head which gently sucks (pulls) on the baby while the mother pushes.
vernix	A white, milky looking substance that coats and protects the baby's skin in utero.

Resources

The following resources were compiled by the author in July 2010. Please be aware that while every care has been taken in providing accurate and non-judgemental links, website contents do change. In most instances, the last reference listed is for an online forum, which has specific pages related to the topic in question.

In addition to the websites and help lines listed below, you can also try contacting your local hospital (ask to speak to someone in the social work department) for support, information and advice. Further information is also provided in the References and further reading section.

Conception

Pregnancy counselling and crisis services

Please be aware that some crisis services are non-directive and/or misleading. This means that the service has an ulterior agenda (if you want to know more about this, download this article written by the Abortion Rights Coalition of Canada at <www.arcc-cdac.ca/action/CPC-brochure.pdf>). Unfortunately, this is a common practice worldwide. As such, some of the countries listed below only have termination counselling services listed, as genuine pregnancy crisis services could not be found. The services listed below are, to the author's knowledge, non-directive.

Australia

The National Pregnancy Support Helpline	www.health.gov.au/pregnancyhelpline 1800 422 213
birth.com.au	http://forum.birth.com.au/

Canada

Canadians for Choice	www.canadiansforchoice.ca 1 888 642 2725
Canadian Parents	www.canadianparents.com

Ireland

Positive Options Crisis Pregnancy Services	www.positiveoptions.ie Free text LIST to 50444
Roller Coaster	www.rollercoaster.ie

New Zealand

Abortion Services in New Zealand	www.abortion.gen.nz
OHbaby!	www.ohbaby.co.nz

United Kingdom

Marie Stopes International	www.mariestopes.org.uk 0845 300 8090
Pregnancy Forum	www.pregnancyforum.org.uk

United States

National Abortion Federation	www.prochoice.org 1 800 772 9100
Mad Mums	www.madmums.com

Adoption services

Australia

Attorney-General's Department	www.ag.gov.au (click on 'Intercountry adoption') 1800 422 213
Community Information and Services for Australians	www.community.gov.au (type 'adoption' in the search box) 1300 653 227
Intercountry Adoption Resource Network (ICARN)	www.icarn.com.au 1800 422 213
The Bub Hub Forum	www.bubhub.com.au/community/forums

Canada

Adoption Council of Canada	www.adoption.ca 1 888 54 ADOPT
Canada Adopts!	www.canadaadopts.com (click on 'Discuss Adoption')

Ireland

The Adoption Authority of Ireland	www.adoptionboard.ie 01 2309 300
International Adoption Association Ireland (IAA)	www.iaaireland.org 01 4992 206
Adoption Support Network of Ireland (ASNI)	www.adoption.ie

New Zealand

Child, Youth and Family	www.cyf.govt.nz (click on 'Adoption') 0508 326 459
Inter Country Adoption New Zealand (ICANZ)	www.icanz.gen.nz 9 623 9365
OHbaby!	www.ohbaby.co.nz

United Kingdom

Adoption UK	www.adoptionuk.org 01 295 752240
Intercountry Adoption Centre (IAC)	www.icacentre.org.uk 0870 516 8742
After Adoption	http://forums.afteradoption.org.uk

United States

Child Welfare Information Gateway	www.childwelfare.gov/adoption 800 394 3366
adoption.com	http://forums.adoption.com/adoptive-parents

Foster care services

Australia

Australian Foster Care Association (AFCA)	www.fostercare.org.au
Raising Children Network	http://raisingchildren.net.au/forum (click on 'Parents Like Me', then 'Adoptive and foster parents')

Canada

Foster Care Council of Canada	www.afterfostercare.ca
	1 613 220 1039
Canadian Parents Forum	http://forum.canadianparents.com

Ireland

Irish Foster Care Association (IFCA)	www.ifca.ie
	01 459 9474
Roller Coaster	www.rollercoaster.ie

New Zealand

New Zealand Family and Foster Care Federation	www.fostercarefederation.org.nz
	0800 69 33 23
OHbaby!	www.ohbaby.co.nz

United Kingdom

Fostering Information Line	www.fostering.org.uk
	0800 783 4086
UK Adoption and Fostering Forums	http://ukaff.org.uk

United States

National Foster Parent Association (NFPA)	www.nfpainc.org
	253 683 4246
After Adoption	www.forums.afteradoption.org.uk

Assisted reproductive technology

Australia

Australia's National Infertility Network	www.access.org.au
	02 9737 0158
IVF Friends	www.ivffriends.com.au

Canada

Assisted Human Reproduction Canada	www.ahrc-pac.gc.ca
Infertility Awareness Association of Canada (IAAC)	www.iaac.ca
	1800 263 2929
IVF.ca Forums	www.ivf.ca/forums/

Ireland

National Infertility Support and Information Group (NISIG)	www.nisig.ie 1890 647 444
Irish Infertility Support Forums	www.irishinfertilitysupportforums.ie
Roller Coaster	www.rollercoaster.ie

New Zealand

Fertility New Zealand	www.fertilitynz.org.nz
OHbaby!	www.ohbaby.co.nz

United Kingdom

Fertility Friends	www.fertilityfriends.co.uk www.fertilityfriends.co.uk/forum

United States

Infertility in America	www.ivfinamerica.com 253 683 4246
IVF Connections	www.ivfconnections.com

Assisted reproductive technology for LGBT individuals

Australia

Ethical Surrogacy	www.ethicalsurrogacy.blogspot.com
Gay Dads Australia	www.gaydadsaustralia.com 02 9737 0158
Rainbow Families Council	www.rainbowfamilies.org.au 02 9737 0158
Work, Love and Play	www.work-love-play.blogspot.com
birth.com.au	http://forum.birth.com.au/

Canada

Family Pride Canada	www.uwo.ca/pridelib/family 519 661 2111 ext. 85828
LGBTQ Parenting Connection	www.lgbtqparentingconnection.ca 416 324 4100
Canadian Parents Forum	http://forum.canadianparents.com

Ireland

Citizens Information	www.citizensinformation.ie (click on 'Birth, family and relationships', then 'Same-sex couples') 1890 777 121
Gay and Lesbian Equality Network (GLEN)	www.glen.ie/law/parenting.html 01 672 8650
LGBT Helplines	www.lgbt.ie/

New Zealand

Rainbow Families New Zealand	www.rainbowfamiliesnz.org www.rainbowfamiliesnz.org/forum.html

United Kingdom

Pink Parents	www.pinkparents.org.uk 01380 727 935
Rainbow Surrogacy Support UK	www.rainbowsurrogacysupport.com

United States

Circle Surrogacy	www.circlesurrogacy.com
Gay Parent Magazine	www.gayparentmag.com 718 380 1780
Proud Parenting	www.proudparenting.com 253 683 4246

Genetic counselling and testing

Please note that most major (teaching) hospitals around the world provide genetic testing. These resources are for additional information only.

Australia

Sydney Genetics	www.sydneygenetics.com 02 9229 6444
Raising Children Network	http://raisingchildren.net.au/articles/disabilities_genetic_counselling.html http://raisingchildren.net.au/forum

Canada

Canadian Association of Genetic Counsellors	www.cagc-accg.ca 905 847 1363
Parents Canada Forum	http://forums.parentscanada.com

Ireland

National Centre for Medical Genetics (NCMG)	www.genetics.ie/clinical 01 409 6902
Roller Coaster	www.rollercoaster.ie

New Zealand

Birthright Healthy Beginnings	www.birthright.co.nz/preg_tests.html
Mums on Top	http://friends.mumsontop.co.nz/forum

United Kingdom

The British Society for Human Genetics (BSHG)	www.bshg.org.uk 0121 627 2634
Baby and Bump	www.babyandbump.com

United States

American Board of Genetic Counselling (ABGC)	www.abgc.net 913 895 4617
American Pregnancy Association Forums	www.americanpregnancy.org/forums

Legal advice

Australia

Find Law Australia	www.findlaw.com.au
Legal Aid	www.legalaid.nsw.gov.au (For other states, swap 'nsw' for 'wa', 'qld', etc.)

Canada

Legal Line	www.legalline.ca

Ireland

Legal Aid Board	www.legalaidboard.ie 1890 615 200

New Zealand

New Zealand Law Society	www.lawsociety.org.nz (click on 'For the public', then 'Find a lawyer')

United Kingdom

The Law Society	www.lawsociety.org.uk (click on 'Find a solicitor')

United States

Lawyers Dot Com	www.lawyers.com

Pregnancy

Australia

Pregnancy, Birth and Beyond	www.pregnancy.com.au
Prescribing Drugs in Pregnancy	www.tga.gov.au/docs/html/medpreg.htm 1800 020 653
The Royal Women's Hospital	www.thewomens.org.au/PregnancyandBirth
birth.com.au	http://forum.birth.com.au/

Canada

Mother Risk	www.motherisk.org/women/drugs.jsp 416 813 6780
Women's Health Matters	www.womenshealthmatters.ca
Canadian Parents Forum	http://forum.canadianparents.com

Ireland

EU Mom	www.eumom.com
St James's Hospital (National Medicines Information Centre)	www.stjames.ie (click on 'Departments', then 'NMIC') 1850 727 727
Roller Coaster	www.rollercoaster.ie

New Zealand

Drug Safety in Pregnancy	www.druginformation.co.nz/pregnancy.htm
Treasures	www.treasures.co.nz
OHbaby!	www.ohbaby.co.nz

United Kingdom

Baby Centre	www.babycentre.co.uk
NHS Evidence: Medication in pregnancy	www.patient.co.uk/pdf/pilsL671.pdf
The NHS Pregnancy Care Planner	www.nhs.uk (search 'pregnancy care planner')
Pregnancy Forum	www.pregnancyforum.co.uk

United States

American Pregnancy Association	www.americanpregnancy.org 972 550 0140
Drugs in Pregnancy and Lactation	www.safefetus.com 1-800-772-9100
Baby Center Community	http://community.babycenter.com

Pregnancy loss

Australia

Bonnie Babes Foundation	www.bonniebabes.org.au 1300 266 643
National Twin Loss Support	www.murraylandstwinloss.org.au 0419 039 194
Stillbirth and Neonatal Death Support (SANDS)	www.sands.org.au 03 9899 0217
Sydney IVF Miscarriage Management	www.miscarriage.com.au 02 9229 6420
birth.com.au	http://forum.birth.com.au
Essential Baby	www.essentialbaby.com.au/forums

Canada

Many websites that support parents who have lost a baby or child are US-based. If you need someone to talk to, call your local hospital and ask to speak to the social worker. You might also like to try <www.griefshare.org> for a list of support groups in your area.

Canadian Foundation for the Study of Infant Deaths	www.sidscanada.org 905 688 8884
Canadian Parents	www.canadianparents.com/pregnancy/pregnancy-loss
Lost Dream	www.lostdream.ca
Canadian Parents Forum	http://forum.canadianparents.com

Ireland

Irish Stillbirth & Neonatal Death Society	www.isands.ie 01 872 6996
Miscarriage Association of Ireland	www.miscarriage.ie 01 873 5702
Roller Coaster	www.rollercoaster.ie

New Zealand

Miscarriage Support Auckland	www.miscarriagesupport.org.nz
Twin Loss NZ	www.twinloss.org.nz
Stillbirth and Newborn Death Support (SANDS)	www.sands.org.nz 04 478 0895
The Lost Ones Forum	www.thelostones.co.nz
OHbaby!	www.ohbaby.co.nz

United Kingdom

The Miscarriage Association	www.miscarriageassociation.org.uk 01924 200 799
Stillbirth and Neonatal Death Charity (SANDS)	www.uk-sands.org 020 7436 5881
Babyloss	www.babyloss.com

United States

Centering Corporation	www.centering.org 1 866 218 0101

The Compassionate Friends	www.compassionatefriends.org 877 969 0010
A Heartbreaking Choice	www.aheartbreakingchoice.com
M.I.S.S. Foundation	www.missfoundation.org 1 623 979 1000
Pregnancy Loss	www.pregnancyloss.info

Birth

Australia

Australian College of Midwives	www.midwives.org.au 1300 360 480
Australian Doula College	www.australiandoulacollege.com.au 1300 139 507
Caesarean Awareness Network Australia	www.canaustralia.net 07 3878 7915
Homebirth Australia	www.homebirthaustralia.org
Royal Australian and NZ College of Obstetricians and Gynaecologists	www.ranzcog.edu.au 03 9417 1699
birth.com.au	www.birth.com.au http://forum.birth.com.au/
Belly Belly	www.bellybelly.com.au/forums
Essential Baby	www.essentialbaby.com.au/forums

Canada

Canadian Association of Midwives	www.canadianmidwives.org 514 807 3668
Canadian Parents	www.canadianparents.com
Doula Care	www.doulacare.ca 888 879 3199
Homebirth in Canada Information	www.babycenter.ca/pregnancy
The Society of Obstetricians and Gynaecologists of Canada	www.sogc.org 1800 561 2416

Baby Center Birth Clubs	www.babycenter.ca/community/birthclubs
Canadian Parents Forum	http://forum.canadianparents.com
Parents Canada	http://forums.parentscanada.com

Ireland

Association for Improvements in the Maternity Services Ireland (AIMS)	www.aimsireland.com 01 660 3499
Doula Ireland	www.doulaireland.com 087 057 2500
Home Birth Association of Ireland	www.homebirth.ie 090 649 3596
Institute of Obstetricians and Gynaecologists	www.rcpi.ie/faculties/pages/ obstetriciansandgynaecologists.aspx 01 863 9700
School of Nursing and Midwifery (Trinity College Dublin)	www.nursing-midwifery.tcd.ie 01 896 2692
AIMS Forum	www.aimsireland.com/phpbb
Roller Coaster	www.rollercoaster.ie

New Zealand

Birthworks New Zealand	www.birthworks.org.nz 09 6300 962
Homebirth Aotearoa	www.homebirth.org.nz
New Zealand College of Midwives	www.midwife.org.nz 03 377 2732
Royal Australian and New Zealand College of Obstetricians and Gynaecologists	www.ranzcog.edu.au +61 3 9417 1699
Kidspot.com.au Forums	http://social.kidspot.com.au/iforum.php
OHbaby!	www.ohbaby.co.nz

United Kingdom

Association for Improvements in the Maternity Services (AIMS)	www.aims.org.uk/ 0300 365 0663
Birth Choice	www.birthchoiceuk.com
Birth Trauma Association	www.birthtraumaassociation.org.uk

Doula UK	www.doula.org.uk
	0871 4333 103
Home Birth Reference Site	www.homebirth.org.uk
Royal College of Midwives	www.rcm.org.uk
	020 7312 3535
Royal College of Obstetricians and Gynaecologists	www.rcog.org.uk
	020 7772 6200
Baby Centre Community	http://community.babycentre.co.uk/
Ask a Mum	www.askamum.co.uk

United States

American Congress of Obstetricians and Gynecologists (ACOG)	www.dona.org
	888 788 3662
DONA International (Doulas)	www.mana.org
	888 923 6262
Midwives Alliance of North America (MANA)	www.acog.org
	202 638 5577
VBAC	www.vbac.com
	310 375 3141
Baby and Bump	www.babyandbump.com
Baby Center	www.babycenter.com
Baby Corner	www.babycorner.com

Babies

Breast and bottle-feeding

It is accepted that breastfeeding is best for baby. However, many mothers cannot breastfeed, or choose not to do so. Additionally, if childcare is the father's mandate, bottle-feeding may be essential.

Australia

| Australian Breastfeeding Association | www.breastfeeding.asn.au |
| | 1800 686 2686 |

Raising Children Network	http://raisingchildren.net.au/articles/bottle-feeding_and_formula_-_facts.html/context/205
birth.com.au	http://forum.birth.com.au/

Canada

Baby Center Formula Feeding	www.babycenter.ca/baby/formula
Breastfeeding Committee for Canada	www.breastfeedingcanada.ca
Baby Center Canada Community	www.babycenter.ca/community

Ireland

Breastfeeding Ireland	www.breastfeeding.ie
Feeding for Life (This is a commercial formula website)	www.feedingforlife.ie (click on '0-3 months', then 'Bottlefeeding')
Roller Coaster	www.rollercoaster.ie

New Zealand

Kiwi Families	www.kiwifamilies.co.nz/Topics/Babies/Feeding-Your-Baby.html (click on 'Bottle Feeding')
La Leche League New Zealand	www.lalecheleague.org.nz 04 471 0690
OHbaby!	www.ohbaby.co.nz

United Kingdom

NHS Bottle feeding	www.nhs.uk/conditions/bottle-feeding
NHS Breastfeeding	www.breastfeeding.nhs.uk 0300 100 0212
Baby Centre	www.babycentre.co.uk

United States

Baby Center: Bottle-feeding basics	www.babycenter.com/0_bottle-feeding-basics_752.bc
Kelly Mom	www.kellymom.com
La Leche League International	www.llli.org 877 452 5324
Parents Connect	www.parentsconnect.com

Playgroups

Please note that most playgroups are aimed at mothers. To find father's groups, see page 260.

Australia

Playgroup Australia	www.playgroupaustralia.com
	1800 171 882
Mothersgroup.com.au	www.mothersgroup.com.au

Canada

| Mom's Club Worldwide Directory | www.newcomersclub.com |
| Canadian Moms Online | www.canadianmomsonline.com |

Ireland

| Irish Preschool Play Association (IPPA) | www.ippa.ie |
| Cuidiú | www.cuidiu-ict.ie |

New Zealand

| Playgroups | www.playgroups.co.nz |
| Mums on Top | http://friends.mumsontop.co.nz |

United Kingdom

| Up My Street | www.upmystreet.com |
| | (click on 'find my nearest', then type 'playgroups' in the search field) |

United States

| Social Toddler | www.socialtoddler.com |

Safe sleeping

General resources for safe sleeping can be found through Dr James McKenna <www.nd.edu/~jmckenn1/lab> and Dr Howard Chilton <www.babydoc.com.au>.

Australia

| SIDS and Kids | www.sidsandkids.org |
| | 1300 308 307 |

Canada

| Canadian Foundation for the Study of Infant Deaths | www.sidscanada.org
1 800 363 7437 |

Ireland

| National Paediatric Mortality Register | www.sidsireland.ie
01 878 8455 |

New Zealand

| SIDS New Zealand | www.sids.org.nz
0800 164 455 |

United Kingdom

| The Foundation for the Study of Infant Deaths (FSID) | www.fsid.org.uk
0808 802 6868 |

United States

| Attachment Parenting International | www.attachmentparenting.org |
| American SIDS Institute | www.sids.org
770 426 8746 |

Parenting

Australia

Raising Children Network	http://raisingchildren.net.au
Tresillian Family Care Centres	www.tresillian.net 1800 637 357
Triple P Positive Parenting Program	www1.triplep.net
birth.com.au	http://forum.birth.com.au/
Essential Baby	www.essentialbaby.com.au/forums

Canada

Healthy Beginnings Hotline	1800 637 357
Today's Parent	www.todaysparent.com
Triple P Positive Parenting Program	www9.triplep.net
Canadian Parents Forum	http://forum.canadianparents.com

Ireland

Barnardos Parent Training Database	www.barnardos.ie/training_and_resources/parenting.html
Parent Line	www.parentline.ie 1890 927 277
Roller Coaster	www.rollercoaster.ie

New Zealand

Kiwi Families	www.kiwifamilies.co.nz
Parent Help Line	www.parenthelp.org.nz 0800 568 856
Triple P Positive Parenting Program	www33.triplep.net
OHbaby!	www.ohbaby.co.nz

United Kingdom

Parentline Plus	www.parentlineplus.org.uk 0808 800 2222
Positive Parenting	www.parenting.org.uk 0845 643 1939
Triple P Positive Parenting Program	www8.triplep.net
Baby Centre	www.babycentre.co.uk

United States

Parent Help Line	www.st-johns.org/services/parenthelpline 1 888 727 5889
Parenting	www.parenting.com
Triple P Positive Parenting Program	www5.triplep.net
Parents Connect	www.parentsconnect.com

Child safety

Have a look at the first aid and safety demonstration video clips at the Raising Children Network here: <http://raisingchildren.net.au/safety/newborns_safety.html>.

Australia

Child Safety Awareness	www.childsafetyawareness.com

| St John Ambulance First Aid Courses | www.stjohn.org.au |

Canada

| Canadian Red Cross | www.redcross.ca |
| Safe Kids Canada | www.safekidscanada.ca |

Ireland

| Child Safety Awareness Programme | www.hse.ie (search for 'Child safety awareness programme') |
| Irish Red Cross | www.redcross.ie |

New Zealand

| Child Safety Foundation | www.childsafety.co.nz |
| St John | www.stjohn.org.nz/education |

United Kingdom

| Safe Kids | www.safekids.co.uk |
| St John Ambulance | www.sja.org.uk |

United States

| American Safety Zone | www.americansafetyzone.com |
| Medic First Aid International | www.medicfirstaid.com |

Babies and children with extra needs

Australia

Association for Children with a Disability	www.acd.org.au 1800 654 013
Children with Disability Australia	www.cda.org.au 1800 222 660
Gifted Children Australia	www.gifted-children.com.au

Canada

| Special Need Child Canada | www.special-need-child-canada.com 888 248 6658 |

World Council for Gifted and Talented Children	https://world-gifted.org

Ireland

Enable Ireland	www.enableireland.ie 01 872 7155
Gifted Kids	www.giftedkids.ie
Inclusion Ireland	www.inclusionireland.ie 01 855 9891

New Zealand

Disability Action	www.ccsdisabilityaction.org.nz 0800 227 200
New Zealand Association for Gifted Children (NZAGC)	www.giftedchildren.org.nz

United Kingdom

Contact a Family	www.cafamily.org.uk 0808 808 3555
The Children's Trust Tadworth	www.thechildrenstrust.org.uk 01 737 365 000
National Association for Gifted Children (NAGC)	www.nagcbritain.org.uk 0845 450 0295

United States

National Association for Gifted Children (NAGC)	www.nagc.org
National Dissemination Center for Children with Disabilities (NICHCY)	www.nichcy.org 800 695 0285
Support for Families of Children with Disabilities	www.supportforfamilies.org

Anger resources

Every parent experiences angry feelings at some point. Feeling angry does not make you a bad parent. However, if there is a lot of expressed anger in the home (such as shouting or other physical manifestations of anger), it can be very damaging to children. The resources below will help you to identify why you are feeling angry, as well as ways to deal with that anger. Also listed are ways to find psychologists or family counselling services in your area.

IMPORTANT: If you become so angry that you feel you might hurt your child (or yourself), you need to put your child somewhere safe and seek help urgently. Treat the situation as an emergency and call a help line immediately. All help lines listed below, to the best of the author's knowledge, are open 24 hours a day, 7 days a week.

Australia

Parentline	www.parentline.com.au ACT: 02 6287 3833 NSW: 1300 1300 52 NT/QLD: 1300 30 1300 SA: 1300 364 100 TAS: 1300 808 178 VIC: 13 22 89 WA: 1800 654 432
Raising Children Network	http://raisingchildren.net.au/articles/feeling_angry.html/context/303
Relationships Australia (counselling)	www.relationships.com.au 1300 364 277

Canada

Child, Youth and Family Crisis Line	www.icrs.ca/ In Ottawa: 613 260 2360 Long distance: 1 877 377 7775
Public Health Agency of Canada	www.phac-aspc.gc.ca (click on 'Health Promotion', 'Childhood and Adolescence', 'Family/Parenting') 204 789 2000

Ireland

1Life Helpline	1800 247 100
AIM Family Services (counselling)	www.aimfamilyservices.ie 01 670 8363

New Zealand

LifeLine	www.lifeline.co.nz 0800 543 354
Relationship Services	www.relate.org.nz

United Kingdom

Samaritans Helpline	www.samaritans.org 08457 90 90 90
Counselling Directory	www.counselling-directory.org.uk

United States

Crisis Clinic Helpline	866 461 3222
American Family Therapy Academy (counseling)	www.afta.org 202 483 8001

Mental health

Australia

Beyond Blue	www.beyondblue.org.au 1300 22 4636
Black Dog Institute	www.blackdoginstitute.org.au 02 9382 4523
Mental Illness Fellowship of Australia	www.mifa.org.au 1800 985 944
Post and Antenatal Depression Association (PANDA)	www.panda.org.au 1300 726 306
BlueBoard Forum	http://blueboard.anu.edu.au
Reach Out	http://au.reachout.com

Canada

Canadian Network for Mood and Anxiety Treatments (CANMAT)	www.canmat.org
Mental Health Commission of Canada	www.mentalhealthcommission.ca
Pacific Postpartum Support Society	www.postpartum.org 604 255 7999
Mood Disorders Society of Canada Forum	www.mooddisorderscanada.ca/forum

Ireland

Aware	www.aware.ie 1890 303 302
Mental Health Ireland	www.mentalhealthireland.ie 01 284 1166
Post Natal Depression Ireland	www.pnd.ie 021 492 3162
Roller Coaster	www.rollercoaster.ie

New Zealand

Mental Health Foundation of New Zealand	www.mentalhealth.org.nz 09 300 7010
Postnatal Distress Support Network Trust	www.postnataldistress.org.nz 09 836 6967
OHbaby!	www.ohbaby.co.nz

United Kingdom

Meet a Mum Association (MAMA—for mothers who have experienced depression)	www.mama.co.uk
Mind	www.mind.org.uk 0845 766 0163
The Royal College of Psychiatrists	www.rcpsych.ac.uk 020 7235 2351
Depression Forums	www.depressionforums.co.uk

United States

American Psychiatric Association: Healthy Minds Healthy Lives	www.healthyminds.org 1 800 273 8255
American Psychological Association	www.apa.org/topics/depress
National Alliance on Mental Illness (NAMI)	www.nami.org 800 950 6264
Postpartum Support International (PSI)	http://postpartum.net 800 944 4773
Blue People Forum	www.bluepeople.com

Fathers

Australia

Dads at Home	www.dadsathome.net
Dads Club	www.dadsclub.com.au
Dads in Distress	www.dadsindistress.asn.au 1300 853 437
Gay Dads Australia	www.gaydadsaustralia.com.au
Single Fathers Australia	www.singlefather.com.au
Dads Club Forum	www.dadsclub.com.au/forum

Canada

Caring Dads	www.caringdadsprogram.com
Dads Canada	www.dadscanada.com 416 410 3237
Father Involvement Research Alliance (FIRA)	www.fira.ca
Fatherhood Dreams	www.fatherhooddreams.com (click on the 'resources' link for information on gay parenting)
Canadian Parents Forum	www.canadianparents.com

Ireland

Dad	www.dad.ie www.dad.ie/chat 021 492 3162
Marriage Equality Network	www.marriagequality.ie

New Zealand

Auckland Single Parent's Trust	http://singleparents.org.nz
Fathers of New Zealand	http://fathers.orconhosting.net.nz 09 479 5016
Hey Dads	www.heydads.com 021 135 4972
OHbaby!	www.ohbaby.co.nz

United Kingdom

Dad	www.dad.info
Dad at Home	www.dadathome.co.uk
Dads UK	http://dads-uk.co.uk http://dads-uk.co.uk/forums
Gay Dad Support	www.gaydadsupport.net
Separated Dads	www.separateddads.co.uk

United States

At Home Dad	www.athomedad.org 888 35 77924
The Good Men Project	www.goodmenproject.org 800 950 6264
Great Dad	www.greatdad.com
Proud Parenting	www.proudparenting.com
Single Dad	www.singledad.com
Brand New Dad Forum	www.brandnewdad.com/forums/

Other useful resources

Domestic violence and abuse

Australia

Another Closet: Domestic Violence in Gay and Lesbian Relationships	http://ssdv.acon.org.au
Australian Domestic & Family Violence Clearinghouse	www.austdvclearinghouse.unsw.edu.au 1800 75 33 82
Domestic Violence Line	1800 656 463
The Immigrant Women's Domestic Violence Service	www.iwdvs.org.au 1800 755 988
The Line	www.theline.gov.au 1800 200 526

Canada

Domestic Abuse Must Stop	www.domesticabusemuststop.org
National Domestic Violence Hotline	800 799 7233
Same Sex Abuse	www.womanabuseprevention.com/html/same-sex_partner_abuse.html

Ireland

AMEN: Confidential Help for Male Victims	www.amen.ie 086 7941 880
Gay Men's Health Service	www.gaymenshealthservice.ie
Safe Ireland	www.safeireland.ie 090 647 9078
Women's Aid	www.womensaid.ie 1800 341 900

New Zealand

Domestic Violence in New Zealand: A Masculinist Perspective	www.menz.org.nz/Information/domestic.htm
Lesbian and Gay Domestic Violence	www.menz.org.nz/Information/dvlesbian.htm
The New Zealand Violence Clearing House	www.nzfvc.org.nz
Preventing Violence	www.2shine.org.nz 0508 384 357

United Kingdom

Broken Rainbow (Domestic violence support for LGBT individuals)	www.broken rainbow.org.uk 0300 999 5428
ManKind Initiative	www.mankind.org.uk 01823 334 244
Women's Aid	www.womensaid.org.uk 0808 2000 247

United States

Anti-Violence Project (for LGBTQ individuals)	www.avp.org 212 714 1141
Battered Men	www.batteredmen.com

| The National Domestic Violence Hotline | www.ndvh.org
1800 799 7233 |
| Stop Abuse for Everyone (SAFE) | www.safe4all.org |

Single parents

Australia

Parents Without Partners Australia	www.pwpaustralia.net
Single Fathers Australia	www.singlefather.com.au
Single Mum	www.singlemum.com.au

Canada

| Parents Without Partners Canada | www.pwpcanada.com |
| Support to Single Parents | www.supporttosingleparents.ca
506 858 1303 |

Ireland

One Family	http://onefamily.ie
OPEN : Lone Parent Groups in Ireland	www.oneparent.ie 01 814 8860
SOLO: Support for People Parenting Alone	www.solo.ie

New Zealand

| Auckland Single Parent's Trust | http://singleparents.org.nz
09 424 6388 |

United Kingdom

Gingerbread	www.gingerbread.org.uk 0808 802 0925
Only Dads	www.onlydads.org 01803 868 683
Only Mums	www.onlymums.org 01803 868 683

United States

Single Black Parents	www.singleblackparents.com
Single Dad	www.singledad.com
Single Mom	www.singlemom.com
Single Parent Center	www.singleparentcenter.net

References and further reading

All of the articles, books, and websites referred to in the body of this book are listed here. Further reading has been included in some cases. Some good general guides can be found below:

Baby Love, Robin Barker, 2009, Macmillan, Sydney.

Birth Day, Mark Sloan, 2009, Ballantine Books, New York.

Conceptions and Misconceptions, Arthur Wisot & David Meldrum, 2004, Hartley & Marks Publishers, Vancouver.

Dream Babies, Christina Hardyment, 2007, Frances Lincoln Press, London.

Everything Conceivable, Liza Mundy, 2008, Anchor Books, New York.

I Was a Really Good Mom Before I Had Kids, Trisha Ashworth & Amy Nobile, 2007, Chronicle Books, San Francisco.

It Gets Easier (And Other Lies We Tell New Mothers), Claudine Wolk, 2008, New Buck Press, Philadelphia.

Kidwrangling, Kaz Cooke, 2010, Viking, Melbourne.

Misconceptions, Naomi Wolf, 2003, Anchor Books, New York.

Motherless Mothers, Hope Edelman, 2006, Harper, New York.

The Birth Wars, Mary-Rose MacColl, 2009, University of Queensland Press, Brisbane.

The Bitch in the House, Cathi Hanauer (Ed), 2003, Perennial HarperCollins, New York.

The Mask of Motherhood, Susan Maushart, 1997, Penguin Books, New York.

The Mommy Myth, Susan Douglas & Meredith Michaels, 2004, Free Press, New York.

Towards Parenthood, Jeanette Milgrom et al., 2009, ACER Press, Melbourne.

Up the Duff, Kaz Cooke, 2009, Viking, Melbourne.

Chapter 1: Conception isn't always straightforward

Bach R 1998, *Illusions: The adventures of a reticent messiah* (p. 65), Dell Publishing: NY.

Galpern E 2007, 'Gender and justice: Assisted reproductive technologies—overview and perspective using as reproductive justice framework', *Reproductive Health and Human Rights Gender and Justice Program*, Center for Genetics and Society Canada, <http://geneticsandsociety.org/downloads/ART.pdf>, accessed July 2010.

International Committee for Monitoring Assisted Reproductive Technology (ICMART): de Mouzon J, Lancaster P, Nygren KG, Sullivan E, Zegers-Hochschild F, Mansour R, Ishihara O & Adamson D 2009, 'World collaborative report on assisted reproductive technology, 2002', *Human Reproduction*, 24(9): 2310-2320.

Pawelski JG, Perrin EC, For JM, Allen CE, Crawford JE, Del Monte M, Kaufman M, Klein JD, Smith K, Springer S, Tanner JL & Vickers DL 2006, 'The effects of marriage, civil union, and domestic partnership laws on the health and wellbeing of children', *Pediatrics*, 118(1): 349-364.

Siegel S, Dittrich R & Vollman J 2008, 'Ethical opinions and personal attitudes of young adults conceived by in vitro fertilisation', *Journal of Medical Ethics*, 34: 236-240.

United Nations 1948, 'The Universal Declaration of Human Rights', <www.un.org/en/documents/udhr/>, accessed July 2010.

van Londen WM, Juffer F & van Ijzendoorn MH 2007, 'Attachment, cognitive, and motor development in adopted children: Short-term outcomes after international adoption', *Journal of Pediatric Psychology*, 32(10): 1249-1258.

Common causes of infertility

Higgins IL 2006, *Creating life against the odds: The journey from infertility to parenthood*, Xlibris Corporation: Bloomington, IN.

Wisot AL & Meldrum DR 2004, *Conceptions and misconceptions: The informed consumer's guide through the maze of in vitro fertilization and other assisted reproduction techniques*, Hartley & Marks: Vancouver.

When to seek help getting pregnant

Higgins IL 2006, *Creating life against the odds: The journey from infertility to parenthood*, Xlibris Corporation: Bloomington, IN.

What is third party reproduction? Unravelling the terminology

American Society for Reproductive Medicine 2006, 'Third party reproduction (sperm, egg, and embryo donation and surrogacy): A guide for patients', <www.asrm.org/uploadedFiles/ASRM_Content/Resources/Patient_Resources/Fact_Sheets_and_Info_Booklets/thirdparty.pdf>, accessed July 2010.

Same sex parenting: ART, adoption and fostering

Ethics Committee of the American Society for Reproductive Medicine 2009, 'Access to fertility treatment by gays, lesbians, and unmarried persons', <www.asrm.org/uploadedFiles/ASRM_Content/News_and_Publications/Ethics_Committee_Reports_and_Statements/fertility_gaylesunmarried.pdf>, accessed July 2010.

Jones HW 2010, 'Same-sex parentage and ART', in SL Crockin & HW Jones (eds), *Legal conceptions: The evolving law and policy of assisted reproductive technologies*, The Johns Hopkins University Press: Baltimore, MD.

Sauer MV, Wang JD, Douglas NC, Nakhuda GS, Vardhana P, Jovanovic V & Guarnaccia MM 2009, 'Providing fertility care to men seropositive for human immunodeficiency virus: Reviewing 10 years of experience and 420 consecutive cycles of in vitro fertilization and intracytoplasmic sperm injection', *Fertility and Sterility*, 91(6): 2455-2460.

United Nations 1948, 'The Universal Declaration of Human Rights', <www.un.org/en/documents/udhr/>, accessed July 2010.

Legislation

Australia

The Commonwealth of Australia does not currently legislate for reproductive technology practice or the legal consequences, however a uniform national set of laws is being developed (see <www.scag.gov.au/lawlink/SCAG/ll_scag.nsf/pages/scag_meetingoutcomes>, click on 'Summary of Decisions November 2009', scroll down to 'Surrogacy'). Therefore, each state and territory is responsible for implementing its own legislation.

Following is a list of Acts and Bills that cover reproductive technology in Australia. For a discussion on same sex parenting reforms in Australia, please see 'Federal Same-Sex Parenting Reforms' by the Gay and Lesbian Rights Lobby, <http://glrl.org.au/index.php/Rights/Parenting/Federal-Same-Sex-Parenting-Reforms>.

Australian Capital Territory

Parentage Act 2004, <www.legislation.act.gov.au/a/2004-1/current/pdf/2004-1.pdf>, accessed July 2010.

New South Wales

Assisted Reproductive Technology Act 2007, <www.legislation.nsw.gov.au/maintop/view/inforce/act+69+2007+cd+0+N>, accessed July 2010.

Status of Children Act 1996, <www.legislation.nsw.gov.au/fragview/inforce/act+76+1996+pt.3-div.1-sec.14+0+N?tocnav=y>, accessed July 2010.

Northern Territory

Status of Children Act 1979,
> <http://notes.nt.gov.au/dcm/legislat/legislat.nsf/d989974724db65b1482561cf0017
> cbd2/2c0bd4a258cca8a469256ecb001a34c3>, accessed July 2010.

Queensland

Surrogacy Act 2010,
> <www.legislation.qld.gov.au/LEGISLTN/CURRENT/S/SurrogacyA10.pdf>, accessed
> July 2010.

South Australia

Family Relationships Act 1975,
> <www.legislation.sa.gov.au/LZ/C/A/FAMILY%20RELATIONSHIPS%20ACT%201975/
> CURRENT/1975.115.UN.PDF>, accessed July 2010.

Reproductive Technology (Clinical Practices) Act 1988,
> <www.legislation.sa.gov.au/LZ/C/A/REPRODUCTIVE%20TECHNOLOGY%20
> %28CLINICAL%20PRACTICES%29%20ACT%201988/CURRENT/1988.10.UN.PDF>,
> accessed July 2010.

Tasmania

Status of Children Act 1974,
> <www.thelaw.tas.gov.au/tocview/index.w3p;cond=;doc_id=36%2B%2B1974%2BAT
> %40EN%2B20100221210000>, accessed July 2010.

Surrogacy Contracts Act 1993,
> <www.thelaw.tas.gov.au/tocview/index.w3p;cond=;doc_id=4%2B%2B1993%2BAT%
> 40EN%2B20100221210000>, accessed July 2010.

Victoria

Assisted Reproductive Treatment Act 2008,
> <www.legislation.vic.gov.au/Domino/Web_Notes/LDMS/PubLawToday.nsf/
> a12f6f60fbd56800ca256de500201e54/a8005e3c7c1e23c2ca2576930008026f>,
> accessed July 2010.

Status of Children Act 1974,
> <www.legislation.vic.gov.au/Domino/Web_Notes/LDMS/PubLawToday.nsf/
> a12f6f60fbd56800ca256de500201e54/cad97ab5147f5e6cca257695007eb2e6>,
> accessed July 2010.

Western Australia

Human Reproductive Technology Act 1991,
> <www.slp.wa.gov.au/legislation/statutes.nsf/main_mrtitle_435_homepage.html>,
> accessed July 2010.

Canada

Canada does not have an all-encompassing law that covers same sex parents and reproductive technology. For a full discussion of the legal issues and implications, please see 'Same Sex Spousal and Family Rights in Canada' by

CanadianLawyers,<www.canadian-lawyers.ca/Understand-Your-Legal-Issue/ Family-Law/Same-Sex-Spousal-and-Family-Rights-in-Canada.html>.

In 2004, the Canadian Senate approved the Assisted Human Reproduction Act legislation that covers commercial surrogate contracts.

Assisted Human Reproduction Act (Bill C-13),
>   <www2.parl.gc.ca/HousePublications/Publication.aspx?pub=bill&doc=c-13&parl= 37&ses=2&language=E&File=19#1>, accessed July 2010.

Europe

For extensive coverage of same sex rights in Europe, country-by-country, please refer to International Lesbian, Gay, Bisexual, Trans and Intersex Association (ILGA)'s highly recommended website at <www.ilga-europe.org/ europe/guide/country_by_country>.

India

India is emerging as a leader in terms of international surrogacy due to the commercial status of surrogacy, which was made legal in India in 2002. While many people fully support women's right to be paid for surrogacy and for gay men to access surrogacy services, the nature of world politics and poverty in India means the potential for women's bodies to be exploited needs sensitive consideration.

Ethical Surrogacy, an Australian-based organisation run by two gay fathers, has been established to support others going through the process by sharing their own story of ART in India—see 'Resources' on page 242 for further information.

National guidelines for accreditation, supervision and regulation of ART clinics
>   *in India,* Indian Council for Medical Research and National Academy of Medical
>   Sciences (India), <www.icmr.nic.in/art/art_clinics.htm>, accessed July 2010.

New Zealand

Human Assisted Reproductive Technology Act 2004,
>   <www.legislation.govt.nz/act/public/2004/0092/latest/whole.html>, accessed
>   July 2010.

United Kingdom

There have been dramatic improvements to legislation in the UK for same sex parents, who now enjoy similar rights to those of heterosexual parents. For a review of the relevant legislation, see 'Rights for Same Sex Parents' by the Union of Shop, Distributive and Allied Workers, <www.usdaw.org.uk/ equality/resource_library/files/RLF372/372RightsForSameSexParentsLft. pdf>.

Human Fertilisation and Embryology Act 1990,
<www.dh.gov.uk/en/Publicationsandstatistics/Publications/
PublicationsLegislation/DH_080205>, accessed July 2010.

Surrogacy Arrangements Act 1985,
<www.opsi.gov.uk/RevisedStatutes/Acts/ukpga/1985/cukpga_19850049_en_1>,
accessed July 2010.

United States

Like Australia and Canada, laws differ for same sex parents and ART depending on the State in which you live. For a quick breakdown of laws, look at The American Surrogacy Center's 'Legal overview of surrogacy laws by state', <www.surrogacy.com/legals/map.html>.

The World

The best updates on same sex laws and ART can be found in the highly recommended International Lesbian and Gay Association's 'LGBT world legal wrap up survey', at <www.gaylawnet.com/ezine/crime/ILGA_2009.pdf>.

Chapter 2: Pregnancy

Bagamary T & Iglesias M 2008, *Oh baby, I'm having a baby: Wise, witty, warm and wildly wry quotes for mothers-to-be* (p. 20), CCC Books: Westfield, MA.

Maushart S 1997, *The mask of motherhood*, Random House Australia: Sydney.

What is Intrauterine Growth Restriction?

Collins S, Asulkumaran S, Hayes K, Jackson S & Impey L 2008, *Oxford handbook of obstetrics and gynaecology*, Oxford University Press: London.

Srinivas SK, Edlow AG, Neff PM, Sammel MD, Andrela CM & Elovitz MA 2009, 'Rethinking IUGR in preeclampsia: Dependent or independent of maternal hypertension?', *Journal of Perinatology*, 29: 680-684.

Walid MS & Pomortsev AV 2008, 'Early screening for IUGR: Comparison of two related echographic markers', *Archives of Gynecology and Obstetrics*, 297(4): 551-556.

Can men get postnatal depression?

Condon JT, Boyce P & Corkindale CJ 2004, 'The first-time fathers study: A prospective study on the mental health of men during the transition to parenthood', *Australian and New Zealand Journal of Psychiatry*, 38: 56-64.

Goodman SH, Brogan D, Lynch ME, Fielding B 1993, 'Social and emotional competence in children of depressed mothers', *Child Development*, 64: 516-531.

Seimyr L, Edhborg E, Lundh W & Sjorgen B 2004, 'In the shadow of maternal depressed mood: Experiences of parenthood during the first year after childbirth', *Journal of Psychosomatic Obstetrics and Gynaecology*, 25: 23–34.

Can finding out the sex of the baby affect women?

de Tychey C, Briancon S, Lighezzolo J, Spitz E, Kanuth B, de Luigi V, Messembourg C, Girvan F, Rosati A, Thockler A & Vincent S 2008, 'Quality of life, postnatal depression and baby gender', *Journal of Clinical Nursing*, 17(3): 312–322.

What is stillbirth and how common is it?

Bhutta ZA, Darmstadt GL, Haws RA, Yakoob MY & Lawn JE 2009, 'Delivering interventions to reduce the global burden of stillbirths: Improving service supply and community demand', *BMC Pregnancy and Childbirth*, 9(Supp 1): S7.

Hughes P, Turton P, Hopper E & Evans CDH 2002, 'Assessment of guidelines for good practice in psychosocial care of mothers after stillbirth: A cohort study', *The Lancet*, 360(9327): 114–125.

International Stillbirth Alliance, <www.stillbirthalliance.org/modules.php?name= Content&pa=showpage&pid=14>, accessed July 2010.

Lawn JE, Yakoob MY, Haws RA, Soomro T, Darmstadt GL & Bhutta ZA 2009, '3.2 Million stillbirths: Epidemiology and overview of the evidence review', *BMC Pregnancy and Childbirth*, 9(Supp 1): S2.

Stanton C, Lawn JE, Rahman H, Wilczynska-Ketende K & Hill K 2006, 'Stillbirth rates: Delivering estimates in 190 countries', *The Lancet*, 367(9521): 1487–1494.

Tveit JV, Saastad E, Stray-Pedersen B, Bordhal PE, Flenady V, Fretts R & Froen JF 2009, 'Reduction of late stillbirth with the introduction of fetal movement information and guidelines: A clinical quality improvement', *BMC Pregnancy and Childbirth*, (22): 9–32.

Yakoob MY, Menezes EV, Soomro T, Haws RA, Darmstadt GL & Bhutta ZA 2009, 'Reducing stillbirths: Behavioural and nutritional interventions before and during pregnancy', *BMC Pregnancy and Childbirth*, 9(Supp 1): S3.

How can the loss of a baby affect subsequent pregnancies and birthing decisions?

Armstrong DS, Hutti MH & Myers J 2009, 'The influence of prior loss on parents' psychological distress after the birth of a subsequently healthy infant', *Journal of Obstetric, Gynecologic and Neonatal Nursing*, 38(6): 654–666.

Côté-Arsenault D & Donato KL 2007, 'Restrained expectations in late pregnancy following loss', *Journal of Obstetric, Gynecologic & Neonatal Nursing*, 36(6): 550–557.

Côté-Arsenault D & Marshall R 2000, 'One foot in, one foot out: Weathering the storm of perinatal loss', *Research in Nursing and Health*, 23: 473–486.

Côté-Arsenault D & Morrison-Beedy D 2001, 'Women's voices reflecting changed expectations for pregnancy after perinatal loss', *Journal of Nursing Scholarship*, 33(3): 239-244.

DeBackere KJ, Hill PD & Kavanaugh KL 2008, 'The parental experience of pregnancy after perinatal loss', *Journal of Obstetric, Gynecologic and Neonatal Nursing*, 37(5): 525-537.

Klier CM, Geller PA & Ritsher JB 2002, 'Affective disorders in the aftermath of miscarriage: A comprehensive review', *Archives of Women's Mental Health*, 5: 129-149.

Wright PM 2005, 'Childbirth education for parents experiencing pregnancy after perinatal loss', *Journal of Perinatal Education*, 14(4): 9-15.

Bleeding in pregnancy

Harlev A, Levy A, Zaulan Y, Koifman I, Mazor M, Wiznitzer A, Faizayev E & Sheiner MD 2008, 'Idiopathic bleeding during the second half of pregnancy as a risk factor for adverse perinatal outcomes', *Journal of Maternal-Fetal and Neonatal Medicine*, 21(5): 331-335.

Koifman A, Levy A, Zaulan Y, Harlev A, Mazor M, Wiznitzer A & Sheiner E 2008, 'The clinical significance of bleeding during the second trimester of pregnancy', *Archives of Gynecology and Obstetrics*, 278(1): 47-51.

Poulose T, Richardson R, Ewings P & Fox R 2006, 'Probability of early pregnancy loss in women with vaginal bleeding and a singleton live fetus at ultrasound scan', *Journal of Obstetrics and Gynaecology*, 26(8): 782-784.

Smith N 2006, *Understanding pregnancy*, British Medical Association: London.

Yang J, Hartmann K, Savitz DA, Herring AH, Dole N, Olsham AF & Thorp JM 2004, 'Vaginal bleeding during pregnancy and preterm birth', *American Journal of Epidemiology*, 160(2): 118-125.

Is it safe to exercise during pregnancy?

American Congress of Obstetricians and Gynecologists (ACOG) 2003, *Exercise during pregnancy*, <www.acog.org/publications/patient_education/bp119.cfm>, accessed July 2010.

Clapp JC 2005, 'Exercise during pregnancy: A clinical update', *Clinics in Sports Medicine*, 19(2): 273-286.

Food cravings

Corbett RW, Ryan C & Weinrich S 2003, 'Pica in pregnancy: Does it affect pregnancy outcomes?', *American Journal of Maternal Child Nursing*, 28: 183-189.

How soon after delivery can I have sex?

Baksu B, Davas I, Agar E, Akyol A & Varolan A 2007, 'The effect of mode on delivery on postpartum sexual function in primiparous women', *International Urogynecology Journal*, 18(4): 401-406.

Cunningham F, Leveno K, Bloom S, Hauth J, Rouse D & Spong C 2009, *Williams obstetrics*, McGraw-Hill: United States.

Hill BF & Jones JS 1993, 'Venous air embolism following orogenital sex during pregnancy', *The American Journal of Emergency Medicine*, 11(2): 155-157.

Truhlar A, Cerny V, Dostal P, Solar M, Parizkova R, Hruba I & Zabka L 2007, 'Out-of-hospital cardiac arrest from air embolism during sexual intercourse: Case report and review of the literature', *Resuscitation*, 73(3): 475-484.

Chapter 3: Birth and post-partum

Maushart S 2000, *The mask of motherhood: How becoming a mother changes our lives and why we never talk about it*, Penguin Books: New York.

NSW Department of Health 2009, *New South Wales Mothers and Babies 2006*, <www.health.nsw.gov.au/pubs/2009/pdf/mothers_babies.pdf>, accessed July 2010.

Can fear affect childbirth?

Alehagen S, Wijma B & Wijma K 2006, 'Fear of childbirth before, during, and after childbirth', *Acta Obstetricia et Gynecologica Scandinavia*, 85(1): 56-62.

Hofberg L 2000, 'Tokophobia: An unreasoning dread of child birth', *British Journal of Psychiatry*, 176: 83-85.

Saistao T & Halmesmaki E 2003, 'Fear of Childbirth: A neglected dilemma', *Acta Obstetricia et Gynecologica Scandinavia*, 82: 201-208.

Wijma K 2003, 'Why focus on fear of childbirth?', *Journal of Psychosomatic Obstetrics and Gynecology*, 24(3): 141-143.

What are the risks and side effects of epidurals?

Cook TM, Counsell D & Wildsmith JAW 2009, 'Major complications of central neuraxial block: Report on the Third National Audit Project of the Royal College of Anaesthetists', *British Journal of Anaesthesia*, 102(2): 179-190.

Lain S, Ford J, Hadfield R, Blyth F, Giles W & Roberts C 2008, 'Trends in the use of epidural analgaesia in Australia', *International Journal of Gynecology & Obstetrics*, 102(3): 253-258.

McGrady E & Litchfield, K 2004, 'Epidural analgesia in labour', *Continuing Education in Anaesthesia, Critical Care & Pain*, 4(4): 114-117.

Queensland Health 2008, *Epidural pain relief for your labour*, <www.health.qld.gov. au/consent/documents/anaesthetic_05.pdf>, accessed July 2010.

Ravishankar S, Angram M, Douglas J, Gunka V & McTaggart R 2005, 'Inadequate epidural study', *Canadian Journal of Anesthesia*, 52: A141.

What will happen to my vagina?

Mayo Clinic 2009, Postpartum care: *What to expect after a vaginal birth*, <www. mayoclinic.com/health/postpartum-care/PR00142>, accessed July 2010.

Royal College of Obstetricians and Gynaecologists 2007, *The management of third- and fourth-degree perineal tears*, <www.rcog.org.uk/files/rcog-corp/uploaded-files/GT29ManagementThirdFourthDegreeTears2007.pdf>, accessed July 2010.

Sultan AH, Kamm MA & Hudson CN 1993, 'Anal sphincter disruption during vaginal delivery', *New England Journal of Medicine*, 329: 1905–1911.

What is a TENS machine?

Collins S, Arulkumaran S, Hayes K, Jackson S & Impey L 2008, *Oxford handbook of obstetrics and gynaecology*, Oxford University Press: Oxford.

Hofmeyr GJ, Neilson JP, Alfirevic Z, Crowther CA et al. 2008, *Pregnancy and childbirth: A Cochrane pocketbook*, Wiley Blackwell: London.

van der Spank JT, Cambier DC, De Paepe HMC, Danneels LAG, Witvrouw EE & Beerens L 2000, 'Pain relief in labour by transcutaneous electrical nerve stimulation (TENS)', *Archives of Gynecology and Obstetrics*, 264(3): 131–136.

Mother guilt in birth

Bort J, Pflock A & Renna D 2005, *Mommy guilt: Learn to worry less, focus on what matters most and raise happier kids*, AMACOM Press: New York.

Vaginal births: At home

Boucher D, Bennett C, McFarlin B & Freeze R 2009, 'Staying home to give birth: Why women in the United States choose homebirth', *Journal of Midwifery and Women's Health*, 54(2): 119–126.

de Jonge A, van der Goes BY, Ravelli ACJ, Amelink-Verburg MP, Mol BW, Nijhuis JG, Bennebroek Gravenhorst J & Buitendijk SE 2009, 'Perinatal mortality and morbidity in a nationwide cohort of 529 688 low-risk planned home and hospital births', *BJOG*, 116(9): 1177–1184.

Are homebirths safe?

Australian Society of Independent Midwives 2008, 'To the maternity services review committee Canberra', <www.health.gov.au/internet/main/publishing.nsf/ Content/maternityservicesreview-326>, accessed July 2010.

National Institute for Health and Clinical Excellence 2007, *Intrapartum care: NICE guidance*, <www.nice.org.uk/Guidance/CG55>, accessed July 2010.

Royal Australian and New Zealand College of Obstetricians and Gynaecologists 2008, *Maternity services review*, <www.health.gov.au/internet/main/publishing.nsf/Content/maternityservicesreview-214>, accessed July 2010.

The business of being born 2008, motion picture, Barranca Productions: New York. Distributed by Red Envelope Entertainment and New Line Home Entertainment.

VBAC: What are my chances?

American College of Obstetricians and Gynecologists (ACOG) 2004, 'Vaginal birth after previous caesarean delivery', *Clinical Management Guidelines for Obstetrician-Gynecologists*, 54, <www.acog.org/acog_districts/dist9/pb054.pdf>, accessed July 2010.

Dodd, JM, Crowther CA, Hiller, JE, Haslam RR & Robinson JS 2007, 'Birth after caesarean study—planned vaginal birth or planned elective repeat caesarean for women at term with a single previous caesarean birth: Protocol for a patient preference study and randomised trial', *BMC Pregnancy and Childbirth*, 7: 17.

Dodd J, Pearce E & Crowther C 2004, 'Women's preferences and experiences following Caesarean birth', *Australian and New Zealand Journal of Obstetrics and Gynaecology*, 44: 521-524.

Mayo Clinic 2008, *Vaginal birth after C-section (VBAC)*, <www.mayoclinic.com/health/vbac/VB99999/PAGE=VB00001>, accessed July 2010.

Women and Newborn Health Service 2000, *Care of a woman with a previous caesarean section: Antepartum preparation*, <www.kemh.health.wa.gov.au/development/manuals/O&G_guidelines/sectionb/1/b1.1.10.pdf>, accessed July 2010.

Caesarean births: Elective and emergency

Todman D 2007, 'A history of caesarean section: From ancient world to the modern era', *Australian and New Zealand Journal of Obstetrics and Gynaecology*, 47: 357-361

Are caesarean sections safe?

Brown S & Lumley J 1998, 'Maternal health after childbirth: Results of an Australian population based survey', *British Journal of Obstetrics and Gynaecology*, 105(2): 156-161.

Brown S & Lumley J 2000, 'Physical problems after childbirth and maternal depression at six to seven months postpartum', *British Journal of Obstetrics and Gynaecology*, 107(10): 1194-1201.

National Institute for Clinical Excellence 2004, *Caesarean Section: Understanding NICE guidance—Information for pregnant women, their partners and the public*, <www.nice.org.uk/nicemedia/live/10940/29336/29336.pdf>, accessed July 2010.

National Institutes of Health 2006, *Cesarean delivery on maternal request*, <http://consensus.nih.gov/2006/cesarean.htm>, accessed July 2010.

Shiliang L, Robert ML, Joseph KS, Heaman M, Sauve R & Kramer MS 2007, 'Maternal mortality associated with low-risk planned caesarean delivery versus planned vaginal delivery at term', *Canadian Medical Association Journal*, 176(4): 455-461.

What is pre-eclampsia?

Bhattacharya S, Campbell DM & Smith NC 2009, 'Pre-eclampsia in the second pregnancy: Does previous outcome matter?', *European Journal of Obstetrics, Gynaecology, and Reproductive Biology*, 144(2): 130-134.

Collins S, Arulkumaran S, Hayes K, Jackson S & Impey L 2008, *Oxford handbook of obstetrics and gynaecology*, Oxford University Press: Oxford.

Haddad B & Sibai BM 2009, 'Expectant management in pregnancies with severe pre-eclampsia', *Seminars in Perinatology*, 33(3): 143-151.

Hernández-Díaz S, Toh S & Cnattingius S 2009, 'Risk of pre-eclampsia in first and subsequent pregnancies: Prospective cohort studies', *British Medical Journal*, 338: b2255.

Does the number of caesareans you have increase your risk of danger?

The Royal Australian and New Zealand College of Obstetricians and Gynaecologists 2008, 'Maternity Services Review', submission to the Australian Government Maternity Services Review, <www.health.gov.au/internet/main/publishing.nsf/Content/maternityservicesreview-400>, accessed July 2010.

What is a post-partum haemorrhage?

Balki M, Dhumne S, Kasodekar S, Saeward G & Carvalho JC 2008, 'Blood transfusion for primary post partum hemorrhage: A tertiary hospital review', *Canadian Journal of Obstetric Gynaecology*, 30(11): 1002-1007.

Collins S, Arulkumaran S, Hayes K, Jackson S & Impey L 2008, *Oxford handbook of obstetrics and gynaecology*, Oxford University Press: Oxford.

Geller SE, Adams MG & Miller S 2008, 'A continuum of care model for postpartum hemorrhage', *International Journal of Fertility and Women's Medicine*, 52(2-3): 97-105.

Gulmezoglu AM, Widmer M, Merialdi M, Qureshi Z, Piaggio G et al. 2009, 'Active management of the third stage of labour without controlled cord traction: A randomized non-inferiority controlled trial', *Reproductive Health*, 21: 6-12.

Chapter 4: Babies

Kids: Websters' quotations, facts and phrases (2008, p. 4), Icon Group International: San Diego, CA.

What are breastfeeding rates in developed countries?

Australian Bureau of Statistics 2001, *Breastfeeding in Australia*, <www.abs.gov.au/ausstats/abs@.nsf/mf/4810.0.55.001>, accessed July 2010.

Cattaneo A, Yngve A, Koletzko B & Guzman R 2005, 'Protection, promotion and support of breast-feeding in Europe: Current situation', *Public Health Nutrition*, 8(1): 39-46.

Department of Health and Human Services, Centers for Disease Control and Prevention 2009, *Breast Feeding Report Card United States 2009*, <www.cdc.gov/breastfeeding/pdf/2009BreastfeedingReportCard.pdf>, accessed July 2010.

International Labour Organization 2005, *Recommendations related to breastfeeding and employed mothers*, <www.cdph.ca.gov/programs/breastfeeding/documents/mo-ilo-recommendemployment.pdf>, accessed July 2010.

Public Health Agency of Canada 2008, *Canadian perinatal health report 2008*, <www.publichealth.gc.ca/cphr/>, accessed July 2010.

Scientific Advisory Committee on Nutrition 2008, *Infant feeding survey 2005: A commentary on infant feeding practices in the UK*, Her Majesty's Stationery Office: Norwich.

World Health Organization 2003, *Global strategy for infant and young child feeding*, <www.who.int/nutrition/publications/gs_infant_feeding_text_eng.pdf>, accessed July 2010.

Breastfeeding is 'natural', so it must always be easy, right?

Crossley M 2009, 'Breastfeeding as a moral imperative: An autoethnographic study', *Feminism and Psychology*, 19(1): 71-87.

Locke A 2009, 'Natural versus taught: Competing discourses in antenatal breastfeeding workshops', *Journal of Health Psychology*, 14(3): 435-446.

Mattar CN, Chong YS, Chan YS, Chew A, Tan P, Chan YH & Rauff M 2007, 'Simple antenatal preparation to improve breastfeeding practice: A randomized controlled trial', *American College of Obstetrics and Gynecologists*, 109(1): 73-80.

McCarter-Spaulding D 2008, 'Is breastfeeding fair? Tensions in feminist perspectives on breastfeeding and the family', *Journal of Human Lactation*, 24: 206-212.

Su LL, Chong YS, Chan YH, Chan YS, Fok D, Tun KT, Ng F & Rauff M 2007, 'Antenatal education and postnatal support strategies for improving rates of exclusive breast feeding: Randomised controlled trial', *British Medical Journal*, 335: 596.

Wilkinson RB & Scherl FB 2006, 'Psychological health, maternal attachment and attachment style in breast- and formula-feeding mothers: A preliminary study', *Journal of Reproductive and Infant Psychology*, 24(1): 5-19.

Breastfeeding, formula-feeding and bonding

Britton JR, Britton HL & Gronwaldt V 2006, 'Breastfeeding, sensitivity and attachment', *Pediatrics*, 118: 1436-1443.

Wilkinson RB & Scherl FB 2006, 'Psychological health, maternal attachment and attachment style in breast- and formula-feeding mothers: A preliminary study', *Journal of Reproductive and Infant Psychology*, 24(1): 5-19.

Sleeping and settling

Balter L (ed) 2000, *Parenthood in America: An encyclopedia, Volume 2*, Greenwood Publishing Group: Santa Barbara, CA.

Ding K 2009, *New parenthood and sleep deprivation*, <www.ahealthyme.com/topic/sleepdeprive>, accessed July 2010.

How much sleep does my baby need?

Raising Children Network, *Baby sleep: In a nutshell*, <http://raisingchildren.net.au/articles/babies_sleep_nutshell.html/context/316>, accessed July 2010.

What is comfort settling?

Barker R 2009, *Baby love*, Pan Macmillan: Sydney.

Cooke K 2003, *Kid wrangling*, Penguin Books: Melbourne.

Green G 2001, *New toddler taming: The guide to your child from one to four*, Random House: Sydney.

Sunderland M 2006, *The science of parenting*, DK Publishing: New York.

Is there a link between poor infant sleep and postnatal depression?

Armstrong KL, Van Haeringen AR, Dadds MR & Cash R 1998, 'Sleep deprivation or postnatal depression in later infancy: Separating the chicken from the egg', *Journal of Paediatrics and Child Health*, 34: 260-262.

Barr JA 2006, 'Postpartum depression, delayed maternal adaption, and mechanical infant caregiving: A phenomenological hermeneutic study', *International Journal of Nursing Studies*, 45: 362-369.

Bayer JK, Hiscock H, Hampton A & Wake M 2007, 'Sleep problems in young infants and maternal mental and physical health', *Journal of Paediatrics and Child Health*, 43: 66-73.

Boyce P & Stubbs JM 1994, 'The importance of postnatal depression', *Medical Journal of Australia*, 161(8): 471-472.

Buist A 1998, 'Child abuse, post partum depression and parenting difficulties: A literature review of associations', *Australian and New Zealand Journal of Psychiatry*, 32(3): 370-378.

Dennis C-L & Ross L 2005, 'Relationships among infant sleep patterns, maternal fatigue, and development of depressive symptomatology', *Birth: Issues in Perinatal Care*, 32(3): 187-193.

Fisher JR 2009, 'Brief behavioural intervention for infant sleep problems reduces depression in mothers', *Evidence-Based Mental Health*, 12(2): 46-57.

Hiscock H, Bayer J, Hampton A, Ukoumunne OC & Wake M 2008, 'Long-term mother and child mental health effects of a population-based infant sleep intervention: Cluster-randomized, controlled trial', *Pediatrics*, 122: 621-627.

Martin J, Hiscock H, Hardy P, Davey B & Wake M 2007, 'Adverse associations of infant and child sleep problems and parent health: An Australian population study', *Pediatrics*, 119: 947-955.

Morgan JF 2009, 'Mothers were less likely to be depressed after a structured behavioural intervention for infant sleep problems', *Evidence Based Medicine*, 14(2): 45-52.

Murray L & Cooper PJ 1997, 'Effects of postnatal depression on infant development', *Archives of Disease in Childhood*, 77: 99-101.

Paris R, Bolton RE & Weinberg MK 2009, 'Postpartum depression, suicidality, and mother-infant interactions', *Archive of Women's Mental Health*, 12: 309-321.

Paulson JF, Dauber S & Leiferman JA 2006, 'Individual and combined effects of postpartum depression in mothers and fathers on parenting behavior', *Pediatrics*, 118(2): 659-668.

Wisner KL, Chambers C & Sit DK 2006, 'Postpartum depression: A major health problem', *The Journal of the American Medical Association*, 296(21): 2616-2618.

Where can I find extra support?

Hiscock H, Bayer J, Hampton A, Ukoumunne OC & Wake M 2008, 'Long-term mother and child mental health effects of a population-based infant sleep intervention: Cluster-randomized, controlled trial', *Pediatrics*, 122: 621-627.

How to cope with persistent crying

Barr R, Trent B & Cross J 2006, 'Age-related incidence curve of hospitalized Shaken Baby Syndrome cases: Convergent evidence for crying as a trigger to shaking', *Child Abuse & Neglect*, 30(1): 7-16.

Lee C, Barr R, Catherine N & Wicks A 2007, 'Age-related incidence of publicly reported Shaken Baby Syndrome cases: Is crying a trigger for shaking?', *Journal of Developmental & Behavioral Pediatrics*, 28(4): 288-293.

Co-sleeping safely

McKenna JJ & McDade T 2005, 'Why babies should never sleep alone: A review of the co-sleeping controversy in relation to SIDS, bedsharing and breast feeding', *Paediatric Respiratory Reviews*, 6(2): 134-152.

Sobralske MC & Gruber M 2009, 'Risks and benefits of parent/child bed sharing', *Journal of the American Academy of Nurse Practitioners*, 21: 474-479.

Task Force on Sudden Infant Death Syndrome 2005, 'The changing concept of Sudden Infant Death Syndrome: Diagnostic coding shifts, controversies regarding the sleeping environment, and new variables to consider in reducing risk', *Pediatrics*, 116(5): 1245-1255.

Chapter 5: Motherhood

Choi P, Henshaw C, Baker S & Tree J 2005, 'Supermum, superwife, supereverything: Performing femininity in the transition to motherhood', *Journal of Reproductive and Infant Psychology*, 23(2): 167-180.

Douglas SJ & Michaels MW 2004, *The mommy myth* (p. 27), Free Press: New York.

Nelson A 2003, 'Transition to motherhood', *Journal of Obstetric, Gynecologic & Neonatal Nursing*, 32(4): 465-477.

Priel B & Besser A 2002, 'Perceptions of early relationships during the transition to motherhood: The mediating role of social support', *Infant Mental Health Journal*, 23: 343-360.

Is it normal to feel so overwhelmed?

Ahlborg T & Strandmark N 2001, 'The baby was the focus of attention: First time parents' experiences of their intimate relationship', *Scandinavian Journal of Caring Sciences*, 15: 318-325.

Barclay L, Everitt L, Rogan F, Schmied C & Wyllie A 1997, 'Becoming a mother: An analysis of women's experiences of early motherhood', *Journal of Advanced Nursing*, 25: 719-728.

Hall W 1992, 'Comparison of the experience of women and men in dual-earner families following the birth of their first infant', *Journal of Nursing Scholarship*, 24: 33-38.

Lupton D 2000, 'A love/hate relationship: The ideals and experiences of first-time mothers', *Journal of Sociology*, 36: 50-63.

McVeigh C 1997, 'Motherhood experiences from the perspective of first-time mothers', *Clinical Nursing Research*, 6: 335-348.

Nyström K & Öhrling K 2004, 'Parenthood experiences during the child's first year: Literature review', *Journal of Advanced Nursing*, 46(3): 319-330.

Olsson P, Jansson L & Norberg A 1998, 'Parenthood as talked about in Swedish ante- and postnatal midwifery consultations', *Scandinavian Journal of Caring Sciences*, 12: 205-214.

Rogan F, Shmied V, Barclay L, Everitt L & Wylie A 1997, 'Becoming a mother: Developing a new theory of early motherhood', *Journal of Advanced Nursing*, 25: 877-885.

Sethi S 1995, 'The dialectic in becoming a mother: Experiencing a postpartum phenomenon', *Scandinavian Journal of Caring Sciences*, 9: 235-244.

White M, Wilson ME, Elander G & Persson B 1999, 'The Swedish family: Transition to parenthood', *Scandinavian Journal of Caring Sciences*, 13: 171-176.

Working mums and stay-at-home mums

Stone P & Lovejoy M 2004, 'Fast-track women and the "choice" to stay home', *Annals of the American Academy of Political and Social Sciences*, 596: 62-83.

Zaslow J 2002, 'Moving on: Good mother/bad mother: The debate over staying home with kids gets ugly', *Wall Street Journal*, September 5, D1.

Zimmerman TS, Aberle JT, Krafchick JL & Harvey AM 2008, 'Deconstructing the "Mommy Wars": The battle over the best mum', *Journal of Feminist Family Therapy*, 20(3): 203-219.

How much money is a stay-at-home mum worth?

Hanrahan M 2008, *Six-figure moms*, Salary.com, <www.salary.com/Articles/ArticleDetail.asp?part=par901>, accessed July 2010.

Tips for returning to work

Cooksey E, Joshi H & Verropoulou G 2009, 'Does mothers' employment affect children's development? Evidence from the British 1970 birth cohort and the American NLSY79', *Longitudinal and Life Course Studies*, 1(1): 95-115.

Raising Children Network 2006, *Tips for returning to work*, <http://raisingchildren.net.au/articles/tips_for_returning_to_work.html/context/848>, accessed July 2010.

When guilt has a purpose

Menesini E & Camodeca M 2008, 'Shame and guilt as behaviour regulators: Relationships with bullying, victimization and prosocial behaviour', *British Journal of Developmental Psychology*, 26(2): 183-196.

Postnatal depression

Halbreich U & Karkun S 2006, 'Cross-cultural and social diversity of prevalence of postpartum depression and depressive symptoms', *Journal of Affective Disorders*, 91: 97-111.

Morrell CJ, Slade O, Warner R, Paley G, Dixon S, Walters SJ, Brugha T, Barkham M, Parry GJ & Nicholl J 2009, 'Clinical effectiveness of health visitor training in psychologically informed approaches for depression in postnatal women: Pragmatic cluster randomised trial in primary care', *British Journal of Medicine*, 338: a3045.

Seimyr L, Edhborg M, Lundh W & Sjögren B 2004, 'In the shadow of maternal depressed mood: Experiences of parenthood during the first year after childbirth', *Journal of Psychosomatic Obstetric Gynecology*, 25: 23-34.

Chapter 6: Fatherhood

Allen S & Daly K 2007, *The effects of father involvement: An updated research summary of the evidence*, Centre for Families, Work & Well Being, University of Guelph: Canada, <www.fira.ca/cms/documents/29/Effects_of_Father_Involvement.pdf>, accessed July 2010.

Deave T & Johnson D 2008, 'The transition to parenthood: What does it mean for fathers?', *Journal of Advanced Nursing*, 63(6): 626-633.

Eggebeen DJ & Knoester C 2001, 'Does fatherhood matter for men?', *Journal of Marriage and Family*, 63: 381-393.

Henley K & Pasley K 2005, 'Conditions affecting the association between father identity and father involvement', *Fathering*, 3(1): 59-80.

Palkovitz R & Palm P 2009, 'Transitions within fathering', *Fathering*, 7(1): 3-22.

Schiller F 1781, *The robbers* (Act 1, Scene 1), <www.gutenberg.org/files/6782/6782.txt>, accessed July 2010.

How many dads choose to stay at home?

Randall K 2008, *Honey, I'm home: Stay-at-home dads' psychological well-being gauged in new study*, The University of Texas at Austin, <www.utexas.edu/features/2008/fathers/>, accessed July 2010.

Rochlen AB, McKelly RA, Suizzo M & Scaringi V 2008a, 'Predictors of relationships satisfaction, psychological well-being, and life satisfaction among stay-at-home-fathers', *Psychology of Men and Masculinity*, 9(1): 17-28.

Rochlen AB, Suizzo M, McKelly RA & Scaringi V 2008b, 'I'm just providing for my family: A qualitative study of stay-at-home fathers', *Psychology of Men and Masculinity*, 9(4): 193-206.

Andre's story

Institute for Women's Policy Research 2007, *Maternity leave in the United States: Paid parental leave is still not standard, even among the best US employers*, <www.iwpr.org/pdf/parentalleaveA131.pdf>, accessed July 2010.

Chapter 7: Families Come in All Shapes and Sizes

Australian Bureau of Statistics 2010, '3236.0 - Household and family projections, Australia, 2006 to 2031', <www.abs.gov.au/ausstats/abs@.nsf/Latestproducts/F32FD FD19296EC55CA25773B0017C628?opendocument> and <www.abs.gov.au/ausstats/ abs@.nsf/Latestproducts/9A3339CA258E1ACACA25773B0017C824?opendocument>, accessed August 2010.

Howard J 1999, *Families* (p. 234), Transaction Publishers: New Brunswick, NJ.

Koons JE 2005, 'Just married? Same-sex marriage and a history of family plurality', *Michigan Journal of Gender and Law*, 12(1): 1-87.

Murdock G 1949, *Social Structure*, Macmillan: New York.

Office for National Statistics UK 2005, *Focus on families*, <www.statistics.gov.uk/ downloads/theme_compendia/fof2005/families.pdf>, accessed July 2010.

US Census Bureau 2008, *Household, families, subfamilies and married couples: 1980 to 2008*, <www.census.gov/compendia/statab/2010/tables/10s0059.pdf>, accessed July 2010.

Domestic abuse: What it is and what you can do about it

Ellsberg M, Jansen HA, Heise L, Watts CH & Garcia-Moreno C 2008, 'Intimate partner violence and women's physical and mental health in the WHO multi-country study on women's health and domestic violence: An observational study', *The Lancet*, 371(9619): 1165-1172.

Garcia-Moreno C, Jansen HA, Ellsberg M, Heise L & Watts CH 2006, 'Prevalence of intimate partner violence: Findings from the WHO multidisciplinary-country study on women's health and domestic violence', *The Lancet*, 368(9551): 1260-1269.

Mayo Clinic 2009, *Domestic violence against women: Recognize patterns, seek help*, <www.mayoclinic.com/health/domestic-violence/WO00044>, accessed July 2010.

Smith M, Davies P & Segal J 2009, *Domestic violence and abuse: Signs of abuse and abusive relationships*, <www.helpguide.org/mental/domestic_violence_abuse_ types_signs_causes_effects.htm>, accessed July 2010.

Smith M & Segal J 2009, *Help for abused and battered women: Domestic violence shelters, support and protection*, <www.helpguide.org/mental/domestic_ violence_abuse_help_treatment_prevention.htm>, accessed July 2010.

Same sex parents

American Academy of Pediatrics 2002, 'Coparent or second-parent adoption by same-sex parents', *Pediatrics*, 109(2): 339-340.

American Society for Reproductive Medicine 2006, 'Access to fertility treatment by gays, lesbians, and unmarried persons', *Fertility & Sterility*, 86: 1333-1335.

International Conference on LGBT Human Rights 2006, *Declaration of Montréal*, <www.declarationofmontreal.org/declaration/DeclarationofMontreal.pdf>, accessed July 2010.

Millbank J 2003, 'From here to maternity: A review of the research on lesbian and gay families', *Australian Journal of Social Issues*, 38: 541-600.

Short E, Riggs DW, Perlesz A, Brown R & Kane G 2007, *Lesbian, gay, bisexual and transgender (LGBT) parented families*, The Australian Psychological Society, <www.psychology.org.au/Assets/Files/LGBT-Families-Lit-Review.pdf>, accessed July 2010.

LGBT parenting

Armesto JC 2002, 'Developmental and contextual factors that influence gay fathers' parental competence: A review of the literature', *Psychology of Men and Masculinity*, 3(2): 67-78.

Biblarz T & Stacey J 2009, 'How does the gender of parents matter?', *Journal of Marriage and Family*, 72: 3-22.

Bos HMW, Van Balen F & Van Den Boom D 2003, 'Planned lesbian families: Their desire and motivation to have children', *Human Reproduction*, 18: 2216-2224.

Chan RW, Raboy B & Patterson C 1998, 'Psychosocial adjustment among children conceived via donor insemination by lesbian and heterosexual mothers', *Child Development*, 69(2): 443-457.

Donovan C & Wilson A 2008, 'Imagination and integrity: Decision-making among lesbian couples to use medically provided donor insemination', *Culture, Health and Sexuality*, 10: 649-665.

Gartrell N, Rodas C, Deck A, Peyser H & Banks A 2006, 'The USA national lesbian family study: Interviews with mothers of 10-year-olds', *Feminism and Psychology*, 16: 175-192.

Golombok S, Perry B, Burston A, Murray C, Mooney-Somers J, Stevens M & Golding J 2003, 'Children with lesbian parents: A community study', *Developmental Psychology*, 39: 20-33.

Lindsay J, Perlesz A, Brown R, McNair R, de Vaus D & Pitts M 2006, 'Stigma or respect: Lesbian-parented families negotiating school settings', *Sociology*, 40: 1059-1077.

McNair R 2004, *Outcomes for children born of ART in a diverse range of families*, Victorian Law Reform Commission: Melbourne.

Patterson C 1998, 'The family lives of children born to lesbian mothers', in C Patterson & A D'Augelli (eds), *Lesbian, gay and bisexual identities in families: Psychological perspectives*, Oxford University Press: New York.

Patterson C, Fulcher M & Wainwright J 2002, 'Children of lesbian and gay parents: Research, law and policy', in B Bottoms, M Kovera & B McAuliff (eds), *Children, social science and the law*, Cambridge University Press: Cambridge.

Perlesz A, Brown R, Lindsay J, McNair R, deVaus D & Pitts M 2006, 'Family in transition: parents, children and grandparents in lesbian families give meaning to "doing family"', *Journal of Family Therapy*, 28: 175-199.

Riggs D 2008, 'Lesbian mothers, gay sperm donors, and community: Ensuring the wellbeing of children and families', *Health Sociology Review*, 17: 226-234.

Appendix A: Research

BBC News 2006, 'First measles death for 14 years', 3 April, <http://news.bbc.co.uk/2/hi/uk_news/england/4871728.stm>, accessed July 2010.

Bruce RR (ed.) 1994, *Seeing the unseen: Dr Harold E. Edgerton and the wonders of strobe alley*, MIT Press: Cambridge, MA.

Deer B 2010, *Nailed: Dr Andrew Wakefield and the MMR-autism vaccine fraud: Summary of Brian Deer's investigation into a threat to children's health*, <http://briandeer.com/mmr/lancet-summary.htm>, accessed July 2010.

Holt LE 1894, *The care and feeding of children: A catechism for the use of mothers and children's nurses*, Appleton & Company: New York.

Horton R 2004, 'A statement by the editors of *The Lancet* [regarding allegations of misconduct concerning an article published by Dr Andrew Wakefield]', *The Lancet*, <http://image.thelancet.com/extras/statement20Feb2004web.pdf>, accessed July 2010.

Kelleher O 2010, 'Vaccine Plea over measles outbreak', *The Irish Times*, 1 February, <www.irishtimes.com/newspaper/ireland/2010/0201/1224263502520.html>, accessed July 2010.

Kellett C 2010, 'Medicos fear measles timebomb', *Brisbane Times*, 11 February, <www.brisbanetimes.com.au/travel/travel-news/medicos-fear-measles-timebomb-20100210-ns70.html>, accessed July 2010.

Park M 2010, *Medical journal retracts study linking autism to vaccine*, CNN, <http://edition.cnn.com/2010/HEALTH/02/02/lancet.retraction.autism/index.html?hpt=T2>, accessed July 2010.

Public Health Agency of Canada 2010, *Global measles activity*, <www.phac-aspc.gc.ca/tmp-pmv/2010/meas-roug-012610-eng.php>, accessed July 2010.

Spock B 1946, *The common sense book of baby and child care*, Duell, Sloan & Pearce: New York.

Wakefield AJ, Murch SH, Anthony A, Linnell J, Casson DM, Malik M, Berelowitz M, Dhillon MP, Thomson MA, Harvey P, Valentine A, Davies SE & Walker-Smith JA 1998, 'Ileal-lymphoid-nodular hyperplasia, non-specific colitis, and pervasive developmental disorder in children', *The Lancet*, 351: 637-641.

Appendix B: How to start a support group

Kelly B 2003, *Worth repeating: More than 5,000 classic and contemporary quotes* (p. 168), Kregel Publications: Grand Rapids, MI.

Reay-Young R 2001, 'Support groups for people living with a serious mental illness: An overview', *International Journal of Psychosocial Rehabilitation*, 5: 56–80.

Schizophrenia Fellowship of New South Wales 2007, *Leading groups: A guide to leadership, support groups and SFNSW*, Schizophrenia Fellowship of NSW: Gladesville.

Index

A

acid reflux 118-19, 230
active labour 69, 230
adoption 2, 12, 16, 17-22, 239-40
age and IVF 6-9
anger resources 256-8
anovulation 3, 230
antenatal 230
  care 43
  checks 81, 82
  classes 71, 85, 99, 100, 106, 108, 181
anxiety 42, 115, 149-56, 201, 219
  see also postnatal depression (PND)
artificial insemination 11, 12, 230
assisted reproductive technology (ART)
    2, 230, 241
  for LGBT individuals 16, 242-3
  resources for 241-2
autism 200, 213-14
  and the MMR vaccine 220, 222-4

B

babies
  bonding with 105, 127-8
  see bottle feeding; breastfeeding;
    premature babies; settling; sleeping
baby blues 123, 149, 152, 230
Baby-Friendly Hospital Initiative
    (BFHI) 97, 231
birth 59-93, 248-50
  and mother guilt 71
  partners' perspectives 87-92
  and recovery 92-3
  water 67-9

see also caesarean section; vaginal
    births
birth centres 67-72, 231
birthing decisions and previous loss of
    a baby 42
birthing stool 76
blastocysts 7
bleeding
  in pregnancy 42-7
  subchorionic 45-6, 236
body image and pregnancy 47-52
bonding with baby 105, 127-8
bottle feeding 95-105, 251-2
  and bonding 105
  formula feeding by choice 103-5
breastfeeding 95-105, 250-1
  bonding 105
  and expressed milk 96-7, 99
  grief of discontinuing 98-9
  rates in developed countries 97-8
  support 99-100
breech position 81

C

caesarean section 8, 60, 63, 65
  elective and emergency 77-84, 96,
    199, 213
  number and risk 87
  requested 85-7
  risks to mother 87
  safety of 79-80
  vaginal births after (VBAC) 75-7, 237
'camping out' method 107, 115, 116, 232
cervix 3, 11, 231
child safety 254-5

chlamydia 3, 231

clomid 5, 43, 231

colostrum 96, 232

comfort settling 95, 105, 107, 108, 109, 112-14, 115, 116, 232

conceiving and same sex relationships 10-12

controlled crying 95, 106, 109, 110-11, 112, 113-15, 232

coping

  with persistent crying 120

  with sick or premature babies 118-23

  with sleep deprivation 123-8

  support groups 12, 80, 97, 225-9

  without support 117-18

co-sleeping 97, 106, 107, 113, 124-5, 232

crying

  controlled 95, 106, 109, 110-11, 112, 113-15, 232

  coping with persistent 120

D

delivery suites in hospitals 61-7, 232

depression 32-5, 258-9

  see also postnatal depression (PND)

domestic violence and abuse 201-2, 261-3

donor conception 9-12

doula 69

drugs and pregnancy 47

E

ectopic pregnancy 3, 232

endometriosis 85

episiotomy 66, 232

expressed milk 96-7, 99

F

families 197-216

  large 209-11

  only child 205-7

  same sex parents 206-9

  and separation 180-2

when traditional roles cause strain on 211-13

  and work, balancing 175-8

fatherhood 165-96

  and identity 167-71

  reflections on 187-96

  stay-at-home dads 171-8

  working dads 171-8

fathers

  and parenting 260-1

  and postnatal depression 32-5

  on relationships 186-7

  resources for 260-1

  tips for single or divorced 186

feeding *see* bottle feeding; breastfeeding

feelings during pregnancy 28-43

fibroids 3, 232

first aid 120-2

food cravings 52

forceps delivery 78

foster care services 240-1

fostering 2, 16-17, 23-6, 241

G

gender roles 172-5

general anaesthetic 83-4

genetic counselling and testing 243-4

gestational carrier 13, 233

guilt, mother 71, 142-9

H

health risks and pregnancy 43-7

home birthing 72-5, 249, 250

hypnobirthing 69

hysteroscopy 7, 233

I

identity

  and fatherhood 167-71

  and motherhood 131-7

Implanon 35, 233

infertility, common causes 3-4

Intrauterine Growth Restriction
(IUGR) 29, 30, 234
in-vitro fertilisation (IVF) 2, 4-9, 234,
241, 242

L

laparoscopic surgery 7, 234
legal advice 244-5
lesbian, gay, bisexual and transgender
(LGBT) 1-2
and assisted reproductive technology
(ART) 16, 242-3
lobby groups 17
let-down reflex 98, 234
linea nigra 47, 48, 51, 234
live-in service 114, 234
lobby groups 17, 225-6, 229
low-lying placenta 84
luteal phase 3, 234

M

male postnatal depression 32-5
marriage, when traditional roles cause
strain on 211-13
medications and pregnancy 47
mental health 258-9
see also anxiety; depression; postnatal
depression (PND); post partum
psychosis
miscarriage 6, 40, 41-3, 45, 247
MMR vaccine and autism (research)
220, 222-4
mother guilt 142-9
in birth 71
motherhood 129-64
and identity 131-7
reflections on 156-64
stay-at-home mums 136-41
tips for returning to work 141
working mums 136-41
see also postnatal depression (PND)
mothering, motherless 160-3
mothers, single 198-205

O

ovarian reserve testing 3
ovulation 3, 4, 5, 11, 21, 29, 235

P

palpation 3, 235
pap smears 3, 235
parenting
a child with different abilities 213-15
and fathers 260-1
live-in service 114, 234
and research 218-24
resources for 253-4
same sex 13-17, 207-9
pelvic floor exercises 66
perineum 66, 80, 235
placenta accreta 87, 235
placenta praevia 79, 80, 87, 235
playgroups 252
polycystic ovarian syndrome (PCOS)
43, 235
Post and Antenatal Depression
Association (PANDA) 258
postnatal depression (PND) 37, 114, 136,
258-9
and dads 32-5
and mums 149-56
and poor infant sleep 115-16
support 152
symptoms/treatment 154-6
post-partum 59-93, 150
post-partum haemorrhage 88, 89-90,
236
post-partum psychosis 150, 152
pre-eclampsia 81, 82
pregnancy 27-58
and age 6-9
and bleeding 42-7
and body image 47-52
counselling and crisis services 238-9
and drugs 47
feelings during 28-43
and health risks 43-7

loss 38-43, 246-8
 and medications 47
 miscarriage 6, 40, 41-3, 45, 247
 resources 245-8
 and sex 33, 36, 52-7
 and sex of the baby 35-8
 stillbirth 38-41
pregnant, seeking help to get 9
premature babies
 coping with 119-22
 and expressed milk 96-7

R

reflux apnoea 122, 236
relationships 178-86
 breakdown of 31-2, 35-7, 166, 180-2,
  184-6, 203-5, 209
 LGBT 2, 9-12, 13-17, 18, 137-8, 166, 201,
  206-9
 when traditional roles cause strain
  on 211-13
research 218-24
 autism and the MMR vaccine 222-4
 evaluating 220-1
 fatally flawed 221-2
 studies 219-20

S

sacroiliac pain 29, 236
safe sleeping 252-3
same sex
 parents 206-9
 relationships and conceiving 10-12
settling 105-16
 comfort 95, 105, 107, 108, 109, 112-14,
  115, 116, 232
sex
 after delivery 54, 56, 57, 66-7, 178-80,
  181, 182-3, 195
 oral 55
 and pregnancy 33, 36, 52-7, 181
sex of the baby 35-8
sick babies, coping with 118-23

single parents 184-6, 263-4
sleep deprivation, coping with 123-8
sleeping 105-16
 'camping out' method 107, 115, 116, 232
 commonly used methods 107
 co-sleeping 97, 106, 107, 113, 124-5, 232
 and postnatal depression 115-16
sperm ducts 3, 236
stay-at-home dads 171-8
stay-at-home mums 136-41
stillbirth 38-41
subchorionic bleed 45-6, 236
support, coping without 117-18
support groups 12, 80, 97, 225-9
surrogacy 13-17, 242, 243

T

TENS machine 68, 69, 236
third party reproduction 12, 13, 266
transverse position 84
trauma, past 83

U

uterine atony 89, 237

V

vagina 66-7
vaginal births
 after caesareans (VBAC) 75-7, 237
 birth centres 67-72, 231
 delivery suites in hospitals 61-7, 232
 at home 72-5, 249, 250
 when things don't go to plan 69-72

W

water birth 67-9, 236
work and families, balancing 175-8
working dads 171-8
working mums 136-41